RURAL BEHAVIORAL

HEALTH CARE

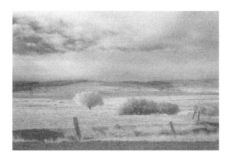

RURAL BEHAVIORAL HEALTH CARE

An Interdisciplinary Guide

Edited by B. Hudnall Stamm

American Psychological Association • Washington, DC

Published by
American Psychological Association
750 First Street, NE
Washington, DC 20002
www.apa.org

To order
APA Order Department
P.O. Box 92984
Washington, DC 20090-2984

Tel: (800) 374-2721, Direct: (202) 336-5510
Fax: (202) 336-5502, TDD/TTY: (202) 336-6123
Online: www.apa.org/books/
E-mail: order@apa.org

In the U.K., Europe, Africa, and the Middle East, copies may be ordered from
American Psychological Association
3 Henrietta Street
Covent Garden, London
WC2E 8LU England

Typeset in Century Schoolbook by NOVA Graphic Services, Jamison, PA

Printer: Port City Press, Baltimore, MD
Cover Designer: Naylor Design, Washington, DC
Project Manager: NOVA Graphic Services, Jamison, PA

The opinions and statements published are the responsibility of the authors, and such opinions and statements do not necessarily represent the policies of the American Psychological Association.

Library of Congress Cataloging-in-Publication Data
Rural behavioral health care : an interdisciplinary guide / edited by B. Hudnall Stamm.—1st ed.
 p. cm.
 Includes bibliographical references and index.
 ISBN 1-55798-983-4 (alk. paper)
 1. Rural health. 2. Rural health services. 3. Primary care (Medicine) 4. Mental health services. 5. Social medicine.   I. Stamm, B. Hudnall, 1958-

RA771.R875 2003
362.1'04257—dc21   2002043752

British Library Cataloguing-in-Publication Data
A CIP record is available from the British Library.

Printed in the United States of America
First Edition

This book is dedicated to Gil Hill
in grateful recognition for
a lifetime of commitment to
making the world a better place.

Contents

Contributors

Robert K. Ax, PhD, Federal Correctional Institution, Petersburg, VA

S. Megan Berthold, PhD, LCSW, CTS, Program for Torture Victims, Los Angeles, CA

James Boulger, PhD, Center for Rural Mental Health Studies, School of Medicine, University of Minnesota, Duluth

Marlene S. Buchner, MS, School of Nursing, University of North Dakota, Grand Forks

Catherine Campbell, PhD, Department of Psychology, University of Southern Mississippi

Tony Cellucci, PhD, Department of Psychology, Idaho State University, Pocatello

Stuart A. Copans, Department of Psychiatry, Dartmouth Medical School, Hanover, NH; Monadnock Family Services, Peterborough, NH

Byron Crouse, MD, Center for Rural Mental Health Studies, School of Medicine, University of Minnesota, Duluth

Joseph Davenport III, PhD, MSSW, Consultant, Columbia, MO

Judith A. Davenport, PhD, LCSW, School of Social Work, University of Missouri, Columbia

Gary Davis, PhD, Center for Rural Mental Health Studies, School of Medicine, University of Minnesota, Duluth

Patrick H. DeLeon, PhD, past president, American Psychological Association, Washington, DC

Ronald D. Deprez, PhD, MPH, Public Health Resource Group, Portland, ME

Garret D. Evans, PhD, National Rural Behavioral Health Center, University of Florida, Gainesville

Thomas J. Fagan, PhD, Randolph Macon College, Ashland, VA

Steven W. Friedrichsen, DDS, Department of Dental Sciences, Idaho State University, Pocatello

John A. Gale, MS, Public Health Resource Group, Portland, ME

Renee V. Galliher, PhD, Department of Psychology, Utah State University, Logan

Sister Anthony Marie Greving, FSE, BA, Idaho Area V Agency on Aging, Pocatello, ID

Susan Guralnick, MA, North West Geriatric Education Center, University of Washington, Seattle

Corey Habben, PsyD, Institute for Personal Development, Morris, IL

Angela Hager, PhD, Department of Psychology, Marshall University, Huntington, WV

Kristofer J. Hagglund, PhD, Robert Wood Johnson Foundation, Princeton, NJ

David S. Hargrove, PhD, Department of Psychology, University of Mississippi, Oxford

Craig Higson-Smith, MA, South African Institute of Traumatic Stress, Johannesburg, South Africa

Gil Hill, independent consultant

Shelia M. B. Holton, PsyD, Federal Correctional Institution, Waseca, MN

Alison Howard, BS, Offices of Rural Health and Substance Abuse, Practice Directorate, American Psychological Association, Washington, DC

Amy C. Hudnall, MA, *NWSA Journal*, a Publication of the National Women's Studies Association and the Department of History, Appalachian State University, Boone, NC

Bette A. Ide, PhD, RN, School of Nursing, University of North Dakota, Grand Forks

Kathy Kemele, MS, PA-C, Department of Family Practice, Mercer University School of Medicine, Macon, GA

Mary Beth Kenkel, PhD, School of Psychology at Florida Institute of Technology, Melbourne

Bradley D. Kuper, PhD, Kaiser-Permanente, Sacramento, CA

Ronald F. Levant, EdD, Nova Southeastern University, Ft. Lauderdale, FL

Helen Linkey, PhD, Department of Psychology, Marshall University, Huntington, WV

Judith A. Lyons, PhD, G.V. (Sonny) Montgomery Veterans Affairs Medical Center, University of Mississippi Medical Center, Jackson

Carol A. Markstrom, PhD, Family and Consumer Sciences, Child Development and Family Studies, West Virginia University, Morgantown

Susan L. Metrick, PsyD, Institute for Graduate Clinical Psychology, Widener University, Chester, PA; the Center for Psychological Services, Paoli, PA

Pamela L. Mulder, PhD, Department of Psychology, Marshall University, Huntington, WV

Ted Nirenberg, PhD, Department of Psychiatry and Human Behavior, Brown University School of Medicine, Providence, RI

Katherine C. Nordal, PhD, The Nordal Clinic, P.A., Vicksburg, MS

Neill F. Piland, DrPH, Medical Group Management Association Center for Research, Englewood, CO; Institute of Rural Health, Idaho State University, Pocatello

Sarah D. Richie, Department of Psychology, University of Mississippi, Oxford

Paulette Running Wolf, EdD, Department of Educational Leadership and Counseling Psychology, Washington State University, Pullman; ORC Macro, Atlanta, GA

Amy Watson Ruth, BA, *NWSA Journal*, a Publication of the National Women's Studies Association, Appalachian State University, Boone, NC

Morgan T. Sammons, PhD, U.S. Naval Hospital, Keflavik, Iceland; Mental Health Department, Naval Medical Center, Annapolis, MD

Samuel F. Sears, Jr., PhD, University of Florida, Gainesville

B. Hudnall Stamm, PhD, Institute of Rural Health and Department of Psychology, Idaho State University, Pocatello

Henry E. Stamm IV, PhD, Wind River History Center, Dubois, WY

Kathy Tidwell, MSW, School of Social Work, Boise State University, Boise, ID

Peter Vik, PhD, Department of Psychology, Idaho State University, Pocatello

Morton O. Wagenfeld, PhD, Department of Sociology, Western Michigan University, Kalamazoo; Health Services Program, Walden University, Naples, FL

Mary Wakefield, PhD, Center for Health Policy, Research, and Ethics, George Mason University, Fairfax, VA; Center for Rural Health, School of Medicine and Health Sciences, University of North Dakota, Grand Forks

Donald L. Weaver, MD, National Health Service Corps, Bureau of Health Professions, Health Resources, and Services Administration, U.S. Department of Health and Human Services, Washington, DC

Acknowledgments

This book was written with the help of the American Psychological Association Committee on Rural Health. In particular, Gil Hill, former director of the Office of Rural Health in the Practice Directorate of the American Psychological Association, has been a constant support. Gil's knowledge of Washington, DC and his ever-present vigilance to its vicissitudes kept the members of the Committee on the cutting edge. The U.S. Department of Health and Human Services, Health Resources and Services Administration Bureau of Health Professions contract number HRSA 99-BHPR-A70703, provided funding for managing the manuscript.

The staff of the Idaho State University Institute of Rural Health supported me throughout the process. I thank Sally A. Kreilach, Barbara J. Cunningham, Debbie Dahlquist, Joann Anderson, John Ahedor, Steven Lore, and Karen Johnson as well as members of the Institute's Idaho Community HealthCorps, an AmeriCorps program. Sheila Margiotta, Sheri Taylor, and Susie Metrick made untold contributions. I am forever indebted to Amy C. Hudnall and Amy Watson Ruth of Ink River Associates for their assistance with editing. Without the kindness of Robin C. Bonner of NOVA Graphic Services, I would not have made it through the final stages of publishing this book.

My quest to understand policy and practice was launched and continues to be supported by my then student and now friend, Joseph M. Rudolph. Craig Higson-Smith, a friend and colleague from South Africa, and I spent hours via e-mail and in cabins in the woods during our too infrequent visits passionately trying to understand the meaning of *rural*. Beth Hilgartner inspired me to keep writing. Both of my mothers have loved me through yet another book, showing me what strong women can do. My spouse, the other Dr. Stamm, is well-known for his unflagging and mostly freely given assistance with this book; it could not have been done without him.

RURAL BEHAVIORAL
HEALTH CARE

Introduction

B. Hudnall Stamm, Susan L. Metrick, Mary Beth Kenkel, Judith A. Davenport, Joseph Davenport III, Amy C. Hudnall, Amy Watson Ruth, Craig Higson-Smith, and Carol A. Markstrom

Overview

Rural areas represent a significant part of the United States, in terms of both quantitative proportion and qualitative contribution to the national identity. In this introduction, we briefly acquaint the reader with issues expanded in the book, including the ongoing struggle to define *urban*, *rural*, and *frontier*. This struggle is remarkably no less difficult than differentiating between behavioral and mental health. Unlike the common solution to the latter problem, which is using the term *mental* or *behavioral* health to represent all things related to both, there are a significant number of times when a clear definition of rural is needed. This book does not provide a simple answer but it does examine many of the issues associated with living rural.

Few people have specific understanding of what *rural*, much less *frontier*, entails. The definitions of *rural* are nearly as diverse as the places and populations they are meant to classify and may vary depending on the purpose of the definition (Boyd, 1997). Generalizing across definitions, the rural portions of the United States contain just over 80% of the land and about 20% (55 million) of the population (U.S. Department of Agriculture, Economic Research Service [USDA-ERS], 2000). These 55 million people, although increasing in number, represent a decreasing percentage of the population.

There is a lack of consensus regarding the definition of *rural* (Rourke, 1997). The definitions are so problematic that the U.S. Office of Rural Health Policy (ORHP) issued a publication on the definitions of *rural* (Ricketts, Johnson-Webb, & Taylor, 1998), later expanded to a full text (Ricketts, 1999). No approach to defining *rural* is entirely satisfactory; such definitions are always arbitrary, and any one definition may not take into account other important variables. Perhaps, as Cordes (1990) noted, the only thread that ties rural areas together is their lower population densities.

Dr. Stamm may be reached at Campus Box 8174, Institute of Rural Health, Idaho State University, Pocatello, ID 83209. E-mail: bhstamm@isu.edu

Population density is the basis for the most typical type of definition. In older definitions used by the Bureau of the Census, the label *rural* was applied to areas with 2,500 or fewer persons or to open countryside and the label *urban* to cities (and the closely settled areas around them) with 50,000 or more inhabitants. These clusters of 50,000 or more people, composed of a population nucleus and adjacent communities with a high degree of economic and social integration, are called metropolitan statistical areas (MSAs; U.S. Bureau of the Census, 1994). Some theorists believe that these definitions are outdated and prefer a definition of 50 or fewer people per square mile for *rural*. Other theorists believe definitions should reflect a rural–urban continuum (Conger, 1997; Ricketts, 1999).

Population density models also refer to frontier areas, which contain six to seven people per square mile. These remote communities are usually protected from large-scale settlement by harsh climate, difficult terrain, lack of water, distance from metropolitan areas, or lack of exploitable resources (Duncan, 1993; Popper, 1986). These areas, mostly west of the 98th meridian, constitute 45% of the U.S. land mass but contain less than 1% of the population.

Rural Issues: Sometimes a "Tough Row to Hoe"

Despite definitional differences, a general characterization of rural settings emerges from the literature (Bushy, 1994; Human & Wasem, 1991; Weinert & Long, 1990). Substance abuse rates are probably similar to those in urban areas, but it is generally more difficult to get treatment (see chapter 4). Obtaining treatment for people with serious mental disorders is a particular problem (see chapter 16). The technological infrastructure, which could hold promise for ameliorating other problems, falls short of expectations (see chapter 11). Rural economies are fragile. Younger individuals migrate out, seeking education or work and leaving behind a greater proportion of elderly and dependent individuals (see chapter 15). Rural residents have less formal education, higher unemployment rates, and more poverty than urban residents (see chapter 3). In the remainder of this introduction, we briefly highlight some key rural issues.

Agribusiness and Changing Economies

In 1998, 14% of people in the United States living outside of metropolitan areas were in poverty and saw a greater income decline—58% of rural families living at or below 300% of the poverty level compared with 46% of urban families—than did their urban counterparts (USDA-ERS, 2000b). Farm workers seem to fare the worst, earning just over half of the national average for wage earners. More than one third of farm workers have annual family incomes of less than $15,000 (USDA-ERS, 2000b). Rural poverty seems to be durable. For example, between 1980 and 1999, national poverty rates averaged 13.9% ($SEM = 0.67$). The mean poverty rate for the five poorest states (Alabama, Arkansas, Louisiana, Mississippi, and West Virginia), all which have large rural populations, averaged 22.1% ($SEM = 0.19$). The five states with the lowest poverty rates (Connecticut, Maryland, Massachusetts, New Hampshire, and New Jersey) had a poverty rate of 8.7% (*SEM* = 2.1). Only one of the lowest five, New Hampshire, has a sizable rural population (U.S. Bureau of the Census, 2000).

For centuries, agriculture has been the rural economic mainstay. The rise of corporate agriculture, which is rapidly displacing family farms and causing economic dislocations in agriculture-dependent communities, presents new problems for rural communities and mental health practitioners (Dannerbeck, Davenport, & Davenport, 1999). Some towns have rapidly declined, and others have seen rapid shifts in their cultural makeup. Although the largely culturally and ethnically different newcomers bring a strong work ethic, family values, and religious beliefs, all of which are usually prized in small-town America, the differences in culture, language, and race are not easily overcome. Small towns typically have few mental health services, and workers in those fields often experience difficulty in reaching out, particularly when newcomers speak a variety of languages and come from a variety of different cultures (see chapter 18).

The *farm crisis* is the culmination of a century-old trend. Small farmers and ranchers find it increasingly difficult to compete with corporate farms that have access to huge amounts of capital and the latest technology. Government policies, research, tax laws, and subsidy programs are aimed at large producers. Each year, fewer family farms survive and small towns wither as fewer stores, churches, and schools are required for the reduced population. Social and behavioral problems, such as alcohol abuse, domestic violence, and suicide, increase, whereas there are decreasing resources to deal with them (Davenport & Davenport, 1999).

Data from the USDA-ERS (2000a) indicate a reduction in the number of midsized farms (those with earnings of $10,000–$99,000 per year), down 2.3% (31,400 farms) over 2 years. Most of these farms appear to be dropping into the small-farm class, which increased by 26,860 farms over 2 years. The others appear to have been absorbed into large corporate farms earning more than $100,000 per year, which increased by 8,010 farms over 2 years. This 16% of large, often corporate farms accounted for 57% of land in farms, with an average size of 1,720 acres. Among the 3% of farms earning more than $500,000, the average size was 2,501 acres.

Federal Policies: Improvement and Disappointment

National interest in rural health care, including the issues of mental health and substance abuse, arose in the early 1990s with the activities of the ORHP (Human & Wasem, 1991). The development reflected concern over economic downturns and problems in rural health care access. This interest continues, particularly in serving the underserved (Chavez & DeLeon, 1997). Because governments do not always adequately attend to their rural constituents, problems in rural areas may go unrecognized and untreated; others are created where they did not exist previously or are worsened by the lack of attention.

Since the 1970s, health providers, health researchers, policymakers, and the general public have recognized the importance of promoting health and of reducing the risks of acute and chronic disease and disability. *Healthy People 2000,* developed by the U.S. Department of Health and Human Services (DHHS; 1995), contained goals and a framework for significantly reducing death and disability and for promoting health and quality of life. Attention was also drawn to the disparities in health status among special populations, as well as goals to reduce these differences. *Healthy People 2010* (DHHS, 2000) contains national health objectives that are even more comprehensive, with particular attention to increasing the quality and years of life and to eliminating health disparities, including those that result from living in rural localities and those correlated with gender, race, ethnicity, education, income, disability, and sexual orientation. Particular targets include the higher rates of injury-related deaths (40% higher in rural areas than in urban areas), heart disease, cancer, and diabetes; decreased use of preventive screening; less timely access to emergency services and specialists; and lower percentages of persons who are medically insured.

These initiatives are encouraging signs of the government's intent to improve quality of life in rural communities. However, there are still many areas in which government support is lacking. Many national policies do not address the uniqueness of rural places. Further research is warranted to understand the needs of these communities so that policies may be more effectively implemented. General and governmental lack of knowledge of these issues can be alarming and may reflect apathy, but certainly points toward the possibility of what has been termed *urbancentrism* (Stamm, 2000).

Possible sources of urbancentrism may include myths popularly held by those who lack knowledge of the reality of rural living. Struthers and Bokemeier (2000) reported assumptions that may lead to shortcomings in effective policies, programming, and services: (a) Rural residents are rugged, self-sufficient people with an individualistic orientation; (b) rural communities are better for families because they are cleaner and safer, with a family orientation that provides a safety net; and (c) rural families are close-knit, nuclear, unchanging, and stereotypically *traditional.*

Providing Services

As noted previously, some access issues are driven by inadequate or absent federal and state policies. Some factors are independent of legislative intervention and may reflect distinctly rural properties. In approaches to health promotion and disease prevention, investigators should recognize that lifestyle choices and adoption of healthy behaviors are influenced not only by governmental policies but also by individual, social, geographical, and climatological factors.

On the individual level, changes in health behaviors require the belief that change will produce a desired outcome, the knowledge of what to do, the skills to make the change, and the confidence in one's ability to perform the behavior (Bandura, 1977, 1986). Rural communities must find methods that provide health education and support for behavior change, and they must find dissemination methods to get information to people over large geographical and climatologically powerful areas. Distributing the information through primary care providers is a logical alternative. However, rural health professionals, often understaffed and overtaxed with the demands of acute care, find little time to assess health behaviors and provide information on healthier lifestyles. Media outlets, particularly local newspapers, are another source that has been used effectively in some locales, but some members of very poor rural populations do not have televisions and do not receive (and in some cases, cannot read) newspapers.

Health behaviors are also influenced by social context. The attitudes, values, and health practices of family and friends influence the adoption of healthy behavior. Behaviors that have social approval and conform to social norms are more likely to be adopted. A homogeneous value system emerges and exerts much control. Deviations from the norm are met with strong social disapproval, even ostracism. Rural women in particular are strongly influenced by these social values and attitudes in the choices they make and the behaviors they adopt (Hemard, Monroe, Atkinson, & Blalock, 1998; Mulder et al., 2000; see also chapter 14).

Shame, fear, and stigma can keep rural residents from seeking help for problems that are deemed socially unacceptable, such as mental illness, human immunodeficiency virus (HIV) infection, acquired immunodeficiency syndrome (AIDS), and domestic violence. On the positive side, a tight-knit community engenders a strong informal support network in which neighbors and friends come to one another's aid. Many services provided in urban areas through formal systems of care are handled by the informal systems in rural areas.

Rural Hospitals

There were 5,134 hospitals in the United States in 1996, of which 2,226 were rural (Hirsch & Harriman, 2000). The majority of the small (fewer than 100 beds) rural hospitals are heavily dependent on Medicare revenues for support (Hirsch & Harriman, 2000). The decade of the 1980s was extremely difficult for rural hospitals; an average of 30 rural hospitals closed every year. The rate slowed in the 1990s but only to 10–15 hospital closures per year (U.S. Office of Inspector General, DHHS, 1999). These closures occurred at the same time the rural population was growing in size.

The Balanced Budget Act of 1997 (Public Law 105-33) established the Medicare Rural Hospital Flexibility Program (RHFP) to bolster the flagging rural hospitals. The program (a) allows small hospitals to be designated as critical access hospitals (CAHs); (b) under Medicare, provides for cost-based reimbursement for acute inpatient (Part A) and outpatient (Part B) services; (c) encourages health network development that focuses on rural health needs; and (d) provides block grants to states to help strengthen the rural healthcare infrastructure. Most hospitals that have gained the CAH designation also are sole community hospitals, located in isolated areas and deemed essential to the community. Although cost-based reimbursement seemed to be the perfect solution for sustaining rural hospitals, cost-based reimbursement, by definition, does not allow for profit. Because most rural hospitals are operating at a very small profit, if any at all, cost-based reimbursement some-times hinders expansion of services and makes it difficult to tolerate the ever-growing costs of health care. Medicaid's expansion to a prospective payment system (PPS) for nonacute care settings further challenges rural hospitals (Dalton, Howard, & Slifken, 2000). For ongoing information about the status of rural hospitals, consult the Rural Policy Research Institute's Rural Hospital tracking program (http://www.rupri.org/rhfp-track/).

Provider Recruitment and Retention Issues

People living in rural and frontier areas need health care, but it can be diffi-cult to recruit and retain professionals to provide that care. Utilization and misdistribution of primary care physicians have been at the center of health workforce policy in the United States (Kohrs & Mainous, 1996). An area is des-ignated as having a primary health care shortage when providers are over-utilized and the ratio of full-time equivalent caregivers to patients is fewer than 1:3500. Nationally, more than 2,000 physicians are needed to remove federal Health Professions Shortage Areas (HPSA) designations. Regardless of whether a particular area meets HPSA criteria, rural and frontier regions have fewer physicians per 100,000 people than do urban areas. In rural and frontier areas, the ratio of provider to patient is 30–68:100,000, in comparison with an urban ratio of 180:100,000 (Ciarlo, Wackwitz, Wagenfeld, Mohatt, & Zelarney, 1996; Pion, Keller, & McCombs, 1997).

Programs such as the NHSC influence the choice to practice in a rural area. The locations of both undergraduate and graduate medical education are also important in determining practice location; 39% of physicians practice in the state in which they received their undergraduate training, and 51% practice in the state where they received their graduate training. General and family practitioners and obstetrician/gynecologists are the most likely to practice in the states where they trained. Time is a major deterrent in choosing or continuing a rural practice; rural providers work more hours and see more patients than do urban providers (Office of Technology Assessment [OTA], 1991). For some rural and frontier providers, this translates to more continuous hours of coverage, fewer opportunities for respite or continuing education, and increased risk of burnout, compassion fatigue, and work-related secondary trauma (OTA, 1991; Stamm, 1999). In short, providers may be dissuaded from choosing a rural practice because of heavy workloads and few professional opportunities or benefits. Unlike their urban counterparts, many rural health professionals do not have easy access to professional col-leagues, consultations and second opinions, medical libraries, or continuing education (OTA, 1991; Stamm, 1999).

Integrated Care and Continuity of Care

Although much has been written about making health services more avail-able, accessible, and acceptable to rural residents, less attention has been directed to finding ways to increase the integration, coordination, and continuity of care. Integrated care includes physical, dental, and mental health care, focusing on promoting and restoring health to the whole person. Coordination among health services and other social service agencies, law enforcement, education, religious communities, and informal support systems is particularly important in rural communities. The scarcity of workforce resources makes coordination imperative to address service gaps and avoid unnecessary duplication (see chapter 8). Providing services across the continuum of care refers to the full range of appropriate interventions, from preventive services to follow-up or aftercare. Rural areas often lack services on both ends of the continuum.

As can be seen, providing or obtaining care in rural and frontier areas can be a tough row to hoe. Some of the policy issues that underlie the provision of service are related to the entirety of rural and frontier life, not just to health care, whereas others are more specific to health care.

References

Bandura, A. (1977). *Social learning theory.* Englewood Cliffs, NJ: Prentice-Hall.

Bandura, A. (1986). *Social foundations of thought and action: A social cognitive theory.* Englewood Cliffs, NJ: Prentice-Hall.

Boyd, G. M. (1997). Introduction. In E. Robertson, Z. Sloboda, G. M. Boyd, L. Beatty, & N. Kozel (Eds.), *Rural substance abuse: State of knowledge and issues* (National Institute on Drug Abuse Research Monograph No. 168, National Institutes of Health Publication No. 97-4177, pp. 131–136). Washington, DC: U.S. Government Printing Office.

Bushy, A. (1994). When your client lives in a rural area. Rural health care delivery issues. *Issues in Mental Health Nursing, 15,* 253–266.

Chavez, N., & DeLeon, P. H. (1997). Serving the underserved: Our societal responsibility. *Professional Psychology: Research and Practice, 28,* 203–204.

Ciarlo, J. A., Wackwitz, J. H., Wagenfeld, M. O., Mohatt, D. F., & Zelarney, P. T. (1996). *Focusing on "frontier": Isolated rural America. Letter to the Field No. 2.* Frontier Mental Health Services Resource Network. Denver, Colorado. Retrieved March 19, 2000, from http://www.du.edu/frontier-mh/letter2.html

Conger, R. D. (1997). The societal context of substance abuse: A developmental perspective. In E. Robertson, Z. Sloboda, G. M. Boyd, L. Beatty, & N. Kozel (Eds.), *Rural substance abuse: State of knowledge and issues* (National Institute on Drug Abuse Research Monograph No. 168, National Institutes of Health Publication No. 97-4177, pp. 6–36). Washington, DC: U.S. Government Printing Office.

Cordes, S. M. (1990). Come on in, the water's just fine. *Academic Medicine: Journal of the Association of American Medical Colleges, 65*(Suppl. 3), S1–S9.

Dalton, K., Howard, H. A., & Slifken, R. T. (2000). *At risk hospitals: The role of CAH status in mitigating the effects of new prospective payment systems under Medicare.* Chapel Hill, NC: Cecil G. Sheps Center for Health Services Research. Retrieved April 9, 2001, from http://www.shepscenter.unc.edu/research_programs/Rural_Program/wp67.pdf

Dannerbeck, A., Davenport, J. A., & Davenport, J. (1999, March). *The industrialization of agriculture: Impacts on Hispanics and rural communities.* Paper presented at The Changing Face of Rural America, 24th Annual Meeting of the National Institute on Social Work and Human Services in Rural Areas, Salisbury, MD.

Duncan, D. (1993). *Miles from nowhere.* New York: Penguin Books.

Hemard, J. B., Monroe, P. A., Atkinson, E. S., & Blalock, L. B. (1998). Rural women's satisfaction and stress as family health care gatekeepers. *Women and Health, 28*(2), 55–77.

Hirsch, S., & Harriman, J. (2000). *Rural health statistics.* Washington, DC Rural Information Center Health Service (RICHS). Retrieved April 9, 2001, from http://www.nal.usda.gov/ric/richs/stats.htm

Human, J., & Wasem, C. (1991). Rural mental health in America. *American Psychologist, 46,* 232–239.

Kohrs, F. P., & Mainous, A. G. (1996). Is health status related to residence in medically underserved areas? Evidence and implications for policy. *Journal of Rural Health,* 12, 218–224.

Mueller, K. (2001, June). Medicare payment for services in rural communities: Testimony before The Subcommittee on Health, Committee on Ways & Means, U.S. House of Representatives. Retrieved November 5, 2002, from http://www.rupri.org/healthpolicy/index.html.

Mulder, P. L., Kenkel, M. B., Shellenberger, S., Constantine, M., Steiegel, R., Sears, S. F., et al. (2000). *Behavioral healthcare needs of rural women.* Washington, DC: Committee on Rural Health of the American Psychological Association. Retrieved March 19, 2001, from http://www.apa.org/rural/ruralwomen.pdf

Office of Technology Assessment (OTA). (1991). *Health care in rural America* (No PB91-104927). Retrieved November 11, 2000, from http://www.wws.princeton.edu/~ota/disk2/1990/9022_n.html

Pion, G. M., Keller, P., & McCombs, H. (1997). *Mental health problems in rural and isolated areas: Final report of the Ad Hoc Rural Mental Health Provider Work Group* (Substance Abuse and Mental Health Services Administration, Department of Health and Human Services Publication No. SMA-98-3166). Washington, DC: U.S. Government Printing Office.

Popper, F. (1986, Autumn). The strange case of the contemporary American frontier. *Yale Review,* 101–121.

Ricketts, T. C. (Ed.). (1999). *Rural health in the United States.* New York: Oxford University Press.

Ricketts, T. C., Johnson-Webb, K. D., & Taylor, P. (1998). *Definitions of rural: A handbook for health policy makers and researchers.* Rockville, MD: Office of Rural Health Policy, Health Resources and Services Administration, U.S. Department of Health and Human Services.

Rourke, J. (1997). In search of a definition of "rural." *Canadian Journal of Rural Medicine, 2*(3), 113. Retrieved March 19, 2001, from http://www.cma.ca/cjrm/vol-2/issue-3/0113.htm

Stamm, B. H. (1999). Creating virtual community: Telehealth and self-care updated. In B. H. Stamm (Ed.), *Secondary traumatic stress: Self-care issues for clinicians, researchers, and educators* (2nd ed., pp. 179–210). Lutherville, MD: Sidran Press.

Stamm, B. H. (2000, February). *The digital divide in rural America: Public policy and mental health services in rural America.* Invited address presented at the Capitol Area Rural Health Roundtable, a forum sponsored by the George Mason University Center for Health Policy, Research and Ethics, Hart Senate Building, Washington, DC.

Struthers, C. B., & Bokemeier, J. L. (2000). Myths and realities of raising children and creating family life in a rural county. *Journal of Family Issues, 21,* 17–46.

U.S. Bureau of the Census. (1994). *Geographic areas reference manual.* Retrieved March 2, 2001, from http://www.census.gov/geo/www/garm.html

U.S. Bureau of the Census. (2000). *Historical metropolitan area definitions.* Retrieved June 27, 2002, from http://www.census.gov/population/www/estimates/pastmetro.html

U.S. Department of Agriculture, Economic Research Service (USDA-ERS). (2000a). *Rural America.* Retrieved February 25, 2001, from http://www.ers.usda.gov/Topics/view.asp?T=104000

U.S. Department of Agriculture, Economic Research Service (USDA-ERS). (2000b). Rural poverty rate declines, while family income grows. *Rural Conditions and Trends, 11*(2). Retrieved February 25, 2001, from http://www.ers.usda.gov/publications/rcat/rcat112/rcat112j.pdf

U.S. Department of Health and Human Services. (1995). *Healthy people 2000: Review.* Washington, DC: U.S. Government Printing Office.

U.S. Department of Health and Human Services. (2000). *Healthy people 2010: Understanding and improving health* (2nd ed.). Washington, DC: U.S. Government Printing Office. Retrieved March 19, 2001, from http://www.health.gov/healthypeople/Document/tableofcontents.htm

U.S. Office of Inspector General, Department of Health and Human Services. (1999). *Hospital closure.* Atlanta, GA: Author.

Weinert, C., & Long, K. A. (1990). Rural families and health care: Refining the knowledge base. *Marriage and Family Review, 15,* 57–75.

Essays From the Field

B. Hudnall Stamm, with Neill F. Piland (Health Care Administration and Public Health); Byron Crouse, James Boulger, and Gary Davis (Family Medicine); Bette A. Ide and Marlene S. Buchner (Nursing); B. Hudnall Stamm and Renee V. Galliher (Psychology); and Kathy Tidwell (Social Work)

Working well as part of an interdisciplinary team requires people from different fields to learn about and respect each other's knowledge and to build bridges across shared knowledge on behalf of the people and communities they serve. In this section, representatives from five fields—health care administration and public health, family practice, nursing, psychology, and social work—have prepared field-specific essays on rural health. Each essay team was instructed to read the whole manuscript of the book and to select issues that team members believed were particularly important and that their field perspectives could address. These commentaries, which offer glimpses of richer content to come, provide a backdrop for the chapters in this book.

Health Care Administration and Public Health

Rural communities and their residents are exceptionally diverse. Therefore, identifying common problems is essential to proposing solutions that are feasible and policy relevant. The descriptions of rural health history and culture in view of developing policy and practice are certainly relevant. These are greatly enhanced by the presentation of methods of assessing the need for services by particular communities and matching a community's need with the levels of resources that may be available. Distinguishing differences between the need and the effective demand for services is not a trivial or unimportant task. In general, *need* is a concept that is generated by professionals working in a specific field. There is an inherent bias in using professionally determined levels of need for any specific population, service, or disease. The level of need, which will be defined quite differently by medical, public health, and social welfare professionals, is largely independent of the potential effective demand for services.

Effective demand is the quantity of a good or service that will actually be used by a consumer or a population at alternative prices. The gap between levels of professionally determined need and the ability and probability of members of a community to afford and use the proper level of services can be quite large. Residents of most communities, especially rural communities, are incapable of generating and allocating the level of resources necessary to meet professionally defined levels of need. Therefore, planning for rural health care must entail both an assessment of potential demand for care and collaborative planning aimed at addressing the health care problems of the community in relation to the level of resources that members of the community can generate and sustain.

Services must be cost effective in order to remain viable and sustained over time. This is exceptionally difficult in rural communities because of the relatively low number of users and the relatively high capital investment necessary for purchasing and maintaining the systems. It has been difficult to maintain for long even those systems that have been subsidized by federal, state, and private programs without added subsidy.

Rural communities are subject to a variety of health risks associated with poverty, ethnicity, poor sanitation, inadequate housing, transportation shortages, and reduced access to health care. These factors lead to substandard care of both acute and chronic illness. Untreated and inadequately controlled conditions such as diabetes, hypertension, asthma, coronary artery disease, and congestive heart failure result in individual and familial psychological distress, high utilization of expensive emergency and inpatient care, and much poorer health care outcomes.

By any measure, ethnic populations have less access to health services. Within specific ethnic and racial populations, the issues are multiplied by potential discrimination. It is clear that disparities in health status and the utilization of health services do exist. Many of them, however, cannot be explained completely by socioeconomic status, supply, or access to health services. Race and ethnicity—and perhaps discrimination—are explanatory variables. These variables, along with poverty, lack of insurance, and rural health status, are powerful predictors of substandard lifelong health status.

Rural areas are frequently viewed as healthful havens where residents have better health than do their urban counterparts. Some data support this hypothesis. In comparison with urban areas, there is less reported morbidity from acute conditions, and fewer workdays are lost to illness. However, in the case of chronic illnesses, the opposite is true: There is higher prevalence of chronic conditions in rural populations, and these conditions are treated more episodically and less comprehensively. Even the lower reported incidence of acute illness may be an artifact of reduced health care access. The development of organized systems of care through community health centers and rural health clinics have helped provide an infrastructure on which to build more comprehensive programs, but rural areas remain at a disadvantage in generating the resources necessary to make the greatest impact on rural health status.

Federal and state programs are largely community based and therefore require culturally competent community organization and involvement to be effective. Health care can be provided in many types of alternative settings by different types and levels of providers. The effectiveness of the service is the critical outcome. Rural health care systems have been in the forefront of instituting and evaluating the use of nonphysician professionals in providing primary care. Technological innovations such as telehealth and telemedicine have also been launched in rural areas to help bring a broad range of primary and specialty services to rural areas. The use of such innovations must accelerate if rural residents are to receive the same quality of care as nonrural residents.

The continuing drive toward the goals of 100% access and zero health disparities for all people requires the commitment of resources to rural health care services that are not likely to be available without substantial investment from federal and state sources. This can be accomplished only with the continuing commitment from the community.

Family Practice Physicians

Family practice is the medical specialty most often found in rural and frontier regions and is often the only medical specialty found in these regions. The proportion of family practice physicians who work in rural and frontier regions approximates the proportion of the population who live in these regions. Although there are many definitions in rural health care, the definitions of Health Professional Shortage Areas (HPSA) and Medically Underserved Areas (MUA), which are based on the ratio of health care providers to the populations served, are the ones most familiar to family practice physicians (see the introduction in this book).

There are no health problems that are unique to rural and frontier areas; however, there are characteristics of these areas that shape the nature of medical practices. Higher rates of poverty, greater distances to travel for health care, and a higher proportion of the elderly have direct implications for care. Patients often are seen at more advanced stages of illness and with more comorbid conditions. Because of limited access to other medical specialties, family practice physicians in these areas care for patients with more serious and more complex illnesses in comparison with their suburban and urban counterparts. Also because of limited access to emergency services and higher rates of occupational and recreational injuries, rural family practice physicians are more likely to see patients suffering acute, severe trauma, which may have physical and psychological sequelae.

Rural culture presents unique challenges to the family physician. Most established rural residents have a culture of hardiness. This hardiness is supported by residents' will to carry on and an ability to adapt to what life deals them. They also define their health by an ability to work. If patients define health as an ability to work, their refusal to have a cervical Pap test or a screening test for colon cancer is caused not by ignorance of the potential health problem or by defiance of the family physician's recommendation but by a need to work to be healthy.

Further complicating the nature of these medical practices are substance abuse and psychological disorders. Not only do family practice physicians find themselves caring for people with complicated medical conditions but, because of fewer specialists, they also provide most of the mental health care. Finally, because of the factors that shape medical practices in rural areas, family practice physicians have less time available to address issues of health promotion, health behaviors, and lifestyle. All of this occurs in a medical economics context of generally lower reimbursement rates in rural areas than in urban areas.

In a rural setting, the family physician is one of the key entry points to the formal and informal health care network across the life span. Rural mental health and behavioral health care are inefficiently provided today. Family physicians are a natural axis as "conveners" of health care. Family physicians are more predictably available and easier to identify in rural areas than are other member of the health system. Because they provide the majority of mental health care in many rural areas, they have a vested interest in the mental health system's working more effectively and efficiently. This is not to say that family physicians should provide the leadership in maintaining an integrated and collaborative system of mental health care, but they may be in the best position to provide the initial impetus for such collaboration. Technologically advanced but simple innovations such as videophones for electronic house calls will greatly assist in these efforts.

Family practice physicians are increasingly finding that the complexity of their patients' health problems exceeds the physicians' abilities to effectively meet their patients' health needs solely through medical care. Rural and frontier family physicians are often engaged in many aspects of community health that go beyond seeing patients in the hospital or in the office. The Association of American Medical Colleges (www.aamc.org) has emphasized the need to promote more community and population care curricula in medical schools. An interdisciplinary team approach addressing the patient, community, and regional needs is becoming a progressively more salient option for optimizing health and minimizing risk of health provider burnout.

A final issue worthy of comment is the role that the acquisition of prescribing privileges plays in emphasizing even further the need for interdisciplinary collaboration. In their 2000 report "To Err is Human," The Institutes of Medicine noted errors in health care delivery that are staggering in scope. Many of the errors deal with medications and drug interactions. In coming years, providers from multiple professions will prescribe medications for patients. If this were to occur in the current system, it is reasonable to expect that medication errors and adverse reactions would increase accordingly. It is essential that health professionals work together to ensure an integrated and collaborating system of care that will encourage the minimization of medication errors and complications. Pharmacists can serve as an excellent resource to all health professionals with regard to the issues of pharmacotherapy for medical and mental illnesses. They can also be of assistance by tracking refills and monitoring adherence to prescribed medication use.

Efforts to broaden the prescriptive authority of other health professionals (e.g., psychologists, nurse practitioners) have not been well received by many medical professionals; however, this reflects the concerns of physicians regarding the amount and level of training of other health professionals. Changes in some clinical psychology programs giving psychopharmacology greater emphasis do answer some of these concerns, but many physicians are unaware of these increased competencies. Changes in the prescriptive authority for psychologists, a potential boon to rural physicians and patients,will best be achieved with the concurrence and understanding of primary care physicians. A therapeutic alliance will be possible only if interprofessional boundaries can be rationally and educationally eliminated.

The family physician will continue to be a key player in developing a multidisciplinary team approach to the understanding, diagnosis, and treatment of mental illness in rural settings. The unique blend of medical skills of primary care physicians and their ability to work carefully and cooperatively with others on the collaborating team can serve only to improve the comprehensive and high-quality care expected and deserved by the rural population.

Nursing

Time and time again, rural nurses have encountered patients who value their rugged independence, discovering that, frustrating as the conflicts with those values may be, they also offer opportunity for ingenuity and innovation in designing and carrying out programs that are acceptable to the rural community. Nurses can take advantage of the fact that they "see the whole picture": individual, family, and community. From that vantage point, rural nurses can focus on becoming a resource for the community and on building trust before trying to implement new programs. One such program that has been extremely effective in providing much-needed and well-accepted mental health services is that of the parish nurse, wherein the rural church acts as sponsor for educational resources and support services for members.

The rural nurse working in primary care is often the best-accepted provider of mental health services. Rural nurse practitioners, because they are often the ones to whom mentally ill clients turn for help, need to have a stronger background in mental disorders and psychopharmacology. Another area of expanding practice is in telehealth and telemedicine programs. Nurses have long been active in assessing clients and sending photos of the findings to the consulting provider. They also present clients over the network. In some cases, they are the telehealth program managers; however, their role is still seen by the public as that of "handmaiden to the physician," and they have had difficulty in obtaining adequate remuneration. It is hoped that as more nurses with advanced practice credentials enter the arena, the situation will change. Nurses performing telehealth also struggle with licensure and the delivery of services across state boundaries; this problem is shared with other providers: physicians, psychologists, social workers, and so forth. Professional licensure is at once enabling, regulating, and restricting. The growing movement toward multistate licensure of nurses, which will make it easier and, it is hoped, less expensive for a nurse to be licensed in multiple states, should provide at least a partial solution. Moreover, multistate nursing licensure laws may provide models for other health professions.

Nurses are aware of the importance of cultural competency. At the University of North Dakota, employees are making some strides toward filling the gap in culturally based services in regard to the provision of nursing services to American Indians. Created by combining parts of three tracks (nursing, medicine, and psychology) under the Quentin N. Burdick Indian Health Program, the Recruitment/Retention of American Indians Into Nursing (RAIN) program began in 1990. RAIN's goal is to improve the provision of health services to American Indian people by training providers who are from similar cultural backgrounds, are knowledgeable about the socioeconomic realities of reservation living, and are committed to the improvement of health in their home communities. Both academic and nonacademic strategies are used in the program to support the development of a sense of belonging on the part of the students. Academic strategies include staff members working with prenursing students as well as with those admitted to the program; students are given a place to work that has a 24-hour open-door policy and is supplied with computers and study areas. Also, there is extensive monitoring and mentoring in writing and other skills. Nonacademic strategies promote academic and social integration to enhance a feeling of belonging. These strategies include encouraging students to participate in College of Nursing activities, sponsoring students to go to professional conferences, financial support (a major factor), increasing faculty awareness of cultural differences, and special awards (pins, blankets) upon graduation. In the summer of 2002, RAIN admitted its hundredth student. Not only has the program worked to increase cultural diversity within the College of Nursing and the university but also the graduates return to work with their people; 90% of the baccalaureate degree graduates and 83% of the master's graduates have done so.

In rural communities, the nurse is usually reported to be the most trusted of providers. As noted earlier, rural nurses know their communities and the networks of relationships in depth. They are aware of the risk factors and resources and their ramifications. Adverse events affecting the community, such as the farm crisis or a natural disaster, accentuate the needs of the community. The rural nurse has an important role to play in regard to the farm crisis, which is in epidemic proportions in the midwestern states and the "farm belt." There is an increase in stress on the families who remain in farming as well as on those who have had to leave. This stress is manifested in many physical and psychological illnesses. Incidences of domestic abuse, child abuse, violence, drug abuse, alcoholism, and suicide are very high. These situations may go untreated because they are so common that people grow accustomed to their presence, and they become a way of life. Feelings of powerlessness and depression are problems experienced on an individual level and can stem from a loss of pride when farmers are unable to provide for their families.

It is frustrating for these nurses when individuals who are in need of intervention and treatment do not seek help or refuse help when it is offered. For this reason, the rural health nurse must actively reach out to these people and involve other community services to help them. These rural nurses play an important role in assessments in primary care settings and sometimes in residents' homes, carrying out individual or group culturally sensitive pre-vention and community action programs. They also can actively collaborate with violence intervention and abuse centers, providing a holistic approach as rural nurses, who can connect the physical with the psychological needs of these people. Unfortunately, these centers are not always available in small rural farm communities, and support systems can be very weak. Therefore, nurses have a bigger job. They must hold all of this together with limited resources.

Psychology

Psychologists have long been active in the public sector, but their participation at the administrative and policy level has perhaps been eclipsed by the stereotype of a psychologist performing individual psychotherapy. This is not to say that psychologists should perform less psychotherapy; instead psychologists can be, should be, and are active in other areas such as policy development and policy advocacy. Because of the relatively greater number of doctoral-level psychologists than doctoral-level psychiatrists, psychologists as a group have many opportunities to be "in the trenches" in rural communities.

One difficulty for psychologists as they operate in rural communities is the establishment of professional identity. As clinical or community clinical psychologists, are they associated with the medical community as "psychological physicians," or are they associated with social services as members of one of the professions that provide counseling? As community psychologists, are they associated with public health? School psychologists are usually associated with the educational systems but are increasingly looking toward the community for their practice venues. Research psychologists who specialize in health care may be associated with any of the aforementioned fields, or they may serve as administrators, evaluators, or university faculty. With this confusing array of options, how do psychologists define themselves in an interdisciplinary rural environment? The answer, of course, is that psychologists may play any of these roles, and the wide-ranging spirit of the field welcomes this diversity. However, the broad range of skills, interests, and subfields that are second nature to psychologists may be confusing to those who define psychology from less sweeping contexts. The popular stereotype of a psychologist is a clinical psychologist. Thus, psychologists working in rural interdisciplinary teams must educate community members and other professionals about the skills and competencies they bring.

Because of their standard training in the scientist–practitioner model (or its variants), psychologists are likely to have more psychometric and research training than members of many other health professions. This background can help facilitate decision making on the basis of data, a skill often needed for obtaining grants. Psychologists' experiences with psychometrics and research design also provide skills necessary for designing research methods, collecting data, and interpreting the outcome of the activities of the grant.

Psychologists and other practitioners working in rural communities often find themselves "wearing many hats" and providing types of services that their urban counterparts would never consider within their scope of practice. This places an increased burden on professionals working in rural communities. For health professionals working in low-infrastructure areas, it is easy to feel threatened in times of scarce health and social resources. Psychologists, with their training in group processes, can contribute skills for facilitating sharing and reducing the conflicts inherent to scarcity. When professionals feel threatened in their work, it is all too easy to retreat into their professional identities and assume that if one of the other fields went away, there would be more for them.

Psychologists can also bring to bear their knowledge to support programs of professional development, which can help strengthen professional quality of life and reduce the negative effects of burnout and secondary or vicarious traumatization. The risk of burnout faced by professionals working in rural environments is high. The relative scarcity of behavioral health resources places rural professionals in a position of being indispensable, and such pressure can be draining. In addition, the frustration of working with clients, one individual, or one family at a time, when the real roots of the problems appear to be at the community or societal level, can lead to a sense of powerlessness and hopelessness in clinicians. Active participation in community, regional, and national organizations aimed at promoting health and effective service appears to be an integral part of the work of the rural clinician.

Psychologists bring to their work strong individual assessment skills and are well suited to consider the unique characteristics of each client, taking into account both the factors associated with living in a rural environment and other social, cultural, family, and individual characteristics. Strong individual assessment, a hallmark of psychological training, can prevent clinicians from taking stereotypes for granted or applying treatment in a one-size-fits-all manner. Particular research emphasis can then be placed on identifying areas of strength unique to rural communities or to some individuals, families, or cultures within these communities. These interventions should then be evaluated through further outcome-based research. In view of the scarcity of resources in rural communities, psychologists can bring their assessment, clinical, and research skills to help ensure that clinical and programmatic efforts are indeed being channeled in the most productive and effective directions possible.

Social Work

Social work is a profession of collaboration and integration that strives to eliminate poverty, minimize dysfunction, and help vulnerable, oppressed people be included and valued by society. Social work training uniquely combines values, theory, and practice. Training is focused on strengths-based systems perspectives that guide assessment and intervention strategies for individuals, families, and communities. Social work interventions tend to occur at the juncture at which people interact with their social environment. Interventions may be designed to introduce change at the individual, family, or community level or any combination of the three. There is a broad range of social work interventions: from individual psychosocial practice to family psychotherapy to social policy work.

In urban social work, functions and professional relationships tend to be more specialized, allowing for a depth of learning and collaboration within a relatively narrow range. Conversely, rural and frontier social workers depend on many colleagues across agencies, and they serve in a number of capacities. Rural and frontier social workers must have a broader base of skill and knowledge than that of their urban counterparts. This is critical when one professional both functions as a member of the community's multidisciplinary team and effectively represents the social work perspective.

Clinical social workers are often the on-call mental health providers for rural hospitals. The absence of psychiatric support is difficult for emergency room staff, which may include physicians, physician's assistants, nurse practitioners, registered nurses, and even emergency medical technicians. Training and experience for new physicians may not have been adequate to prepare them for psychiatric emergency responses or for the necessity of collaborative interdependence with clinical social workers. Suboptimal treatment outcomes may be the end result: (a) Clients may be sent home with insufficient or no medical intervention, (b) involuntary action that could have been prevented may be initiated, or (c) an unnecessary and potentially long transport to an urban center for treatment may occur. The on-call clinical social worker is likely to be the person expected to facilitate these dispositions.

As with emergency rooms, social workers often are the on-call providers for jails. Jailing people because of their mental illnesses continues even though there are laws prohibiting it. Imprisoning people with mental illnesses represents multiple system failures. All too often, it is more difficult and time consuming to get help from a community mental health center or hospital than it is to charge people with petty crimes and take them to jail. Also, in some rural communities and most frontier communities, there are no mental health centers or hospitals to which law enforcement staff can take people. In some areas, when people are taken to mental health or medical facilities, they are transported handcuffed in a police car rather than in an ambulance.

Services to people in jail are critically important. Without them, persons with mental illness may not be given their medication, are released with no follow-up arrangements, or, even worse, are prosecuted for crimes instead of treated. A liaison relationship that incorporates a legal mechanism for release of information between the jail and the community health center or community mental health center can provide (a) screening and consultation for at-risk inmates identified by the jail, (b) identification of inmates who are already in treatment in the community, (c) information regarding the prescribed medication for a person already in treatment, (d) medication support to augment the jail formulary when needed medicines are unavailable in the jail setting, (e) release planning that includes appointments for follow-up in the community, and (f) advocacy with prosecutors for the dismissal of charges, particularly in the case of petty crimes. This liaison program can accomplish a great deal even though it does not have full-time staff, may not have the resources to provide sentencing diversion, and may not meet the formal definition for jail diversion. Especially in rural areas, the development of liaison protocols, regular communication, and follow-up at the jail may be a workable adaptation of formal jail diversion programs that will yield important benefits.

Clinical social workers, social work advocates, community organizers, and social work managers all struggle with the challenges of service delivery. Although not entirely satisfactory, one model, the local authority model, provides promise. Local authorities for public health, mental health, substance abuse, and behavioral health are typically responsible for funding, prioritizing, and evaluating services to geographical areas that usually include more than one county. Local mental health authorities encompass a variety of stakeholders from all counties in the region, including funders, consumers, families, and providers. Advantages of a local authority model include the ability to customize according to local assets and needs; the inherent collaboration at the policymaking level; the ability for all counties to participate in funding and priority setting decisions; and the potential to pool funds from a variety of sources, which adds further to the encouragement for system integration. The disadvantages of a local authority model include inconsistencies across service and target population priorities and implementation of state mandates; inequities of available resources, which make it difficult for lower level authorities to fund essential core services; and less savings, related to economies of scale, that might be higher in the larger centralized systems. Accomplishment of integrated public health, substance abuse, or mental health services as well as other service integration combinations much more likely with a local model than with a centralized model. Social workers across the spectrum of social work activity can play important roles in bringing successful models to rural regions.

Part I

Behavioral Health Care Needs of Rural Communities

1

The Behavioral Health Care Needs of Rural Communities in the 21st Century

Patrick H. DeLeon, Mary Wakefield,
and Kristofer J. Hagglund

Historical Perspective

In this chapter, we review some of the policy and history of rural health care. We continue with observations on the current system and suggest rural health care policies for the 21st century.

The U.S. Congress, Office of Technology Assessment (OTA), report, *Health Care in Rural America* (OTA, 1990), was a landmark publication. During the 20th century, the rural population of the United States became an increasingly smaller proportion of the total U.S. population: At the beginning the century, 60% of the population was rural (Rockefeller Commission, 1969); near the end of the century, only 20%–27% of the nation was considered rural (OTA, 1990). Older residents, with their chronic health impairments, constitute a greater proportion of rural America than of urban America. Rural residents are characterized by relatively low mortality rates (with the striking exception of injury-related causes) but relatively high rates of chronic disease. The barriers that rural residents often face in obtaining necessary health care are truly unique and impressive. Prolonged distances, adverse weather, and other physical obstacles are commonplace. Economic barriers, including lack of access to health insurance, are significant. Rural hospitals are frequently described as "going broke." Health care providers of all disciplines are insufficient in number, and their ability to readily access relevant scientific advances is questionable at best. The OTA report stressed that no single strategy should be considered appropriate for all rural areas or all rural health care providers. Of interest, the authors of the OTA report also expressly noted that they would not examine the quality of rural health care in any detail, pointing out that, by necessity, such an evaluation would have to be measured against the implications of having no locally available service at all (OTA, 1990).

The 1990 OTA report revealed that rural residents appear to use preventive screening services less often than do urban residents; rural residents have fewer contacts with physicians than do individuals in urban areas; and rural

Dr. DeLeon, past president of the American Psychological Association, can be reached by U.S. mail % the American Psychological Association, 750 First Street, NE, Washington, DC 20002-4242. E-mail: deleon1@erols.com

areas have fewer than half as many physicians per capita providing patient care as urban areas. In view of the significant shortage of physician availability, highly credible public policy arguments have been made for the efficacy of developing expanded roles for nonphysician providers, despite the fact that there are also marked shortages in these disciplines. Enhancing interdisciplinary collaboration is often viewed as crucial to strategies for providing necessary care. The report emphasized that the federal government has a distinct role in protecting the well-being of rural America; for example, the federal government was providing nearly half of the resources for rural health activities (e.g., personnel recruitment). At the time that this report was issued, the states were required (pursuant to Public Law 101-269) to provide Medicaid reimbursement for services provided by pediatric and family nurse practitioners (NPs), with the option of reimbursing for other NP and physician's assistant (PA) services. Not surprisingly, the authors of the OTA publication recommended "Option 18: Require States to reimburse under Medicaid for the services of NPs and PAs in rural areas, as long as these services are permitted by State practice acts" (p. 24).

In recognition of the importance of a centralized focus for rural health policy, the Congressional rural caucuses were instrumental in the establishment of the Office of Rural Health Policy (ORHP) within the Department of Health and Human Services (DHHS) in 1987 (subsequently codified by Public Law 100-203). The backbone of health delivery throughout rural America became federally qualified community health centers (CHCs) and federally recognized rural clinics. The authors of the OTA report noted, however, that the number of these centers receiving federal grants diminished in the 1980s; the rate of decline was much greater for rural community health center grantees than for urban grantees. Nevertheless, the OTA authors were impressed by the inherent ingenuity of rural America:

> Many rural providers have found effective means of adapting to changes in their environment. There are numerous examples of efforts by rural hospitals, CHCs, and other facilities to support effective change. Many have found ways to strengthen facility solvency and stabilize operations in the short term (e.g., renewed fundraising, tougher collection policies). Also, many rural facilities have instituted strategies that reconfigure their organizational and service structure for the longer term. (p. 177)

In our judgment, the underlying policy issue related to which disciplines should be authorized to provide what health services (i.e., scope of practice issues) and how they should be reimbursed is of critical importance for rural America. What should be considered sufficient and necessary training to protect the public, and who should ultimately make this determination? Organized medicine's almost monopolistic control simply does not make good policy sense for rural America when, for example, the number of professionally active physicians per 100,000 residents was more than twice as high in urban areas as in rural areas, with wide variations in rural physician supply among states and regions (see http://bhpr.hrsa.gov/healthworkforce/profiles/default.htm). Without question, professional job satisfaction is a critical factor in retaining

health professionals of all disciplines throughout rural America. It is not difficult to understand why highly educated individuals, who may experience
cultural barriers associated with education, find it difficult to continue practicing in regions where their professional judgment is not respected.

It was interesting that the OTA report contained an entire chapter, as one
of two examples of specific services to be highlighted, that focused on rural
mental health care. Perhaps most telling, however, was the extent to which
verifiable data on the prevalence of mental disorders and the availability of
mental health services were scarce and difficult to obtain, in part because the
states were not required to keep records or report back to the federal government in any detail. The available data did suggest that the differences in
mental health status between rural and urban residents were slight but that
alcohol dependence (unlike drug abuse) was apparently higher among rural
than urban residents. The researchers also documented dramatic differences
between rural and urban areas in the availability of local inpatient mental
health services; two thirds of metropolitan counties possessed some kind of
inpatient services in 1983, whereas only 13% of nonmetropolitan counties had
such facilities. The availability in rural areas of comprehensive mental health
services was believed to be much more difficult to determine. The little
existing evidence again suggested not only that rural areas were less likely to
have such services but also that services, where they existed, were narrower
in scope. Emergency mental health services were seen as particularly crucial
but unavailable in rural areas.

For rural residents, one highly significant service problem was the
apparent lack of awareness that mental health services existed and that they
could actually be helpful. Transportation availability, confidentiality concerns,
and difficulty in recruiting and retaining mental health professionals were
noted as continuing problems. Like other rural health professionals, rural
mental health specialists often must become generalists, but to be effective in
any treatment, they must first become a part of the community. Thus, the
potential overlap between personal and professional roles can lead to burnout
and conflicts between professional impartiality and personal values. Another
rural trend was the interdependence of mental and physical systems. Specialist knowledge in the nuances of mental health care to facilitate that interdependence was often unavailable. Nonpsychiatrist physicians accounted for
almost half of the patient visits that resulted in the diagnosis of mental disorders and for approximately 85% of all psychoactive drug prescriptions.
Primary care physicians referred these patients to mental health professionals in 5% of the episodes. Over one fourth of nonpsychiatrist visits were for
psychological problems.

The 1999 Follow-Up Report

In the late 1990s, the federal Office of Rural Health Policy (ORHP) commis-
sioned a report to follow up the landmark OTA publication. The report suggested that despite efforts to strengthen rural hospitals, enhance the efforts to
place professionals in rural areas, and modify payment systems, "many of the

same problems that confronted rural America in the 1980s remain in the 1990s" (Ricketts, 1999, p. vii).

Not surprisingly, the authors of the report found a continued significant shortage of health professionals of all disciplines. Rural America represents 20% of the nation's population, but only 9% of the nation's physicians practice in rural counties. Like the OTA report, this report revealed that rural patients see doctors less often and usually later in the course of an illness than do their urban counterparts and that specialty services are used significantly less often. These findings clearly have direct implications for the quality and cost effectiveness of the received care.

The 1999 report described how systemic changes occurring within the nation's overall health care system during the previous decade were almost overwhelming in their scope and impact. Public concern regarding the escalating costs of health care have resulted in changes in the financing of medical and public health services, which created new forms of organizations—managed care organizations, provider networks, and so forth—that have come to dominate the urban health care environment but have been slower to develop in rural America. Technological advances potentially brought new tools to rural practitioners (e.g., telehealth), thereby reducing their isolation. The high costs of many of these new technologies resulted in their being concentrated into the more densely populated areas, however. Critical ownership and control are thus often found far from the communities they affect.

Ricketts (1999) stated that "the wealth of a community has a direct relationship to its health status" (p. 2). Rural America is growing more slowly, and its population continues to be older than that of the rest of the nation; both facts hinder any significant economic increases. These economic and demographic changes put the health status and health care resources of rural America at risk. Wide variations, as they are related to poverty, race, and ethnicity, exist in health status within rural places and among population groups. Isolation, rural culture, and small size are essential characteristics of rural life and are the specific descriptors of the rural experience that need special attention. Health and health care are linked closely to the economy and demography of a place; therefore, many of the ills associated with poverty are magnified in rural populations.

From a behavioral science perspective, many of rural America's health care priorities are behaviorally (and not medically) based. Rates of mortality from trauma, especially from motor vehicle crashes and for gun-related reasons, are disproportionately higher in rural areas. Rural areas also report higher rates of chronic disease and infant mortality.

> The quality of life of rural versus urban people is seldom considered. Rural people more often describe their health as poor or fair, and there are indications that the types of care they receive and its timeliness compare unfavorably with those of urban dwellers. (Ricketts, 1999, p. 23)

Rural populations have often been viewed as especially vulnerable with regard to access to health care. This is due to poorly developed and fragile health infrastructures; high prevalence rates of chronic illness and disability; socio-economic hardships; and physical barriers such as distance and availability of transportation, including a lack of public transportation. The key to success-fully addressing many of these underlying issues is a fundamentally organi-zational and behavioral orientation.

As indicated previously, the shortage of rural health professionals of all disciplines is one of the few constants in any description of the U.S. health care system. In the 1999 report, however, it was noted that international medical graduates (IMGs) eventually settle permanently in the United States and are more likely to practice in rural areas. It is particularly satisfying to see that the follow-up report appears to be considerably less physician exclu-sive in its perspective; one of the issues highlighted was that the Idaho Rural Interdisciplinary Training Project (RITP) has had a positive impact in culti-vating nonphysician providers for rural America. In 1994, 54% of the gradu-ates from this program were employed in rural or frontier areas 3 years after their training.

As did the previous report, the 1999 report contained a specific chapter on rural mental health, this time also including a focus on substance abuse. The authors suggested that current policy trends, including consideration of parity legislation, may be breaking down some of the historic barriers between the mental and physical health care delivery systems. However, in their judgment, the concerns of rural mental health and substance abuse service providers and consumers were still often overlooked at the national level. Although primary care professionals demonstrate some success in treating a number of mental health problems, rural residents whose mental health problems are so persistent that they require ongoing professional care must often move to urban areas, where these services are readily available. Most rural areas continue to possess fewer mental health services. Historical short-ages of specialty mental health professionals in most rural areas persist. There was a clear sense in the 1999 follow-up report that the authors had access to considerably more comparative data than did the authors of the OTA study. There was also an evolving appreciation of the clinical importance of addressing the psychosocial aspects of health care.

Evolving Challenges

Although public health visionaries such as Albee (1986) and Lalonde (1974) stressed the importance of the psychosocial and environmental aspects of health care for decades, it is only since the early 1990s that this underlying concept has become an integral component of the United States' health planning process. In *Healthy People 2010,* it was noted that "the health of the individual is almost inseparable from the health of the larger community" (U.S. Department of Health and Human Services, 2000, p. 3).

Without question, this policy statement represents a fundamental shift in the federal government's perspective and priorities. A similarly broad and futuristic vision of the importance of underlying clinical and public policy issues was recently provided by the Robert Wood Johnson Foundation (Institute for the Future, 2000). According to this report, incorporation of information tech-nology into health care will be a "prime catalyst of change" (p. 143). In the report, it was also noted that midlevel practitioners may be critical providers because of their ability to provide cost-efficient health care. In addition,

> [s]ocioeconomic status is the number one predictor of poor health ... ill effects of poverty are particularly ominous in the light of an increasing economic gap between the rich and poor, which is independently associated with a worse health status for the bottom economic tiers of society. (p. 143)

We suggest that policy statements represent the behavioral and psychosocial agendas of the future.

Economic Implications of Health Care for Rural Communities

Beyond the composition and availability of clinicians is a broader policy concern regarding the impact of the presence or absence of health care on rural economies. Much of what is known about economic impact of health care is derived from the work pioneered at Oklahoma State University and the Universities of Nebraska and Kentucky. Exploration of the economic implications of health care has been supported by different federal agencies, including the Agency for Healthcare Research and Quality and the U.S. Department of Agriculture. With federal funding, for example, the project Operation Rural Health Works is under way in 15 states; in this program, local data are collected to demonstrate the multiplier effect of locally spent dollars on services and employment for individual communities. The research has shown that communities with good access to health care can survive and grow. In contrast, communities that lose local health care and good access to services lose their ability to prosper. Access to clinicians and facilities is *essential* for economic survival. In fact, health care in rural communities is as much a cornerstone of the local economy as are schools and businesses. Health care service is an economic engine that generates thousands of dollars in additional revenue for local areas.

There are many substantial reasons for supporting a strong health care system. Data from the Operation Rural Health Works Project Briefing Report (2001) indicate that, on average, the health care industry employs 10%–15% of a rural county's workforce. In addition, schools and health services are the most important quality-of-life factors influencing an industry's choice of business location. Finally, a strong health care system attracts retirees.

The economic impact of individual practitioners is also important to consider. According to another study of the economic impact of National Health Service Corps (NHSC) physicians on rural communities, each physician generates more than five jobs and over $233,000 in income to the local economy (Weisgrau, Sheldon, & McDowell, 1997). Although the reauthorization of the NHSC was delayed from 2001 until 2002, a positive economic impact associated with the presence of these clinicians is clearly a strong argument for its reauthorization. Far less is known about the economic impact of other types of clinicians, including the contribution of psychologists, dentists, pharmacists, and nurses. It is likely that these clinicians also contribute substantially to the local economy.

In spite of health care's positive economic impact on rural areas, significant health care spending continues to take place outside of rural communities. For example, an average rural county of 22,000 residents generates $73 million annually in health care expenditures, but only about $35 million is spent locally (Operation Rural Health Works Briefing Report, 2001). Some of this loss is unavoidable when highly specialized services are needed, but a significant portion could stay in rural areas if the health system were organized to encourage local utilization. The trend in the health care industry to move care from high-cost acute care settings to low-cost outpatient settings could capitalize on lower intensity care available in rural areas and contribute to cost containment. In fact, small communities can provide a broad array of primary, preventive, wellness, home health, and residential care.

Although not every hamlet can afford a hospital, rural communities need, at a minimum, a hospital within reasonable distance to anchor their local primary care, support emergency services, and stabilize the ill and the injured. Many rural hospitals have continued to survive because of a patchwork of special protective policies enacted in the 1990s by Congress. For example, some rural hospitals can apply for payment reclassification to a higher, urban wage rate to enhance their Medicare reimbursement. Some are exempted from the inpatient prospective payment system by virtue of their classification as sole community hospitals or their Medicare-dependent hospital status. In the late 1990s, Congress enacted a limited-service hospital payment policy that supports designated critical access hospitals. This latter option is a welcome opportunity that allows cost-based Medicare reimbursement for inpatient and outpatient services and more flexible staffing requirements. Nevertheless, even with these and other programs, many rural hospitals remain threatened, and the Balanced Budget Act of 1997 enacted new prospective payment systems that have been implemented from 1997 to 2002, so the effects remain largely unknown. Great attention to impact of payment policy changes is needed because rural hospitals have a notably poorer Medicare margin than do their urban counterparts. In fact, 39% of all rural hospitals have negative Medicare inpatient margins.

Because rural Americans number about 61 million, it is essential that national policies not defeat rural economies or compromise rural beneficiaries' access to quality health care services. As policy choices are made, the tremendous investment return related to the health care sector should be kept in mind. Health care providers and policymakers should consider the relationship between rural health care systems and rural economies.

The Business of Policy

Congressional staff members play a critical role in the development of public policy, including health policy. However, because they are not likely to be health care providers, they generally do not understand the roles of nonphysician practitioners delivering care in rural areas. Therefore, they cannot be expected to understand the potential for nonphysician practitioners to improve care if practice restrictions are removed and reimbursement for services is allowed or increased. Too often, Congressional staff members are visited by nonphysician practitioners only when the latter are seeking funding or admission to an existing program, such as the NHSC. Coordinated education about how nonphysician practitioners can improve the quality of rural Americans' lives would lay the foundation for future changes. This education, however, is nonexistent. These errors of commission and omission are as long-standing, as is the maldistribution of providers.

How can NPs, PAs, psychologists, and clinical pharmacists, for example, coordinate services to meet the needs of some of the poorest and sickest people in the United States? The tools to improve care in rural areas include an untapped nonphysician workforce, communications and computer technology, increasingly effective medications, and practice guidelines. Unfortunately, most of these tools remain unused by nonphysician practitioners because the professional groups have not seen fit to use them. It is time for nonphysician practitioners (perhaps including selected physician partners) to share with Congressional staff members examples of service delivery models. Some models are not effective. For example, noting that there are more of a certain type of provider in rural areas than in urban is not generally helpful, because of the urban flight that occurs when restrictions on professions are removed. Instead, innovative models of care, such as telehealth, have gained rapid acceptance and support.

A consortium of practitioners delivering a plan to provide health care to rural America, using the most sophisticated tools available, would be well received by Congress. It is not necessary to present the research documenting the needs and problems of delivering care. Congressional staffs are aware of the problems facing rural America, including the maldistribution of health professionals; the economic, education, and transportation challenges; and the stigma associated with seeing a mental health practitioner. They are also acutely aware that legislative proposals that increase costs of existing health care programs (e.g., Medicare, Medicaid) or increase discretionary spending to improve the rural health care delivery systems are "nonstarters." That is, proposals that require large cost increases will not be considered because of the budget implications on other programs. Interdisciplinary practice models that focus on community health, prioritize community education and involvement, and focus on the constituents are needed. Removing practice restrictions and improving reimbursement will necessarily follow from effective models that meet these criteria.

In many ways, the underlying issues surrounding the provision of quality health care to the residents of the rural United States may represent the "final frontier." We are confident that the nation can and will meet this challenge and that, collectively, health care practitioners will embrace a new vision for the future. In so doing, however, we suggest as a prerequisite that some common ground between the involved parties—including nonphysician practitioners, physicians, and consumers—must be reached before demands of public policy regarding the scope of practice issues and determinations of clinical competency can be made. Objectively psychological and social aspects of health care should become a priority. Decisions regarding this and the use of technology should, foremost, be patient oriented.

The educated consumer is the future. It is the responsibility of the helping professions to provide proactive leadership. We are confident that the next rural health follow-up report, perhaps in 2010, will be rewarding and inspirational.

References

Albee, G. W. (1986). Toward a just society: Lessons from observations on the primary prevention of psychopathology. *American Psychologist, 41,* 891–898.

Institute for the Future. (2000). *Health and health care 2010: The forecast, the challenge.* San Francisco: Jossey-Bass.

Lalonde, M. (1974). *A new perspective on the health care of Canadians: A working document.* Ottawa, Ontario, Canada: Government of Canada.

Operation Rural Health Works Project Briefing Report, *1*(1). Retrieved March 19, 2001, from http://www.rupri.org/pubs/archive/old/health/orhw/orhw11/index.html

Ricketts, T. C. (Ed.). (1999). *Rural health in the United States.* New York: Oxford University Press.

Rockefeller Commission. (1969). *Population and the American future: The report of the Commission on Population Growth and the American Future.* Washington, DC: Author.

U.S. Congress, Office of Technology Assessment (OTA). (1990). *Health care in rural America* (Office of Technology Assessment Publication No. OTA-H-34). Washington, DC: U.S. Government Printing Office.

U.S. Department of Health and Human Services. (2000). *Healthy people 2010: Understanding and improving health* (2nd ed.). Washington, DC: U.S. Government Printing Office. Retrieved March 19, 2001, from http://www.health.gov/healthypeople/Document/tableofcontents.htm

Weisgrau, S., & McDowell, S. 1997. *Economic Impact of National Health Service Corps Physicians of Rural Communities.* Kansas City, MO: National Rural Health Association.

2

A Snapshot of Rural and Frontier America

Morton O. Wagenfeld

In this chapter, I "paint" a brief picture that serves as a backdrop for the other contributions. This chapter addresses difficulties in defining *rural,* in separating fact from myth, and in understanding the heterogeneity of its demography and economic base. I pay particular attention to the most sparsely populated subset of rural areas, what is called *frontier.* The frontier areas are largely concentrated in the western United States with population densities of seven or fewer people per square mile. These areas, along with other rural areas, tend to have unstable economies, which may have an impact on the mental health of its residents.

A great deal has been written about the general category of "rural" (see Goreham, 1997, for a comprehensive treatment) and on its mental health problems (e.g., Keller & Murray, 1982; Wagenfeld, Murray, Mohatt, & DeBruyn, 1994). Rural America is a very heterogeneous entity in terms of its demography and economic base. It is also a part of the United States about which numerous myths exist. It is appropriate to consider some definitions of *rural,* a surprisingly difficult task. Extended discussions were published by Wagenfeld et al. (1994) and Ciarlo, Wackwitz, Wagenfeld, and Mohatt (1996).

The dichotomies *urban–rural* and *metropolitan–nonmetropolitan* are not synonymous. The former, employed by the U.S. Bureau of the Census, refers to population density: an area of 2,500 or fewer persons or open countryside. In contrast, urban areas consist of cities with 50,000 or more inhabitants and the closely settled areas around those cities that are economically tied to them (e.g., a metropolitan statistical area). The concept includes a consideration of the social and economic activity patterns of an area's population. *Nonmetropolitan area* is a residual term: a county or aggregation of counties that are not metropolitan. People can refer variously to rural areas, rural counties, or even rural states. The definition, then, is somewhat elastic.

Hewitt (1989) reviewed nine county-based typologies with regard to population size, density, urbanization, adjacency to an urban area, distance from an urban area, and type of economy. It is easy to see that no approach to

Dr. Wagenfeld can be reached at Department of Sociology, Western Michigan University, Kalamazoo, MI 49008. E-mail: morton.wagenfeld@wmich.edu Dr. Wagenfeld is also affiliated with the Health Services Program, School of Health and Human Services, Walden University.

defining *rural* is entirely satisfactory. Such definitions are always arbitrary, and many important variables are not taken into account if only one definition is used. Perhaps, as Cordes (1990) noted, the only thread that ties rural areas of the United States together is population density: It is invariably lower in rural areas.

Recent census data (U.S. Bureau of the Census, 1993) indicate that more than 54 million Americans live in rural areas, constituting about 20% of the population. During much of the 1990s, the growth rate was greater in rural areas than in urban ones. Johnson and Beale (1999) referred to this as the "rural rebound," noting that most rural areas grew at a rate three times that of the 1980s. Gains were the greatest in the Mountain West, Upper Great Lakes, Ozarks, and rural areas of the South and the Northeast. Areas that were losing population were the Great Plains, Western Corn Belt, and Mississippi Delta. There is no compelling explanation for this growth, but improved quality of life is assumed to be the reason.

Data compiled by the U.S. Department of Agriculture (USDA) National Agricultural Library (USDA, 1999) indicate that rural populations differ from the urban populations in a number of important ways in demographic and health-related characteristics. Rural areas have a larger proportion of elderly persons but a smaller proportion of minorities. Poverty is higher, especially among minorities and children. Rural and frontier areas have lower incomes and a slightly higher unemployment rate. In comparison with urban residents, rural residents have lower levels of insurance coverage, a lower likelihood of receiving prescription drug coverage, a higher likelihood of receiving Medicare, and lesser benefits.

Not surprisingly, their self-reported health status was more likely to be fair or poor, and the prevalence of physician-diagnosed chronic conditions was higher. Also not surprisingly, rural areas had fewer and less well-trained health care providers and greater numbers of suboptimal health care facilities. On the other hand, there has been a noteworthy growth in the number of federally assisted health programs such as rural health clinics (RHCs) and community health centers (CHCs).

A Look at Frontier America

Since 1990, there has been a sharpening of focus on the most isolated and sparsely populated of rural areas: the frontier. Very little has been published about the frontier, and so this is the central focus of this chapter. More specifically, the nature of frontier America, its problems, the values of its residents, and some of the obstacles in providing mental health services are considered.

The word *frontier* conjures up a set of images. Historians have even argued that American character has been shaped by it. People associate the frontier with explorers such as Lewis and Clark, pioneers, hunters, trappers, and Indians. Although the frontier of historic imagination no longer exists, a real frontier does live on, protected from large-scale settlement by harsh climate, difficult terrain, lack of water, distance from metropolitan areas, lack of exploitable resources, and federal land policies (Duncan, 1993; Popper,

1986). It is populated by the EuroAmericans and groups of ethnic and racial minorities. A number of journalists, essayists, and academics have looked at both the historical and contemporary appearance of the frontier (Duncan, 1993; Dyer 1997; Eagan, 1998; Norris, 1993; Popper, 1986; Popper & Popper, 1987; Raban, 1996). Collectively, their vision is not optimistic.

Sociodemographic Aspects of the Frontier

As with *rural*, defining *frontier* can be difficult. For many years, the U.S. Bureau of the Census defined a frontier county as having fewer than two persons per square mile. According to this definition, there are 132 rural counties located in 15 states. For federal planning and policy purposes, a population density of fewer than seven persons per square mile is now used as the definition. Under this rubric, there are 394 rural counties in 27 states. These areas are at the extreme end of a rural–urban continuum. The great majority of these largely contiguous counties lie west of the 98th meridian. As a group, they constitute 45% of the land mass but less than 1% of the population (Popper, 1986). Texas has the greatest number of frontier counties (62), whereas New York has only one.

Ten frontier states (i.e., those in which at least half of the counties are frontier) have been identified: Alaska, Colorado, Idaho, Montana, Nevada, New Mexico, North Dakota, South Dakota, Utah, and Wyoming. According to the 1990 figures for the population living in frontier counties, Montana has the highest frontier population (281,822). However, according to the percentage residing in frontier counties, Wyoming, with over 50%, has the highest (Frontier Mental Health Services Resource Network, 1997).

The sparseness of settlement can be appreciated from the fact that the average population density per square mile of land area for the United States is 72.9. For the 10 frontier states, it ranges from 34.6 for New Mexico to barely 1 for Alaska. It can, however, be argued that Alaska is not the ultimate frontier. Although half of the population of Alaska is in the Anchorage Bowl, which houses about 250,000, the largest city in Wyoming contains only 50,000.

Also, as a group, frontier states are experiencing a rate of population growth that is greater than the average for the country. For the United States as a whole, the population grew by 0.9% during the period 1995–1996; for the frontier states, however, the rate of increase was much higher, at 1.5%. Indeed, Nevada and Utah are, respectively, the first and third fastest growing states. These averages can mask some differences. Some frontier areas, particularly in the Great Plains, are experiencing population declines.

How different are frontier areas from the rest of rural areas or the whole United States? Duncan (1993) suggested that they differ in kind, not just degree:

> People in these regions have always had to adapt to weather and terrain, but the counties of the contemporary frontier have made a further adaptation to their unique paucity of people. Health care, education, religion, politics, law and order, transportation, communication, sense of community, sense of self, even the act of finding a mate—virtually every human institution and activity demonstrates the impact of few people and long miles. The very sparsity of people makes life difficult. (pp. 17–18)

Distances can also be daunting. People may drive 50 to 100 miles for groceries and as many as 200 miles for health care. The frontier is also home to large concentrations of Native Americans and Hispanics (see chapter 18).

Vigorous debate has emerged about the meaning of *frontier* and its future (Duncan, 1993; Popper, 1986; Popper & Popper, 1987). On the one hand, its history and resources make it a vital part of the nation's heritage and future. A number of frontier areas are experiencing growth as recreational areas, whereas others are retirement destinations or refuges for people fleeing urban life. On the other hand, it has been asserted that a significant part of the frontier—the Great Plains—as a result of the "largest, longest running agricultural and environmental miscalculation in American history, has become almost totally depopulated" (Popper & Popper, 1987, p. 12). The remedy that Popper and Popper proposed is to allow the region to revert to a pristine state and become a vast wildlife preserve termed a "Buffalo Commons." Echoing this theme, *U.S. News and World Report* ("Life in the Sand Hills," 1995) carried a story on the economic decline and depopulation of the ranching area of the Sand Hills in Nebraska. With the migration of younger people out of rural areas, the population is becoming increasingly elderly. One resident, aged 67, noted,

> The area has turned elderly. I put up the mail and I know how many get Social Security checks, and that's most of them. Our kids got a good education and they took a good work ethic with them when they left, none of them are slackers. But there's nothing here to hold the young ones. The opportunities are better somewhere else. What it means is that Paul and I are the "young couple" in the church and at the Library Society, and that's so sad. (p. 27)

The Sand Hills, part of the Great Plains, are one of the few areas experiencing a population decline (Johnson & Beale, 1999). Johnson (1999) referred to this as "natural decrease" that is symptomatic of fundamental demographic changes.

I have pointed out elsewhere (e.g., Wagenfeld et al., 1994) that, in general, rural areas tend to be economically unstable and that this may have an impact on the mental health of its residents, especially for those in frontier areas. There is little manufacturing. The major sources of income are tourism, ranching, farming, logging, mineral extraction, or even subsidence economies, which rely on gardens or on hunting and gathering of wild foods (see Stamm & Stamm, 1999).

Economic declines have begun earlier in frontier areas than in the rest of the country. For example, the Great Depression began over a decade earlier in the Great Plains than it did in the cities. During the Depression, the proportion of farm families on relief was highest in many of the frontier states. The infamous Dust Bowl, the result of misguided agricultural policies, came to the Plains earlier than to the rest of the Midwest. The more recent farm crisis of the 1980s was also felt more acutely in this area. Many of these same points can also be made with regard to the petroleum industry. The single industrial base of these areas makes earning a consistent living more difficult, and one of the consequences is frequent migration (National Rural Health Association, 1994).

If the economic base becomes depressed or collapses, a chain reaction occurs. Businesses dependent on the dominant industries experience reverses, public services shrink or disappear, and the quality of life suffers (Popper & Popper, 1987). The mental health consequences are far-reaching.

Dyer (1997) took this point several steps further and tried to establish a link among the economic difficulties of rural and frontier areas, mental health problems, anger against the government, and the rise of the militias—all leading to the Oklahoma City bombing. Although readers may be skeptical about some of the evidence, Dyer did present an apocalyptic picture of conditions in this part of the country. If the Oklahoma City bombing had been an isolated event of civic chaos, the article would not be so compelling. However, with the increasing incidence of violence in rural and frontier areas—Ruby Ridge, Idaho, and Waco, Texas—attention to the relation between mental health care and community health has increasing importance.

The paucity of economic opportunity, coupled with distance from metropolitan centers and low population density, has turned some frontier areas into practice bombing ranges, missile sites, and dumps for nuclear waste. In their zeal for economic stability, communities have actively sought these opportunities (Norris, 1993).

Going beyond demography and economics, Fitchen (1991) wrote about the problems of poverty in rural areas and the implications for mental health. She argued that rural poverty is a persistent and self-perpetuating problem that involves intertwining historical, economic, social, cultural, and psychological factors.

Rural and Frontier Values

The effective delivery of mental health services requires models that are consonant with the values of the consumers. A body of research too large to discuss here indicates that a person's values influence the definition of a problem and the likelihood that he or she will seek either informal or formal help (see Wagenfeld et al., 1994).

A pervasive view, firmly entrenched in literature and the mass media, is that rural persons have values different from those of persons from urban areas. There is considerable disagreement on this point in the professional literature. A number of scholars have suggested that rural values, in contrast to urban ones, stress self-reliance, conservatism, a distrust of outsiders, religion, work orientation, emphasis on family, individualism, and fatalism. On the other hand, it has been argued that the gap between rural and urban values, if it exists, is shrinking. Also, it is not clear whether these differences reflect actual community differences or differences in demographic or socioeconomic composition of the communities. Wagenfeld et al. (1994) provided a summary of both sides.

"Rural" is also a state of mind. A town that is considered small in a relatively urbanized state might be considered large in a less populous state. Ching and Creed (1996) elaborated a distinction that may prove beneficial toward a resolution of this debate. First, over the course of history, the rural–urban distinction has been seen as invidious. In contrast to the salubrity of rural life, cities could be characterized as sinkholes of depravity. At other times, urban areas are the apogees of enlightenment, whereas rural venues are cultural backwaters. These terms have implications far beyond a venue; they are a source of identity. A person can live in a rural area but still hold values that are urban. This rural–rustic distinction, which may have enormous heuristic and service delivery potential, has not been explored in any systematic way. It is important to consider rusticity as a source of identity, as well as a basis for such things as help-seeking behavior. However, if contemporary rural–urban value differences have been exaggerated, can the same be said of the frontier? In other words, how different are the values of frontier residents from those of the rest of America, both urban and rural? Empirical data on this point are in short supply. Duncan (1993), a journalist who traveled extensively through the most remote frontier counties (fewer than two persons per square mile), observed that "in addition to reflecting the violent past that they share, the residents of the sparse places confront life with a fatalism less common in the rest of urban/suburban America" (p. 97). Norris (1993), in describing the western Dakotas, presented several examples of clannishness, a sense of inferiority, and mistrust of outsiders.

The issue of value differences is more than an academic debate, inasmuch as it affects service utilization. There are several reasons why a particular health service is not utilized by clients or consumers: It may not be accessible geographically or in terms of hours of operation; fee structures may make it unaffordable; and even if these barriers do not exist, certain services may not be utilized if there is a lack of fit between the values of the providers and con-sumers. The extent to which this is the case in frontier areas is not clear.

Conclusions and Recommendations

I have noted the importance of rural and frontier areas, and I suggest that scholars pursue several lines of investigation.

Understand Rural and Urban Values

First, although it is an empirical question, I think that there are few differ-ences today between rural and urban values. Having said that, I realize that the issue of whether the values of frontier residents differ from those of their counterparts in more populous rural and urban areas has not been explored. Anecdotal evidence suggests that this may be true.

Understand Perception of "Rurality" and Rusticity

Furthermore, as I have noted, patterns of migration have brought urban resi-dents into rural areas. To call them *rural* simply because they reside there may obscure a very important difference. Although their mailing addresses may be rural, their values may remain firmly urban. From the perspective of research, as well as service delivery, it is important to consider the signifi-cance of rusticity as a source of identity, as well as a basis for such things as help-seeking behavior, provider–patient interaction, and attitudes toward and conceptualization of mental health problems. Again, evidence from a focus group in a frontier area suggests that this may, indeed, be the case (Cooper & Wagenfeld, 1998). As a first step, a scale to measure dimensions of "rurality" is needed.

In a review of the demography of rural and frontier areas, Johnson and Beale (1999) noted a rebound in most regions. In reviews of the demography of rural and frontier areas, data indicated a large rebound in most regions. For the Great Plains, natural decrease seems to be the norm. Because population changes, both growth and decline, affect provision of mental health services, examination of frontier communities that exhibit both would almost provide a natural experiment.

Understand Resiliency

Finally, one of the findings coming out of the research on the mental health consequences of the farm crisis of the 1980s was the amazing degree of resiliency displayed by people in the presence of severe economic adversity. Resilience may be key to understanding the behavior of rural and frontier residents and may serve as the basis for preventive and therapeutic interventions (DeBruyn & Wagenfeld, 1994).

References

Ciarlo, J. A., Wackwitz, J. H., Wagenfeld, M. O., & Mohatt, D. F. (1996). *Focusing on "frontier": Isolated rural America. Letter to the Field No. 2*. Denver, CO: Frontier Mental Health Services Resource Network, Denver University Library. Retrieved February 6, 2000, from http://www.du.edu/frontier-mh/

Ching, B., & Creed, G. (Eds.). (1996). *Knowing your place: Rural identity and cultural hierarchy*. New York: Routledge.

Cooper, S. C., & Wagenfeld, M. O. (1998). *Delivering mental health services to children and adolescents with serious mental illness in frontier areas: Parent and provider views. Letter to the Field No. 17*. Denver, CO: Frontier Mental Health Services Resource Network, Denver University Library.

Cordes, S. M. (1990). Come on in, the water's just fine. *Academic Medicine: Journal of the Association of American Medical Colleges, 65*(Suppl. 3), S1–S9.

DeBruyn, J. C., & Wagenfeld, M. O. (1994). Salutogenesis: A new perspective for rural mental health research. *Human Services in the Rural Environment, 18*(1), 20–26.

Duncan, D. (1993). *Miles from nowhere*. New York: Penguin Books.

Dyer, J. (1997). *Harvest of rage*. Boulder, CO: Westview Press.

Eagan, T. (1998). *Lasso the wind*. New York: Knopf.

Fitchen, J. M. (1991). *Endangered spaces, enduring places: Change, identity, and survival in rural America*. Boulder, CO: Westview Press.

Frontier Mental Health Services Resource Network. (1997). *States with frontier populations*. Retrieved February 1, 2000, from http://www.du.edu/frontier-mh/

Goreham, G. (Ed.). (1997). *Encyclopedia of rural America*. Santa Barbara, CA: ABC-CLIO.

Hewitt, M. (1989, July). *Defining "rural" areas: Impact on health care policy and research*. Health Programs, Office of Technology Assessment, Congress of the United States. Washington, DC: U.S. Government Printing Office.

Johnson, K. M. (1999, August). *The rising incidence of natural decrease in the United States*. Paper presented at the annual meeting of the Rural Sociological Society, Toronto, Ontario, Canada. Retrieved February 6, 2000, from http://www.luc.edu/depts/sociology/johnson/p99webnd.html

Johnson, K. M., & Beale, C. M. (1999). The rural rebound: Recent non-metropolitan demographic trends in the United States. *Wilson Quarterly, 12*(Spring), 16–27. Retrieved February 6, 2000, from http://www.luc.edu/depts.sociology/johnson/p99webn.html

Keller, P., & J. D. Murray (Eds.). (1982). *Handbook of rural community mental health.* New York: Human Sciences Press.

Life in the sand hills. (1995, July 17). *U.S. News and World Report,* 26–29.

National Rural Health Association. (1994, September). *Health care in frontier America: A time for change.* Rockville, MD: Office of Rural Health Policy.

Norris, K. (1993). *Dakota: A spiritual geography.* New York: Ticknor & Fields.

Popper, D. E., & Popper, F. (1987). The great plains: From dust to dust. *Planning, 53*(12), 12–18.

Popper, F. (1986, Autumn). The strange case of the contemporary American frontier. *Yale Review,* 101–121.

Raban, J. (1996). *Bad land.* New York: Pantheon.

Stamm, B. H., & Stamm, H. E. (1999). Trauma and loss in native North America: An ethnocultural perspective. In K. Nader, N. Dubrow, & B. H Stamm (Eds.), *Honoring differences: Cultural issues in the treatment of trauma and loss* (pp. 49–75). New York: Brunner-Routledge.

U.S. Bureau of the Census. (1993). *1990 Census of population and housing unit counts (CPH-2).* Washington, DC: U.S. Government Printing Office.

U.S. Department of Agriculture National Agricultural Library (1999, October). Retrieved February 6, 2000, from http://www.nal.usda.gov.ric/richs/stats.htm

Wagenfeld, M. O., Murray, J. D., Mohatt, D., & DeBruyn, J. C. (1994). *Mental health and rural America: 1980–1993.* Washington, DC: U.S. Government Printing Office

3

Poverty and Rural Mental Health

Catherine Campbell,
Sarah D. Richie, and David S. Hargrove

"It's mighty hard to do psychotherapy with a woman who is worried whether she is going to be able to feed her kids." A rural public health nurse made this observation to one of the authors, who was starting a mental health center in rural Mississippi in the early 1970s.

> It's just as hard to get a man who is not able to get a job and is hungry every day to come in to talk about feeling depressed or angry, or even seeing things that are not there. That's just a part of life when you can't work and provide for your family. Talking about your problems is a luxury.

Her point was made time and again in the development of that mental health center. The center served nine rural counties, all with a substantial proportion of people living below poverty level. Going to school hungry was not unusual for children; being out of work or working at subpoverty pay scales was commonplace for adults. Families in which *every* member was required to work characterized the economic condition of the less populated counties of the region. These characteristics were not then and are still not unusual for rural people and communities. "The poor are still there," wrote Harrington (1984) in his second volume on being poor in America. This observation followed his first treatment of poverty that focused on Appalachia (Harrington, 1963), a work that was instrumental in President John F. Kennedy's community mental health center legislation as well as many other progressive social programs.

The purpose of this chapter is to explore the impact of poverty on the mental health of rural Americans and on the type and quality of mental health services that are available. We address prenatal care and care of children first, followed by care of adolescents, adults, and, finally, the elderly. Each group has different mental health needs that are determined by the developmental stage.

Parents living in poverty experience distress because of their concerns for survival and the physical and mental health of their children. In 1995, 45.7% of all single-mother-headed families with children younger than 18 lived in poverty, and 17.7% of all families with children were poor (Schein, 1995). In addition, 60% of those 17.7% are families headed by single mothers (Schein,

Catherine Campbell can be reached at Finch University of Health Sciences/Chicago Medical School, 3333 Green Bay Road, North Chicago, IL 60064. E-mail: Catherine.Campbell@finchcms.edu

1995). In accordance with these statistics, Halpern (1993) revealed that more than half of all poor infants have parents who have not earned a high school diploma. These poverty-stricken parents endure consistent hardship stemming from the conflict between their desire to provide for their children and their financial means to do so. Even something as seemingly benign as a walk down a busy street, one filled with shops and eateries, provides both parents and children with a glimpse of what is beyond their reach. Holidays and birthdays also present problematic situations for parents and children as they try to find a way to balance their celebration with their survival.

Some parents in poverty, confronted with inadequate physical, mental, and financial resources, are simultaneously thwarted by the inability to provide an adequate physical environment for their children. For example, families that are homeless often lack the ability to provide their children with sufficient food, comfort in terms of temperature regulation, and the security needed to sustain mental health during childhood. Homelessness has detrimental effects not only on single mothers but also on the infants and young children for whom they attempt to care. In one study in which homeless mothers with young children were given the Beck Depression Inventory, more than half these mothers were estimated to have elevated scores (Zeanah, 1993). In explanation of the effects of a homeless environment on young children, Zigler, Hopper, and Hall (1993) found that the children's mental health was compromised as they experience the "transience, insecurity, dangers, and frequent parent–child separations" that permeate the lives of homeless families (p. 482).

Rural Poverty Across the Life Span

Poverty, Prenatal Care, and Infancy

Poor mothers, in comparison with women of higher socioeconomic status, are likely to have high stress levels and inadequate prenatal care during pregnancy, as well as to engage in health-threatening behaviors (e.g., drug and alcohol abuse). Therefore, the unborn babies of these poor mothers are more likely to experience "severe and/or chronic intrauterine stress," which may result in small fetal size during gestation, premature labor, low birth weight, and even neurological damage in the infant (Halpern, 1993, p. 74).

Infants with low birth weight, in comparison with infants of normal birth weight, experience a higher incidence of language disorders and learning disabilities, especially as they reach school age (Prizant, Wetherby, & Roberts, 1993). In addition, Prizant et al. (1993) found that a child's socioeconomic status is associated with a disruption in both receptive and expressive language acquisition. The risk of developmental problems is associated with factors related to poverty, such as poor maternal health during pregnancy, child illnesses left untreated, and "less than optimal child-rearing practices" (Prizant et al., 1993, p. 266).

The Epidemiologic Catchment Area (ECA) data showed that women, children, and minorities at the poverty level were at greater risk for mental health problems because of their poverty (Dore, 1993). The ECA study also showed more severe depression among poor mothers, which is critical because of the potential link between a child's lowered mental and motor development and maternal depression and because of the potential for reduced quality of parent–child attachment.

Psychological theory augments understanding the effects of living in poverty on an infant's mental health. Hunt (1968) explained that a distinctive characteristic of living in poverty is crowding, which could potentially provide an infant with more variety in visual and auditory inputs than a less crowded environment. On the basis of Jean Piaget's theory (see Piaget, 1926, 1969), Hunt believed that this greater degree of auditory and visual stimuli should facilitate the intellectual development of the year-old infant. A distinction should be made, however, between the positive and negative effects of crowding. During the second year of life, the child's development could be restricted by crowding. It is believed that as the child begins to crawl and handle objects, he or she may elicit negative reactions from adults because of space constraints (Hunt, 1968). In the third year, the child may be confronted with the family members who are unable to answer his or her incipient questions, which may result in punishment that, in turn, could inhibit further inquiries. Thus, the environment that had initially provided the infant with a greater variety of input now becomes restrictive and limiting.

Poverty and Children

Erik Erikson (see Erikson, 1950, 1968) also defined stages of psychosocial development that can be used as a model for studying and analyzing the behavior of both infants and children reared in poverty. For example, the first stage that Erikson outlined involves the infant's development of basic trust or distrust during the first year of life. With influence from environmental factors, the infant can develop basic trust for caregivers through the satisfaction of basic needs, such as food, shelter, and love (Glazer & Creedon, 1968). If these basic needs are unmet in a poverty-stricken home lacking proper temperature regulation and the necessary supplies to support the infant, a basic distrust develops between the infant and the caregiver. This distrust extends into childhood, as researchers explain, inasmuch as a child growing up in poverty may develop a distrust that is reinforced by the hostility of an impoverished neighborhood (Glazer & Creedon, 1968).

Another of Erikson's stages of psychosocial development, occurring at the age of 4 or 5 years, involves curiosity and exploration of the world around the child. The child begins to initiate goal-oriented activity and healthy competition with others, but, as Glazer and Creedon (1968) explained, children living in poverty may encounter situations that hinder this initiative. If uneducated parents living in poverty cannot help the child achieve a sense of self-worth, the child may learn there is no place for him or her in the world (Glazer & Creedon, 1968).

Helping a child develop the initiative needed to attain a sense of self-worth and expectations of success is important, but it is also important for parents to take a vested interest in the child's everyday life. Hernandez (1997) explained that "the persons with whom a child lives shape the day-to-day interactions the child experiences in the home, and they make decisions influencing the child's experiences outside the home" (p. 157). In addition, these interactions vary, depending on the family's composition, specifically according to the number and types of parents and siblings living in the home. The number of siblings in the home affects the allotment of parental resources, especially if the family has only one parent to begin with.

Not only does the family makeup influence development, but environmental conditions also have an impact on the maturation process, especially if the child is homeless. Luthar (1999) revealed that homeless mothers are more likely to engage in problem behaviors, such as drug and alcohol use, and that mental health care is provided to fewer than 20% of these individuals. Although these statistics concerning the caregivers of young children are alarming, perhaps more alarming are the effects of homelessness on impoverished children. In educational settings, including preschool, homeless children are rated by teachers as having lower cognitive ability, more problems with adaptive behavior, and higher incidences of depression and social withdrawal than same-aged peers.

When a child is removed from his or her family and placed in foster care because of poverty, several issues confront the child, such as separation from the original caregiver, adapting to a new home environment, and the acceptance of new people and experiences. For example, Minuchin, Colapinto, and Minuchin (1998) suggested that the foster caregiver work with the biological mother to ensure that the separation does not threaten the child's sense of security and attachment felt for those caring for him or her. Even if the child remains with the mother in a single-mother-headed family (i.e., no man is present), the child may be at "significantly greater risk of drug and alcohol addiction, mental illness, suicide, and criminality" (Rodgers, 1996, p. 21).

McLeod and Shanahan (1993) revealed that poor children experience greater psychological distress than do children not living in poverty; specific conditions include conduct disorder, depression, decreased self-confidence, and poor social adaptation. These researchers analyzed data from the 1986 Children of the National Longitudinal Survey of Youth (NLSY), which included interviews with the mothers, interviewer's ratings of the home environment, and assessments of the children's cognitive abilities. The data included ratings of the children by their mothers with the categories "often true," "sometimes true," and "not true" on each item of the following six domains of problematic behavior: antisocial behavior, anxiety or depression, hyperactivity, dependency, peer conflict or withdrawal, and headstrong behavior. Researchers found the length of time in poverty had a significant effect on the children's feelings of dependence, unhappiness, and anxiety, independent of the effect of current economic deprivation. The researchers also found that frequently spanked children exhibit significantly more internalizing and externalizing symptoms than do children who were spanked less often.

Almost 16% of all families with children in America lived in poverty in 1997; this rate is expected to increase (Fujiura & Yamaki, 2000). The authors also reported that living in poverty was linked to a greater probability of being in special education programs and having learning difficulties (Fujiura & Yamaki, 2000). Luthar (1999) analyzed studies specifically devoted to researching the effects of poverty on minority children's mental health. One comparison (McLeod & Edwards, 1995) of African American children and White children living in poverty showed that there is little difference between the two groups in vulnerability for psychopathological disorders. Some research has suggested that, because of the added benefit of kinship support and constructive coping, minority children may be even more capable of handling the ill effects of living in poverty (Luthar, 1999).

Poverty and Adolescents

Social support enhances an adolescent's ability to cope with distressing issues associated with poverty, such as high crime rates, inadequate housing, and high rates of teenage pregnancy. Without support, these issues may hinder adolescents in the development of important tasks, such as forming emotional attachments and developing autonomy and other skills necessary in adulthood (Taylor & Roberts, 1995). Although problems with adolescent delinquency exist in both urban and rural areas, rural adolescents may be more naïve about their effects and consequences; such naïveté results from a lack of rural educational programs targeting such activities (Hagen, 1987). Fitchen (1993) explained that human service providers in rural areas should first be aware of kinship ties and community support networks that are still operative and should suggest that some social work programs may assist family members to rebuild social ties based on kinship or to create other support networks within the rural community.

Other research has shown that such social support of adolescents and their families may buffer distress and enhance the child's and adult's adjustment, as well as the parents' child-rearing practices. Taylor and Roberts (1995) interviewed 51 African American adolescents (31 girls and 20 boys) and their mothers or female guardians to collect data on relationships with kin, parenting practices, and psychological adjustment. Results showed that adolescents whose mothers or female guardians reported receiving more social support had a greater sense of self-reliance and fewer instances of engaging in problem behavior. The results also showed that when mothers have assistance, they are less likely to display adverse behaviors, such as threatening and scolding, and are more likely to display supportive behaviors and attitudes. Furthermore, a higher level of kinship support was associated with higher maternal self-esteem, acceptance of the adolescent, and autonomy granting. However, Taylor and Roberts found that the relation between kinship support and adolescent well-being disappeared when the effects of maternal well-being and parenting practices were controlled. This finding suggests that the benefits of kinship support are somehow mediated by characteristics of the mother or female guardian.

Poverty and Rural Adults

Many Americans are likely to face poverty at some point during adulthood. As many as 60% of adults experience living below the poverty line, 30% of that 60% living in extreme poverty (Rank & Hirschl, 1999). Poverty affects psychological well-being in a number of ways. In a large epidemiological study in the

New Haven area, adults living in poverty were found to be at greater risk for psychiatric disorder regardless of age, gender, or ethnicity (Bruce, Takeuchi, & Leaf, 1991). Furthermore, if an individual has a psychiatric disorder, poverty is a negative influence that manifests in ways such as poorer adjustment to living within a community (Armstrong, 1997). When comparing the psychological well-being of rural and urban adults living below the poverty level, Amato and Zuo (1992) found that the urban poor perceive themselves as having better health than the rural poor, who reported more physical complaints. There were no reported differences for happiness or depression. When other variables such as race, gender, and marital status were considered, differences emerged. Rural poor African Americans self-reported their psychological well-being as higher than that of urban poor African Americans. The opposite was true with White subjects. Gender and marital status interact; single men with no children reported higher levels of depression in rural areas, whereas married women with no children reported lower levels of depression in urban areas.

YOUNG ADULTHOOD (AGES 18–40). The heterogeneity of adulthood is attributable in part to decisions made in early adulthood. These include decisions regarding higher education, career path, relationships, marriage, children, and lifestyle. Both poverty and rural isolation have the potential to exert a profound influence on a young person's choices. For example, a young adult may have had to leave school before getting a high school diploma in order to help run the family farm. Adults who have not gone to college were found to be at increased risk for developing chronic diseases such as hypertension and heart disease, possibly in relation to such variables as lower income, poorer diet, poorer health habits, inadequate health care and prevention, and poorer problem-solving skills (Pincus, Callahan, & Burkhauser, 1987). Furthermore, census data on work disability in southern states revealed that the highest rates of work disability were found for rural residents, women, the elderly, persons with less education, African Americans, and persons living in poverty (Holzer, Nguyen, Goldsmith, & Thompson, 1996).

Limited employment, low incomes, and, perhaps, single parent status may contribute to homelessness. First, Rife, and Toomey (1994) identified five major groups of homeless persons in rural areas: (a) young families unable to afford housing, (b) individuals who are currently employed full or part time who earned too little to pay for housing, (c) women who are unable to work because of lack of child care or poor work skills, (d) older disabled men with little social support, and (e) disabled people without resources for community living. Homelessness and low income can lead to increased victimization and violence (Ingram, Corning, & Schmidt, 1996).

In rural areas, it is commonly believed that young people complain that there is nothing to do and that they "can't wait to get out" of their home town. Some young adults channel this disinterest into activities with negative mental health outcomes. Poverty has been found to relate to high-risk behaviors such as early pregnancy, substance use, and high-risk behavior (with regard to human immunodeficiency virus infection) in young adults (Pritchard, Cotton, Godson, & Weeks, 1993). In addition, teenaged mothers (aged 15–19) experience a higher rate of depressive symptoms than do adult mothers; however, poverty and marital status appear to account for this prevalence (Deal & Holt, 1998). Another behavioral health issue faced by rural residents living in poverty is obesity. Although many young adults have begun exercise programs for the first time in their lives, the risk for being overweight is highest from ages 25 to 34 (Williamson, Kahn, Remington, & Anda, 1990).

Among those who seek treatment for their problems, rural clients were also more likely to work less, or not at all, than are urban clients (Dottl & Greenley, 1997). Owen and Kohutek (1981) also noted that young adults (aged 18–24) in poor, sparsely populated areas dropped out of treatment at a rate higher than what had been anticipated, particularly those who were self-referred and presented problems related to marriage and family or substance abuse.

MIDDLE ADULTHOOD (AGES 40–65). Middle adulthood is characterized by responsibilities to others while battling the Eriksonian notion of stagnation. Possible stressors faced in middle adulthood are characterized by the changing dynamics in the family, such as children leaving home, adult children who do not leave the home or continue to be financially dependent on the middle-aged adult, and the caregiving and death of parents. If employed, the individual may have to stay in an unsatisfying job because of caregiving responsibilities to children, parents, grandchildren, or several of these relatives, which possibly creates occupational stress and burnout. Because of the high incidents of early pregnancies in rural populations, grandparenting, which may include parenting duties for young or financially dependent parents, may become an issue early in middle adulthood.

Middle-aged adults may care not only for their children, grandchildren, or both but also for an elderly parent. One of the authors noticed that a number of women in middle adulthood came to a rural public health unit with diffuse symptoms characterized primarily by depression. These women— separated or divorced with husbands in another city or state—had no means of support for themselves or their children. They sought refuge and economic stability with an ailing, elderly relative. These caregivers have been observed to give good care to the relative but are socially isolated because of geographic isolation and the caregiver's value of duty and responsibility (Reed & Weicherding, 1999). Once the elderly relatives died, however, the women, once again, had no income, no inheritance (because the relatives had no assets), and no plan.

Health issues in middle adulthood, such as menopause, chronic pain, diabetes, and hypertension, present challenges for behavioral health care providers working in rural areas. Preventive efforts targeting symptom severity are on the rise; however, persons living in isolated rural areas may not have access to these programs. Psychoeducation can be a tremendously helpful service in a rural facility. Relying exclusively on printed information may be impractical for those in poverty and with low levels of literacy (Christensen & Grace, 1999).

LATE ADULTHOOD (AGES 65 AND OLDER). Older adults' developmental issues are characterized by adjustment, such as retirement, widowhood, and decreased physical and mental capabilities (see chapter 15). Health care costs, absent or limited retirement benefits, and decreased capacity to work contribute to poverty among the elderly. Many older adults are poor for the first time in their lives, and those who enter older adulthood in poverty have almost no opportunity to increase their incomes. Because of past and present discrimination, minority elderly persons may have experienced poverty and will probably face substandard housing and medical care (Freed, 1992; Grant, 1995; Rank & Hirschl, 1999).

Relocation may also be an issue for older adults. Poverty, health issues, or both may necessitate a move to less expensive housing or to an assisted living environment (for the rural poor, this usually means a Medicaid- or Medicare-subsidized nursing home) or to the home of a relative. In a study on the adjustment of rural elderly persons to relocation, Armer (1996) found that if the individual could predict the move, feel a sense of control, and have social support, the experience was less distressing. Prior life satisfaction and grief were also found to affect relocation adjustment.

Insurance coverage appears to be a limiting factor (Neese, Abraham, & Buckwalter, 1999). Once rural elderly persons have found their way to mental health services, they have lower-than-expected dropout rates (Owen & Kohutek, 1981). Lee (1991) found that hardiness is correlated with an elevated perception of physical, mental, and social health. In a study of Appalachian adults over the age of 65, perceived social support, not family proximity, was found to be related to better mental health (McCulloch, 1995). Affective support appears to be important in reducing the health-related stress, and social contacts and instrumental support have some influence on measures of psychological well-being (Revicki & Mitchell, 1990). Even when mental health services are available, few older rural residents seek these services.

Conclusions and Recommendations

Although both familial and social support have been shown to enhance abilities to cope with living in poverty, social attitudes toward such impoverished families are often judgmental. Minuchin et al. (1998) wrote that

> attitudes toward the poor continue to be pernicious: critical, sometimes subtly racist, and insufficiently attuned to the plight of disadvantaged women who are trying to raise their children against heavy odds. . . . This population is regarded as responsible for their poverty by virtue of laziness and lack of will. (p. 240)

Impoverished families may be seen as an encumbrance to a growing society whose members look down on those who do not provide for themselves. Although such negative perspectives for the plight of the poor remain, Minuchin et al. suggested that some societal support exists for the belief that impoverished families are victims of bad economic times.

Until the equation for eliminating poverty and mental health problems has been solved, mental health care workers must turn to the goal of reducing risk factors through policy and intervention. Viewing poverty and mental health issues as intertwining, cyclical influences of quality of life can yield a number of recommendations within a systems paradigm, which means that affecting any part of the system will directly or indirectly influence the entire system.

Utilize and Strengthen Educational Resources

Education is the key to reducing poverty through job opportunities that lead to increased income, potential decreased mental health issues, and increased access to care. Interventions aimed at increasing the education level of rural residents can be implemented throughout the life span. Rural schools are certainly not immune to the nationwide teacher shortages, increased responsibilities of teachers, and low pay for teachers. Thus, increased job satisfaction for rural teachers in order to increase quality of educational opportunities for students should be a top priority for policymakers. There is no greater investment in the future of this country than in education. Behavioral health care workers can assist schools with mental health interventions and political advocacy. State legislators should examine the cost-effectiveness of pilot programs that expose students to training programs utilizing a multidisciplinary health care team approach to reduce risk factors such as disabilities, substance abuse, teen pregnancy, mental and medical illness, and illiteracy.

Increase People's Options Through Vocational Counseling

Another area of intervention is vocational counseling. Because of the difficulties that schools face, assisting students with vocational choices is often overlooked. However, a student from a poor family probably does not have a parent with a college education or exposure to the numerous job opportunities that a college degree can yield. Such a student may be capable of entering college but may not consider it a viable option. As a society, persons who are financially better off often discourage these students either by not recognizing their potential or by not giving specific information about student financial aid and how to obtain it. Therefore, all professionals who encounter children and adolescents should talk with them about their educational goals, perhaps encourage them to aspire to a better socioeconomic status and provide specific information to help them achieve their goals. Higher education academicians should also make a conscious effort to seek out undergraduates who may be first-generation college students, who may be capable of graduate work but never considered it. Adults of all ages can be encouraged to increase their education, which may benefit them immediately and enable them to serve as role models for their children and grandchildren.

Strengthen and Increase Community-Based Mental Health Resources

When the severity of mental health problems increases beyond what the school can accommodate, adequate resources must be made available in rural communities. A well-documented problem in rural areas, limited access to care necessitates creative restructuring of the service delivery system, particularly for poor residents who are uninsured or underinsured. A promising solution is the integration of medical and mental health services in primary care. The result is increased access to mental health services, decreased health care costs due to addressing contributing mental and behavioral issues, and decreasing administrative costs by combining government-assisted community mental health centers and state departments of public health.

Tailor Prevention and Intervention Activities to Specific Communities

Other directions for future research are to seek effective prevention and intervention programs appropriate to specific communities. Risk factors such as teen pregnancy, substance abuse, chronic illness, and domestic violence continue to necessitate effective solutions. Multiple programs exist but often are not evaluated or produce mixed results. Academic–community partnerships offer a means of bringing together researchers, practitioners, and laypersons in order to design, implement, and evaluate programs for all age groups of rural communities.

References

Amato, P. R., & Zuo, J. (1992). Rural poverty, urban poverty, and well-being. *Sociological Quarterly, 33,* 229–240.

Armer, J. M. (1996). An exploration of factors influencing adjustment among relocating rural elders. *Image: Journal of Nursing Scholarship, 28,* 35–39.

Armstrong, K. H. (1997). Factors associated with community adjustment in a sample of young adults with serious emotional disturbances. *Dissertation Abstracts International, 57*(11B), 7272.

Bruce, M. L., Takeuchi, D. T., & Leaf, P. J. (1991). Poverty and psychiatric status: Longitudinal evidence from the New Haven Epidemiologic Catchment Area Study. *Archives of General Psychiatry, 48,* 470–474.

Christensen, R. C., & Grace, G. D. (1999). The prevalence of low literacy in an indigent psychiatric population. *Psychiatric Services, 50,* 262–263.

Deal, L. W., & Holt, V. L. (1998). Young maternal age and depressive symptoms: Results from the 1988 National Maternal and Infant Health Survey. *American Journal of Public Health, 88,* 266–270.

Dore, M. M. (1993). Family preservation and poor families: When "homebuilding" is not enough. *Families in Society, 74,* 545–556.

Dottl, S. L., & Greenley, J. R. (1997). Rural-urban differences in psychiatric status and functioning among clients with severe mental illness. *Community Mental Health Journal, 33,* 311–321.

Erikson, E. H. (1950). *Childhood and society.* New York: Norton.

Erikson, E. H. (1968). *Identity, youth, and crisis.* New York: Norton.

First, R. J., Rife, J. C., & Toomey, B. G. (1994). Homelessness in rural areas: Causes, patterns, and trends. *Social Work, 39,* 97–108.

Fitchen, J. M. (1993). Rural poverty and rural social work. In L. H. Ginsberg (Ed.), *Social work in rural communities* (2nd ed., pp. 99–117). Alexandria, VA: Council on Social Work Education.

Freed, A. (1992). Minority elderly. *Journal of Geriatric Psychiatry, 25,* 105–111.

Fujiura, G. T., & Yamaki, K. (2000). Trends in demography of childhood poverty and disability. *Exceptional Children, 66,* 187–199.

Glazer, N. Y., & Creedon, C. F. (Eds.). (1968). *Children and poverty: Some sociological and psychological perspectives.* Chicago: Rand McNally.

Grant, R. W. (1995). Interventions with ethnic minority elderly. In J. F. Aponte, R. Y. Rivers, & J. Wohl (Eds.), *Psychological interventions and cultural diversity* (pp. 199–214). Boston: Allyn & Bacon.

Hagen, B. H. (1987). Rural adolescents and mental health: Growing up in the rural community. *Human Services in the Rural Environment, 11,* 23–28.

Halpern, R. (1993). Poverty and infant development. In C. H. Zeanah, Jr. (Ed.), *Handbook of infant mental health* (pp. 73–86). New York: Guilford.

Harrington, M. (1963). *The other America: Poverty in the United States*. Baltimore: Penguin Books.

Harrington, M. (1984). *The new American poverty*. New York: Holt, Rinehart, & Winston.

Hernandez, D. J. (1997). Child development and the social demography of childhood. *Child Development, 68*, 149–169.

Holzer, C. E., Nguyen, H. T., Goldsmith, H. F., & Thompson, W. W. (1996). The demographics of disability in the South. *Community Mental Health Journal, 32*, 431–443.

Hunt, J. M. (1968). Changing psychological conceptions of development. In N. Y. Glazer & C. F. Creedon (Eds.), *Children and poverty: Some sociological and psychological perspectives* (pp. 32–45). Chicago: Rand McNally.

Ingram, K. M., Corning, A. F., & Schmidt, L. D. (1996). The relationship of victimization experiences to psychological well-being among homeless women and low-income housed women. *Journal of Counseling Psychology, 43*, 218–227.

Lee, H. J. (1991). Relationship of hardiness and current life events to perceived health in rural adults. *Research in Nursing Health, 14*, 351–359.

Luthar, S. S. (1999). *Poverty and children's adjustment*. Thousand Oaks, CA: Sage.

McCulloch, B. J. (1995). The relationship of family proximity and social support to the mental health of older rural adults: The Appalachian context. *Journal of Aging Studies, 9*, 65–81.

McLeod, J. D., & Edwards, K. (1995). Contextual determinants of children's responses to poverty. *Social Forces, 73*, 1487–1516.

McLeod, J. D., & Shanahan, M. J. (1993). Poverty, parenting, and children's mental health. *American Sociological Review, 58*, 351–366.

Minuchin, P., Colapinto, J., & Minuchin, S. (1998). *Working with families of the poor*. New York: Guilford.

Neese, J. B., Abraham, I. L., & Buckwalter, K. C. (1999). Utilization of mental health services among rural elderly. *Archives of Psychiatric Nursing, 13*, 30–40.

Owen, P. R., & Kohutek, K. J. (1981). The rural mental health dropout. *Journal of Rural Community Psychology, 2*, 38–41.

Piaget, J. (1926). *The language and thought of the child*. New York: Harcourt, Brace, and World.

Piaget, J. (1969). *The psychology of the child* (H. Weaver, Trans.). New York: Basic Books. (Original work published 1966)

Pincus, T., Callahan, L. F., & Burkhauser, R. V. (1987). Most chronic diseases are reported more frequently by individuals with fewer than 12 years of formal education in the age 18–64 United States population. *Journal of Chronic Diseases, 40*, 865–874.

Pritchard, C., Cotton, A., Godson, M., & Weeks, S. (1993). Mental illness, drug and alcohol misuse and HIV risk behaviour in 214 young adult probation clients. *Social Work and Social Science Review, 3*, 150–162.

Prizant, B. M., Wetherby, A. M., & Roberts, J. E. (1993). Communication disorders in infants and toddlers. In C. H. Zeanah, Jr. (Ed.), *Handbook of infant mental health* (pp. 260–279). New York: Guilford.

Rank, M. R., & Hirschl, T. A. (1999). The likelihood of poverty across the American adult life span. *Social Work, 44*, 201–215.

Reed, D. M., & Weicherding, M. (1999). Factors of caregiver isolation in a rural Midwest area. *Home Health Care Services Quarterly, 17*(4), 13–24.

Revicki, D. A., & Mitchell, J. P. (1990). Strain, social support, and mental health in rural elderly individuals. *Journal of Gerontology, 45*, S267–S274.

Rodgers, H. R., Jr. (1996). *Poor women, poor children: American poverty in the 1990s* (3rd ed.). New York: M. E. Sharpe.

Schein, V. E. (1995). *Working from the margins: Voices of mothers in poverty*. Ithaca, NY: Cornell University Press.

Taylor, R., & Roberts, D. (1995). Kinship support and maternal and adolescent well-being in economically disadvantaged African-American families. *Child Development, 66*, 1585–1597.

Williamson, D. F., Kahn, H. S., Remington, P. L., & Anda, R. F. (1990). The 10-year incidence of overweight and major weight gain in the U. S. adults. *Archives of Internal Medicine, 150*, 665–672.

Zeanah, C. H., Jr. (Ed.). (1993). *Handbook of infant mental health*. New York: Guilford.

Zigler, E., Hopper, P., & Hall, N. W. (1993). Infant mental health and social policy. In C. H. Zeanah, Jr. (Ed.), *Handbook of infant mental health* (pp. 480–492). New York: Guilford.

4

Substance Abuse in the Rural Community

Tony Cellucci, Peter Vik, and Ted Nirenberg

There is a considerable body of literature, particularly epidemiological and conceptual papers, about substance abuse in rural areas, showing that growing up in a rural environment today affords little protection against susceptibility to substance abuse or its attendant health and social consequences. In the early 1990s, the Center for Substance Abuse Treatment (CSAT) and the National Rural Institute of Alcohol and Drug Abuse (NRIADA) began sponsoring an excellence award to disseminate innovative approaches for combating substance abuse in rural settings. The journal *Drugs in Society* devoted a special issue to the problem, including a review by Leukefeld, Clayton, and Myers (1992) that summarized the existing knowledge about rural substance abuse treatment. More recently, the National Institute on Drug Abuse (NIDA) released an extensive monograph on the topic (Robertson, Sloboda, Boyd, Beatty, & Kozel, 1997).

This chapter reviews epidemiological data on drinking and substantive use of illicit drugs by rural residents. The emerging context for intervention and service delivery is discussed, with an emphasis on integrated care. Assessment and evidence-based treatments are described, as are special populations. Recommendations for providers, policymakers, and research are offered.

Definitions and characteristics of rural environments are presented in this volume and elsewhere (Bushy, 1994; Conger, 1997b; Weinert & Long, 1990). Conger (1997a) asserted that social control processes and community networks may vary with population density. Declining economic opportunities and rural poverty could undermine family structure and processes that protect youth from drug involvement (Sloboda, Rosenquist, & Howard, 1997). Robertson and Donnermeyer (1998) found that adult drug users were less likely to be married, had less income, and were more likely to be unemployed. Risk factors may be similar across the rural–urban continuum (Donnermeyer, 1992) but may vary for small towns, which are likely to be individually more homogeneous (Oetting, Edwards, Kelly, & Beauvais, 1997).

The same difficulties (e.g., access, acceptability, isolation, rural conservatism) that affect the delivery of general health care in rural areas apply to substance abuse treatment (Conger, 1997b). It is now possible examine the benefits

Tony Celluci can be reached at Box 8021, Idaho State University, Pocatello, ID 83209. E-mail: cellanth@isu.edu

and risks associated with drinking involvement over the life course (National Institute on Alcohol Abuse and Alcoholism, 2000), and there is interest in providing treatment options for problem drinkers and in improving evaluation of the use and effectiveness of substance abuse services (Tucker, Donovan, & Marlatt, 1999). Investigations in rural areas add to this growing knowledge (Booth, Kirchner, Fortney, Ross, & Rost, 2000; Booth, Ross, & Rost, 1999).

Substance Abuse in Rural Areas

Epidemiology and Problems

National data generally indicate no difference in lifetime alcohol use by high school seniors living in rural and urban communities; some studies suggest an elevated risk of binge drinking among rural students. Rural youth also are somewhat more likely to smoke cigarettes and to use smokeless tobacco (Cronk & Sarvela, 1997; Edwards, 1997). The situation with illicit drugs is more complex. Cronk and Sarvela (1997) examined 1976–1992 data from the Monitoring the Future study, a large survey of high school seniors focusing on substance use in the 30 days before they were questioned. Overall, prevalence rates for most substances declined. Similarly, Conger (1997b) presented cross-sectional data indicating that substance use among nonmetropolitan youth was consistent with that of the general population; the percentage of youth likely to be problem users (i.e., daily use of a substance in the previous 30 days) was quite stable across residence.

Somewhat fewer data are available on adult substance use. Leukefeld et al. (1992) found that rural adults reported less frequent lifetime use of cocaine and marijuana than did urban adults; nonetheless, more than 40% of young and middle-aged rural respondents reported using marijuana. In 1990, similar rates of marijuana use in the previous year were evident, although urban adults reported the highest rate of other drug use (Robertson & Donnermeyer, 1998). The Center on Addiction and Substance Abuse (CASA; 2000) issued a report, *No Place to Hide,* on drug abuse in midsize cities and rural areas. This reanalysis of national data revealed that rural eighth graders were more likely to use methamphetamine and cocaine than were their urban counterparts, but it revealed no differences for adults.

Drinking practices are minimally related to geographical regions and degree of urbanization. In the National Longitudinal Alcohol Epidemiological Study (NLAES), there was a slightly higher proportion of current drinkers in urban than in rural areas but little difference in the proportions of heavy drinkers (i.e., those consuming more than five standard drinks per day; Dawson, Grant, Chou, & Pickering, 1995). A well-designed study of at-risk drinking and use of health services in an adult community sample revealed no rural–urban differences in the maximum number of drinks consumed within the previous year (Booth et al., 1999). Screenings of rural residents were as likely to be positive for alcohol problems, approximately 8%, as were those of urban residents. In this and a later report, there were few differences in severity, although rural at-risk drinkers fulfilled somewhat more substance abuse criteria and had more comorbid chronic medical problems (Booth et al., 2000). Residents of rural areas are more likely to experience greater use and problems related to alcohol bootlegging (Logan, Schenck, Leukefeld, Meyers, & Allen, 1999).

Few studies have specifically addressed the health or social costs of substance abuse in rural settings. The prevalence of drug-related mental health problems (e.g., inability to think clearly, anxiety) appears similar in all geographical regions, be they rural or urban, and such problems were reported by over 40% of users (Robertson & Donnermeyer, 1997). Alcohol-related health problems (Brody, Neubaum, Boyd, & Dufour, 1997) include liver disease, pancreatitis, hypertension, cardiomyopathy, cancer, and fetal alcohol effects. Drinking is strongly related to driving fatalities and other accidental injuries. A negative association between population density and alcohol-related driving was reported in the Monitoring the Future data (O'Malley & Johnston, 1999). Rural youth spend more time in cars and thus are at greater risk for drunk driving and related problems, such as traffic tickets and accidents (Edwards, 1997).

Kelleher and Robbins (1997) provided a thoughtful review of the direct and indirect social costs to rural residents from excessive drinking. In the American Drinking Practices Survey, 65% of heavy-drinking rural residents reported negative social consequences such as difficulties with family and friends, employers, or legal authorities. Arrest rates in rural areas for substance use violations equal or exceed those in nonrural counties. Substance abuse is recognized as a major factor in work-related problems; lost productivity is a major component of indirect economic costs. Rural adult residents are engaged in dangerous occupations (e.g., agriculture, mining) and therefore might be at increased risk for work accidents (Robertson & Donnermeyer, 1998). Rural employers also are less prepared to respond to distressed or impaired workers (Paz, 1998).

Intervention

SERVICE DELIVERY. There is little empirical knowledge about best practices for rural substance abuse services. Current research involves studying the impact of various managed care arrangements and increasing privatization (Rivers, Komaroff, & Kibort, 1999). It is not unusual for rural communities to lack detoxification and psychiatric services; jail is used to observe patients with both substance abuse and psychiatric symptoms. A lack of private providers and adequate funding for substance abuse treatment can result in limited services for those with less severe problems. Ironically, helping those with less severe substance abuse problems may be more cost effective, inasmuch as problem drinkers account for a greater portion of substance-related societal problems and costs (Institute of Medicine, 1990; Sobell, Breslin, & Sobell, 1997).

In their analysis of National Household Survey data, Leukefeld et al. (1992) found that rural residents had the lowest level of seeking help for substance abuse problems, although this did not hold in Booth et al.'s (2000) sample of problem drinkers. Robertson (1997) raised a number research issues regarding the seeking of substance abuse treatment by rural residents, such as their preferences for treatment, access to treatment, and the trade-off between outpatient care in the local community and relocation to a regional treatment center.

The optimal substance abuse and service delivery system would involve a broad range of community-based services along the continuum of care. Ideally, individuals with beginning substance abuse problems would receive less intensive services (i.e., stepped care) on the basis of their needs and motivation (Sobell & Sobell, 1999). Therapist factors, particularly an empathetic manner, are important in the design of effective services (Miller & Willoughby, 1997). Individualized treatment planning is necessary. Within treatment centers, "one size fits all" programming is no longer acceptable, particularly for those in rural and frontier areas who may have little professional support but a great deal of community support. Rather, patients should be provided treatment components according to targeted needs on the basis of assessment data.

Literature on rural substance abuse services (Morris, 1995; Morris, & Hill, 1997) has emphasized integrating services into primary care settings. An estimated 20%–50% of patients receiving general medical care have a substance use problem (Lewis & Chernen, 1998). Emphasizing the connection between a patient's physical health and substance use is likely to increase both compliance with medical interventions and motivation to reduce substance use. Efforts to foster collaborations between primary care providers and behavioral health specialists (Bray & Rogers, 1995; Van Hook & Ford, 1998) need further study. It is important to resolve barriers to such partnerships (e.g., reimbursement policies, communication, and disciplinary differences). Intensive and specialized services will continue to be needed; however, they should be effectively coordinated with ongoing health and community social services.

ASSESSMENT AND EMPIRICALLY SUPPORTED TREATMENTS. A variety of tools are available to reliably and effectively assess substance abuse (Sobell, Toneatto, & Sobell, 1994). Their appropriate use depends on the purpose of the evaluation (e.g., screening vs. treatment planning) and the targeted population. Screening measures such as the Alcohol and Use Disorders Identification Test (AUDIT) and the Short Michigan Alcohol Screening Test (SMAST) have been shown to be effective in a rural primary care setting (Barry & Fleming, 1993). A comprehensive evaluation involving multiple sources of data such as interviews, psychometric measures, physiological tests (e.g., toxicology screens, breathalyzer), and collateral information is recommended for treatment planning. Specifically, the pattern of alcohol and drug use, degree of dependence and problems experienced, and motivation should be assessed. Comorbid psychiatric and neurological problems also need to be assessed.

Assessment should be individualized to meet the clinical needs of the person, although a program may require establishing a core battery for program evaluation. The Addiction Severity Index (ASI; McLellan et al., 1992) has been proposed or adopted by state authorities in several rural states. However, Wertz, Cleaveland, and Stephens (1995) found some difficulties in implementing the ASI in a rural, public sector setting. Assessment in rural settings is also guided by the community context: the types of life problems experienced. As an example, Miller and Willoughby (1997) pointed out that the relevant content of skills training and the available nondrinking alternatives might be unique to a particular cultural context.

Reviews of the alcohol field have emphasized that effective treatments are available (Finney & Moos, 1998), and treatment improvements are comparable with those for other chronic medical conditions (O'Brien & McLellan, 1996). No single treatment is useful for all patients, but some treatments, including brief intervention, skills training, behavioral marital treatment, the community reinforcement approach, and the use of recovery groups, are empirically supported.

A meta-analysis indicated that heavy drinkers exposed to brief interventions were two times more likely than controls to reduce their drinking (Wilk, Jensen, & Havighurst, 1997). A Canadian study with primary care providers showed that 3 hours of cognitive behavioral counseling, provided by a nurse, reduced alcohol-related psychosocial problems, liver enzyme (serum glutamic-oxaloacetic transaminase [SGOT]) elevations, and the number of physician visits in relation to a comparison group (Israel et al., 1996). Sanchez-Craig, Davila, and Cooper (1996) reported that a 30-minute motivational telephone interview and a self-help manual led to reduced alcohol consumption (55% at 1 year), particularly among women. Sitharthan, Kavanagh, and Sayer (1996) found that the use of a correspondence method to deliver a brief training program was effective in reducing drinking. Motivational interviewing (CSAT, 1999; Miller & Rollnick, 2002) is often identified with brief interventions, although it also can serve to prepare a patient for more intensive treatment.

Historically, skills training has been the focus of behavioral treatment for substance abuse. Many individuals who abuse drugs have deficits in assertiveness and other basic communication skills. Substance-abusing patients also need to develop alternatives to their alcohol and drug use and to learn to cope with high-risk relapse situations. Behavioral strategies involve modeling, role playing, and feedback to teach alternatives (Monti et al., 1993). Adapted from the treatment of alcohol dependence, this approach also has been successful in the treatment of cocaine abuse in both urban and rural settings (Monti, Rohsenow, Michalec, Martin, & Abrams, 1997). Leukefeld, Godlaski, Hays, and Clark (1999) described ongoing efforts in rural substance-abusing patients in eastern Kentucky. Focus group findings with rural therapists and program directors suggested modifying the typical group approach so as to recognize rural issues (e.g., unemployment, fundamental religious environment, and less willingness to disclose personal problems) and include individual sessions for motivation and case management (Leukefeld, Godlaski, Hayes, & Clark, 2000).

Although there is general acceptance of the importance of including the family in substance abuse treatment, behavioral couples and family therapy has been underused (Epstein & McCrady, 1998; Rotunda & O'Farrell, 1997). In particular, the structured couples treatment program Counseling for Alcoholics' Marriages (CALM) described by O'Farrell (1993) warrants further dissemination. Preliminary couple sessions are used for initial engagement and therapy preparation, assessment of both drinking and relationship factors, negotiation of a sobriety contract, and provision of feedback. Conjoint group sessions (10–12 members) teach communication and negotiation skills. Over the following year, a series of booster sessions are scheduled to promote continuous recovery and rehearse relapse prevention plans. This protocol has been extended from drinking to other substance abuse. Moreover, research has documented that the program beneficially impacts substance use and relationship measures (Fals-Stewart, Bircher, & O'Farrell, 1996).

The Community Reinforcement Approach is a complex package of treatment procedures organized around an operant analysis of substance abuse behavior. This model was originally developed in rural southern Illinois (Azrin, 1976) and has been replicated and extended as the Community Reinforcement and Family Training (CRAFT) program (Meyers & Smith, 1995). CRAFT increases reinforcement for not using substances by strengthening marital and community support. A sobriety contract and the accompanying use of the drug disulfiram are arranged in the context of behavioral marital treatment, along with provision of individual assistance (e.g., legal, vocational) and social opportunities (e.g., recreational activities) contingent on sobriety. A unique component relevant to the rural environment is the provision of an alcohol-free social club (Mallams, Godley, Hall, & Meyers, 1982). The model also has been adapted for significant others who wish to help a family member with a substance abuse problem (Miller, Meyers, & Tonigan, 1999).

Recovery groups have been important in substance abuse treatment, especially in rural areas (Robertson, 1997). Fox, Merwin, and Blank (1995) included self-help groups in their discussion of the rural de facto mental health system. Evidence from several large national studies now supports the use of treatment procedures directed at facilitating voluntary recovery group participation (Finney & Moos, 1998; Longabaugh, Wirtz, Zweben, & Stout, 1998).

SUBSTANCE ABUSE ISSUES FOR SPECIAL POPULATIONS

Adolescents and substance abuse. Adolescent substance use generally differs from adult use in terms of frequency, quantity, and regularity of use; contexts of use; and motivation for use (Myers, Brown, & Vik, 1998). Normative developmental changes and problem behaviors can obscure the deleterious effects of substance abuse in adolescence. These differences have assessment and treatment implications.

Because of the complexity of adolescent substance abuse problems, a broad-spectrum assessment approach covering various domains of life functioning is needed (Myers et al., 1998). Assessment guides the selection of appropriate treatment components for a particular client. Treatment staff should assess the quality of the teenager's social network, recognize alternative pathways to success, and acknowledge diverse indicators of treatment outcomes. Social pressure precipitates substance abuse relapses in teenagers. Adolescents use a variety of strategies to reduce substance use (Brown, 1993). Younger teenagers found support from non-drug-using family members, whereas older youths engaged in academic or extracurricular activities to reduce use. Like adults, substance-using teenagers make self-change efforts after "treatable moments," such as an emergency room visit (Wagner, Brown, Monti, Myers, & Waldron, 1999).

Substance abuse in the elderly. There is a greater proportion of senior citizens in rural communities (Rodrigue, Banko, Sears, & Evans, 1996).

Drinking generally declines with age, but alcohol abuse and benzodiazepine dependence do occur frequently among the elderly (Holroyd & Duryee, 1997) and may increase as baby boomers mature. Drinking for the effects of alcohol has been associated with both increased alcohol consumption and use of depressant medication (Graham et al., 1996). Diagnosing substance abuse problems in the elderly, however, is often difficult because many diagnostic criteria (e.g., failure to fulfill occupational and childrearing obligations) may not apply and most assessment instruments were standardized on younger age groups (Atkinson, 1990).

Holroyd, Currie, Thompson-Heisteman, and Abraham (1997) reported that 21% of patients in a rural elderly outreach program in Virginia had an alcohol-related disorder. These socioeconomically disadvantaged patients were less likely to have a primary care physician, frequently used emergency services, and generally were depressed. None were receiving alcohol treatment. Elderly people benefit from treatment as much as do younger patients, but they respond best to age-specific groups and outreach programs (Nirenberg, Lisansky-Gomberg, & Cellucci, 1998).

Multiple diagnoses. Individuals with multiple diagnoses (i.e., mental disorders independent of substance abuse) constitute a third special population in planning community services. There is a higher incidence of substance use disorders among people with mental illness (Kessler et al., 1997). Substance use can evoke psychiatric symptoms; therefore, individuals who present with comorbid psychiatric features require careful assessment. Symptoms of an independent psychiatric disorder precede substance abuse and continue during periods of abstinence. The course of mental illness is exacerbated by active substance abuse, as evidenced by worsening of symptoms, noncompliance with medication regimens, and decreased adaptive functioning (Rach-Beisel, Scott, & Dixon, 1999).

Although it is recognized that patients with comorbid conditions require specialized treatment services, few such programs have been evaluated. Howland (1995), focusing on rural communities, summarized the difficulties in treating persons with multiple diagnoses, including limited funding, lack of programming for this population, fragmented services with restrictive regulations, philosophical differences between mental health and substance abuse practitioners, and a shortage of staff that are cross-trained. Weiss, Najavits, and Mirin (1998) identified the following treatment guidelines for dual disorders: (a) providing support for the difficulty of living with multiple disorders, (b) monitoring symptoms of both disorders, (c) teaching skills that apply to both disorders, (d) reinforcing improvements, and (e) expecting occasional setbacks in treatment. Existing data favor integrative approaches with simultaneous treatment for both mental health and substance use disorders from the same treatment staff.

Conclusions and Recommendations

During the 1990s, a body of literature on substance abuse in rural areas emerged. Epidemiological studies have convincingly documented similar rates and problems in rural and urban areas (CASA, 2000; Conger, 1997a). Less is known about treatment access, service delivery, and effectiveness. The following are recommendations for providers, public policymakers, and researchers.

Competence in Substance Abuse Detection and Treatment Is Necessary for Generalist Practice

Psychologists and other behavior health care professionals working in rural areas definitely see substance-abusing patients as part of their practice (Cellucci & Vik, 2001). Basic required competencies include taking a substance abuse history; knowledge of symptoms of intoxication, toxicity, and withdrawal for the major drugs of abuse; and a working knowledge of motivational interviewing techniques and the stages of change. In screening programs in primary care settings, the AUDIT, SMAST-13, and serum tests are recommended. Services should be offered according to a stepped-care model starting with brief interventions for nondependent problem users. Because most rural substance abusers present with problems other than substance use, it is critical that therapists recognize and clarify the interrelations between each patient's substance use and the patient's presenting concerns. Bishop (2001) provided an integrated cognitive–behavioral model for treatment. Providers should also learn at least two empirically supported approaches for working with substance abusing patients and their families.

Adopt a Public Health Model

The issue of public policy and substance abuse service provision is sensitive precisely because the use of psychoactive substances invokes unresolved value issues. Many young adults remain ambivalent about their substance use and are unwilling to adopt a lifelong identity as an alcoholic or addict. Progress occurs only through a public health model that includes patients with neurobehavioral disease but targets the entire population of substance abusers. In substance abuse treatment programming for rural areas, the culture of rural communities must be considered. More research on help seeking and treatment acceptability for alcohol and drug problems in rural populations is specifically needed (Booth et al., 2000; Robertson & Donnermeyer, 1997). For many individuals and communities, a harm reduction perspective may be the most effective in public policy, even though opponents misunderstood the model (Marlatt, 1998).

Develop a Coordinated Plan That Integrates the Services of Private Practitioners With an Adequately Funded Public System

The goal of this policy would be to approximate the continuum of care available in population centers. Assessment, family counseling, and aftercare should be available in outlying areas. In particular, the CRAFT program, implemented by a substance abuse public service agency, would fit in the rural community. Regional psychiatric facilities with the capability to assess and stabilize the patients with dual diagnoses are needed. Special population groups (e.g., adolescents, elderly) should also be included in comprehensive community planning.

Funding Sources Must Be Identified and Sustained

Increased advocacy at the state level can promote access to services. Local and regional studies should document costs (Donnermeyer, 1997) because they can add to community understanding and may convince decision makers of the need for publicly supported treatment. Drug courts, although promising (Inciardi, McBride, & Rivers, 1996), also depend on the availability of community services. Also, individuals should not have to be arrested or incarcerated in order to have access to substance abuse treatment. Restoring reasonable substance abuse benefits in private insurance is part of the solution. Employers and managed care programs can use medical cost offset provisions, but parity should be the goal. Government can also have a role in promoting more training of professionals for rural practice through grant and incentive programs for universities to train rural providers with competencies in rural substance abuse treatment.

Expand the Knowledge Base Regarding Substance Abuse in Rural Areas

Clinical researchers with scientist–practitioner training should contribute their expertise to solutions for the substance abuse problems faced by rural communities. One recurrent theme in the literature has been that rural studies can provide a contextual understanding of etiological factors in substance abuse (Conger, 1997b). Such studies would benefit from efforts to classify rural environments and should address how characteristics of rural communities affect substance abuse risk and protective factors.

Develop Effective Ways to Disseminate Empirically Supported Substance Abuse Treatments

Greater research efforts should be directed toward treatments in rural environments (Leukefeld et al., 1999; Miller & Willoughby, 1997). Innovative methods for delivering services to remote areas should be evaluated. Effective prevention methods such as family interventions and regulatory approaches are available (Jason & Barnes, 1997; Spoth, 1997). Analyses are also needed at the community level to better understand community tolerance of substance abuse and other obstacles to effective intervention programs. Like individuals, communities vary on readiness to change (Plested, Smitham, Jumper-Thurman, Oetting, & Edwards, 1999). Community psychologists are called on to work with rural community coalitions to foster positive change.

References

Atkinson, R. M. (1990). Aging and alcohol use disorders: Diagnostic issues in the elderly. *International Psychogeriatrics, 2,* 55–72.

Azrin, N. H. (1976). Improvements in the community-reinforcement approach to alcoholism. *Behavior Research and Therapy, 14,* 339–348.

Barry, K. L., & Fleming, M. F. (1993). The alcohol use disorders identification test (AUDIT) and the SMAST-13: Predictive validity in a rural primary care sample. *Alcohol and Alcoholism, 26,* 33–42.

Bishop, F.M. (2001). *Managing addictions.* Northvale, NJ: Jason Aronson.

Booth, B. M., Kirchner, J., Fortney, J., Ross, R., & Rost, K. (2000). Rural at-risk drinkers: Correlates and one-year use of alcoholism treatment services. *Journal of Studies on Alcohol, 61,* 267–277.

Booth, B. M., Ross, R. L., & Rost, K. (1999). Rural and urban problem drinkers in six southern states. *Substance Abuse and Misuse, 34,* 471–493.

Bray, J. H., & Rogers, J. C. (1995). Linking psychologists and family physicians for collaborative practice. *Professional Psychology: Research and Practice, 26,* 132–138.

Brody, G. H., Neubaum, E., Boyd, G. M., & Dufour, M. (1997). Health consequences of alcohol use in rural America. In E. Robertson, Z. Sloboda, G. M. Boyd, L. Beatty, & N. Kozel (Eds.), *Rural substance abuse: State of knowledge and issues* (National Institute on Drug Abuse Monograph No. 168, National Institutes of Health Publication No. 97-4177, pp. 137–174). Washington, DC: U.S. Government Printing Office.

Brown, S. A. (1993). Recovery patterns in adolescent substance abusers. In J. S. Baer, G. A. Marlatt, & R. J. McMahon (Eds.), *Addictive behaviors across the lifespan: Prevention, treatment, and policy issues* (pp. 161–183). Newbury Park, CA: Sage.

Bushy, A. (1994). When your client lives in a rural area. *Issues in Mental Health Nursing, 15,* 253–266.

Cellucci, T., & Vik, P. (2001). Training for substance abuse treatment among psychologists in a rural state. *Professional Psychology: Research and Practice, 32,* 248–252.

Center for Addiction and Substance Abuse (CASA). (2000). *No place to hide: Substance abuse in mid-size cities and rural America.* New York, NY: National Center on Addiction and Substance Abuse at Columbia University.

Center for Substance Abuse Treatment (CSAT). (1999). Enhancing motivation for change in substance treatment. In *Treatment improvement protocol, 35* (DHHS publication no. SMA 01-3519). Rockville, MD: Substance Abuse and Mental Health Services Administration, Department of Health and Human Services.

Conger, R. D. (1997a). The social context of substance abuse: A developmental perspective. In E. Robertson, Z. Sloboda, G. M. Boyd, L. Beatty, & N. Kozel (Eds.), *Rural substance abuse: State of knowledge and issues* (National Institutes on Drug Abuse Research Monograph No. 168, National Institutes of Health Publication No. 97-4177, pp. 6–36). Washington, DC: U.S. Government Printing Office.

Conger, R. D. (1997b). The special nature of rural America. In E. Robertson, Z. Sloboda, G. M. Boyd, L. Beatty, & N. J. Kozel (Eds.), *Rural substance abuse: State of knowledge and issues* (National Institute on Drug Abuse Research Monograph No. 168, National Institutes of Health Publication No. 97-4177, pp. 38–52) Washington, DC: U.S. Government Printing Office.

Cronk, C. E., & Sarvela, P. D. (1997). Alcohol, tobacco, and other drug use among rural/small town and urban youth: A secondary analysis of the Monitoring the Future Data Set. *American Journal of Public Health, 87,* 760–764.

Dawson, D. A., Grant, B. F., Chou, S. P., & Pickering, R. P. (1995). Subgroup variation in U.S. drinking patterns: Results of the 1992 National Longitudinal Alcohol Epidemiologic Study. *Journal of Substance Abuse, 7*(3), 331–344.

Donnermeyer, J. F. (1992). The use of alcohol, marijuana, and hard drugs by rural adolescents: A review of recent research. In R. W. Edwards (Ed.), *Drug use in rural American communities* (pp. 31–75). Binghamton, NY: Haworth.

Donnermeyer, J. F. (1997). The economic and social costs of drug abuse among the rural population. In E. Robertston, Z. Sloboda, G. M. Boyd, L. Beatty, & N. Kozel (Eds.), *Rural substance abuse: State of knowledge and issues* (National Institute on Drug Abuse Research Monograph No. 168, National Institutes of Health Publication No. 97-4177, pp. 220–245). Washington, DC: U.S. Government Printing Office.

Edwards, R. W. (1997). Drug and alcohol use among youth in rural communities. In E. Robertson, Z. Sloboda, G. M. Boyd, L. Beatty, & N. J. Kozel (Eds.), *Rural substance abuse: State of knowledge and issues* (National Institute on Drug Abuse Research Monograph No. 168, National Institutes of Health Publication No. 97-4177, pp. 53–78). Washington, DC: U.S. Government Printing Office.

Epstein, E. E., & McCrady, B. S. (1998). Behavioral couples treatment of alcohol and drug use disorders: Current status and innovations. *Clinical Psychology Review, 18,* 689–711.

Fals-Stewart, W., Bircher, G. R., & O'Farrell, T. J. (1996). Behavioral couples therapy for male substance abusing patients: Effects on relationship adjustment and drug using behavior. *Journal of Consulting and Clinical Psychology, 64,* 959–972.

Finney, J. W., & Moos, R. H. (1998). Psychosocial treatments for alcohol use disorders. In P. E. Nathan & J. M. Gorman (Eds.), *A guide to treatments that work* (pp. 156–166). New York: Oxford University Press.

Fox, J., Merwin, E., & Blank, M. (1995). De facto mental health services in the rural South. *Journal of Health Care for the Poor and Underserved, 6,* 434–468.

Graham, K., Clarke, D., Bois, C., Carver, V., Dolinki, L., Smythe, C., et al. (1996). Addictive behavior of older adults. *Addictive Behaviors, 21,* 331–348.

Holroyd, S., Currie, L., Thompson-Heisteman, A., & Abraham, I. (1997). A descriptive study of elderly community-dwelling alcoholic patients in the rural South. *American Journal of Geriatric Psychology, 5,* 221–228.

Holroyd, S., & Duryee, J. J. (1997). Substance use disorders in a geriatric psychiatry outpatient clinic: Prevalence and epidemiologic characteristics. *Journal of Nervous and Mental Disease, 185,* 627–632.

Howland, R. H. (1995). The treatment of persons with dual diagnoses in a rural community. *Psychiatric Quarterly, 66,* 33–49.

Inciardi, J. A., McBride, D., & Rivers, J.E. (1996). *Drug control and the courts.* Thousand Oaks, CA: Sage.

Institute of Medicine. (1990). *Broadening the base of treatment for alcohol problems.* Washington, DC: National Academy Press.

Israel, Y., Hollander, O., Sanchez-Craig, M., Booker, S., Miller, V., Gingrich, R., et al. (1996). Screening for problem drinking and counseling by the primary care physician–nurse team. *Alcoholism: Clinical and Experimental Research, 20,* 1443–1450.

Jason, L. A., & Barnes, H. E. (1997). Substance abuse prevention: Beyond the schoolyard. *Applied and Preventive Psychology, 6,* 211–220.

Kelleher, K. J., & Robbins, J. M. (1997). Social and economic consequences of rural alcohol use. In E. Robertson, Z. Sloboda, G. M. Boyd, L. Beatty, & N. Kozel (Eds.), *Rural substance abuse: State of knowledge and issues* (National Institute on Drug Abuse Research Monograph No. 168, National Institutes of Health Publication No. 97-4177, pp. 196–219). Washington, DC: U.S. Government Printing Office.

Kessler, R. C., Crum, R. C., Warner, L. A., Nelson, C. B., Schutenbert, J., & Anthony, J. C. (1997). Lifetime co-occurrence of *DSM–III–R* alcohol abuse and dependence with other psychiatric disorders in the National Co-morbidity Survey. *Archives of General Psychiatry, 54,* 313–321.

Leukefeld, C., Godlaski, T., Hays, L. & Clark, J. (2000). *Behavioral therapy for rural substance abusers.* Lexington, KY: University Press of Kentucky.

Leukefeld, C. G., Clayton, R. R., & Myers, J. A. (1992). Rural drug and alcohol treatment. *Drugs and Society, 7,* 95–116.

Leukefeld, C. G., Godlaski, T. M., Hays, L. R., & Clark, J. (1999). Developing a rural therapy with big city approaches. *Substance Use and Misuse, 34,* 707–725.

Lewis, D. C., & Chernen, L. (1998). Primary care office management. In R. J. Frances & S. I. Miller (Eds.), *Clinical textbook of addictive disorders* (pp. 574–595). New York: Guilford.

Logan, T. K., Schenck, J. E., Leukefeld, C. G., Meyers, J., & Allen, S. (1999). Rural attitudes, opinions, and drug use. *Substance Use and Misuse, 34,* 545–565.

Longabaugh, R., Wirtz, P. W., Zweben, A., & Stout, R. L. (1998). Network support for drinking, Alcoholics Anonymous and long-term matching effects. *Addiction, 93,* 1313–1333.

Mallams, J. H., Godley, M. D., Hall, G. M., & Meyers, R. J. (1982). A social-systems approach to resocializing alcoholics in the community. *Journal of Studies on Alcohol, 43,* 1115–1123.

Marlatt, G. A. (1998). *Harm reduction.* New York: Guilford.

McLellan, A. T., Kushner, H., Metzger, D., Peters, R., Smith, I., Grissom, G., et al. (1992). The fifth edition of the Addiction Severity Index. *Journal of Substance Abuse Treatment, 9,* 199–213.

Meyers, R. J., & Smith, J. E. (1995). *Clinical guide to alcohol treatment: The community reinforcement approach.* New York: Guilford.

Miller, W. R., Meyers, R. J., & Tonigan, J. S. (1999). Engaging the unmotivated in treatment for alcohol problems: A comparison of three strategies for intervention through family members. *Journal of Consulting and Clinical Psychology, 67,* 688–697.

Miller, W. R., & Rollnick, S. (2002). *Motivational interviewing: Preparing people for change.* New York: Guilford.

Miller, W. R., & Willoughby, K. V. (1997). Designing effective alcohol treatment systems for rural populations: Cross-cultural perspectives. *Bringing excellence to substance abuse services in rural and frontier America* (Center of Substance Abuse Treatment, Technical Assistance Publication No. 20; Department of Health and Human Services Publication No. SMA 97-3134, pp. 83–92). Washington, DC: U.S. Government Printing Office.

Monti, P. M., Rohsenow, D. J., Abrams, D. B., Zwick, W. R., Binkoff, J.A., Munroe, S. M., et al. (1993). Development of a behavior analytically-derived alcohol-specific role-play assessment instrument. *Journal of Studies on Alcohol, 3,* 103–113.

Monti, P. M., Rohsenow, D. J., Michalec, E., Martin, R. A., & Abrams, D. B. (1997). Brief coping skills treatment for cocaine abuse: Substance use outcomes at three months. *Addiction, 92,* 1717–1728.

Morris, J. A. (1995). Alcohol and other drug dependency treatment: A proposal for integration with primary care. *Alcoholism Treatment Quarterly, 13,* 45–56.

Morris, J. A., & Hill, J. G. (1997). Rural hospital addictions screening and treatment. In J. A. Morris (Ed.), *Practicing psychology in rural settings: Hospital privileges and collaborative care* (pp. 127–143). Washington, DC: American Psychological Association.

Myers, M. G., Brown, S. A., & Vik, P. W. (1998). Adolescent substance abuse. In E. J. Mash & R. A. Barkley (Eds.), *Treatment of childhood disorders* (pp. 692–729). New York: Guilford.

National Institute on Alcohol Abuse and Alcoholism (2000). *Alcohol and health: 10th special report to the US Congress* (National Institutes of Health Publication No. 00-1583). Rockville, MD: Author.

Nirenberg, T. D., Lisansky-Gomberg, E. S., & Cellucci, T. (1998). Substance abuse disorders. In M. Hersen & B. Vincent (Eds.), *Handbook of clinical geropsychology* (pp. 147–172). New York: Plenum Press.

O'Brien, C. P., & McLellan, A. T. (1996). Myths about the treatment of addiction. *Lancet, 347,* 237–240.

Oetting, E. R., Edwards, R. W., Kelly, K., & Beauvais, F. (1997). Risk and protective factors for drug use among rural American youth. In E. Robertson, Z. Sloboda, G. M. Boyd, L. Beatty, & N. Kozel (Eds.), *Rural substance abuse: State of knowledge and issues* (National Institute on Drug Abuse Research Monograph No. 168, National Institutes of Health Publication No. 97-4177, pp. 90–130). Washington, DC: U.S. Government Printing Office.

O'Farrell, T. J. (1993). A behavioral marital therapy couples group program for alcoholics and their spouses. In T. J. O'Farrell (Ed.), *Treating alcohol problems: Marital and family interventions* (pp. 170–209). New York: Guilford.

O'Malley, P. M., & Johnston, L. D. (1999). Drinking and driving among U.S. high school seniors, 1984–1997. *American Journal of Public Health, 89,* 678–684.

Paz, J. (1998). The drug free workplace in rural Arizona. *Alcoholism Treatment Quarterly, 16,* 133–145.

Plested, B., Smitham, D. M., Jumper-Thurman, P., Oetting, R., & Edwards, R. W. (1999). Readiness for drug use prevention in rural minority communities. *Substance Use and Misuse, 34,* 521–544.

RachBeisel, J., Scott, J., & Dixon, L. (1999). Co-occurring severe mental illness and substance abuse disorders: A review of recent literature. *Psychiatric Services, 50,* 1427–1434.

Rivers, J. E., Komaroff, E., & Kibort, A. C. (1999). Access to health and human services for drug users: An urban/rural community systems perspective. *Substance Use and Misuse, 34,* 707–725.

Robertson, E. B. (1997). Introduction to mental health service delivery in rural areas. In E. Robertson, Z. Sloboda, G. M. Boyd, L. Beatty, & N. Kozel (Eds.), *Rural substance abuse: State of knowledge and issues* (National Institute on Drug Abuse Research Monograph No. 168, National Institutes of Health Publication No. 97-4177, pp. 413–417). Washington, DC: U.S. Government Printing Office.

Robertson, E., Sloboda, Z., Boyd, G. M., Beatty, L., & Kozel, N. J. (Eds.). (1997). *Rural substance abuse: State of knowledge and issues.* (National Institute on Drug Abuse Research Monograph No. 168, National Institutes of Health Publication No. 97-4177). Washington, DC: U.S. Government Printing Office.

Robertson, E. B., & Donnermeyer, J. F. (1997). Illegal drug use among rural adults: Mental health consequences and treatment utilization. *American Journal of Drug Alcohol Abuse, 23,* 467–484.

Robertson, E. B., & Donnermeyer, J. F. (1998). Patterns of drug use among non-metropolitan and rural adults. *Substance Use and Misuse, 33,* 2109–2129.

Rotunda, R. J., & O'Farrell, T. J. (1997). Marital and family therapy of alcohol use disorders: Bridging the gap between research and practice. *Professional Psychology: Research and Practice, 28,* 246–252.

Rodrigue, J. R., Banko, C. G., Sears, S. F., & Evans, G. (1996). Old territory revisited: Behavior therapists in rural America and innovative models of service delivery. *The Behavior Therapist, 19,* 97–100.

Sanchez-Craig, M., Davila, R., & Cooper, G. (1996). A self-help approach for high-risk drinking: Effects of an initial assessment. *Journal of Consulting and Clinical Psychology, 64,* 694–700.

Sitharthan, T., Kavanagh, D. J., & Sayer, G. (1996). Moderating drinking by correspondence: An evaluation of a new method of intervention. *Addiction, 91,* 345–355.

Sloboda, Z., Rosenquist, E., & Howard, J. (1997). Introduction: Substance abuse in rural America. In E. Robertson, Z. Sloboda, G. M. Boyd, L. Beatty, & N. Kozel (Eds.), *Rural substance abuse: State of knowledge and issues* (National Institute on Drug Abuse Research Monograph No. 168, National Institutes of Health Publication No. 97-4177, pp. 1–5). Washington, DC: U.S. Government Printing Office.

Sobell, L. C., Breslin, F. C., & Sobell, M.B. (1997). Substance-related disorders: Alcohol. In S. M. Turner & M. Hersen (Eds.), *Adult psychopathology and diagnosis* (pp. 128–158). New York: Wiley.

Sobell, L. C., & Sobell, M. B. (1996). *Timeline follow-up: User's guide.* Toronto: Addiction Research Foundation.

Sobell, L. C., Toneatto, T., & Sobell, M. B. (1994). Behavioral assessment and treatment planning for alcohol, tobacco and other drug problems: Current status with an emphasis on clinical applications. *Behavior Therapy, 25,* 533–580.

Sobell, M. B., & Sobell, L. C. (1999). Stepped care for alcohol problems: An efficient method for planning and delivering clinical services. In J. A. Tucker, D. M. Donovan, & G. A. Marlatt (Eds.), *Changing addictive behavior: Bridging clinical and public health strategies* (pp. 331–343). New York: Guilford.

Spoth, R. (1997). Challenges in defining and developing the field of rural mental disorder preventive intervention research. *American Journal of Community Psychology, 25,* 425–449.

Tucker, J. A., Donovan, D. M., & Marlatt, G. A. (1999). *Changing addictive behavior: Bridging clinical and public health strategies.* New York: Guilford.

Van Hook, M. P., & Ford, M. E. (1998). The linkage model for delivering mental health services in rural communities: Benefits and challenges. *Health and Social Work, 23,* 53–60.

Wagner, E. F., Brown, S. A., Monti, P. M., Myers, M. G., & Waldron, H. B. (1999). Innovations in adolescent substance abuse intervention. *Alcoholism: Clinical and Experimental Research, 23,* 236–249.

Weinert, C., & Long, K. A. (1990). Rural families and health care: Refining the knowledge base. *Marriage and Family Review, 15,* 57–75.

Weiss, R. D., Najavits, L. M., & Mirin, S. M. (1998). Substance abuse and psychiatric disorders. In R. J. Frances & S. I. Miller (Eds.), *Clinical textbook of addictive disorders* (pp. 291–318). New York: Guilford.

Wertz, J. S., Cleaveland, B. L., & Stephens, R. S. (1995). Problems in the application of the Addiction Severity Index (ASI) in rural substance abuse services. *Journal of Substance Abuse, 7,* 175–188.

Wilk, A. I., Jensen, N. M., & Havighurst, T. C. (1997). Meta-analysis of randomized control trials addressing brief interventions in heavy alcohol drinkers. *Journal of General Internal Medicine, 12,* 274–283.

5

Needs Assessment, Identification and Mobilization of Community Resources, and Conflict Management

Pamela L. Mulder, Helen Linkey, and Angela Hager

Problem-solving strategies and interventions are useful only when the problems themselves are accurately identified and understood, are issues of actual concern for the people involved, and can be addressed by the use of resources that are currently available. In this chapter, several procedures commonly used to assess and prioritize actual needs, identify community resources, and mobilize community members to take action are presented. Methods used by researchers and behavioral health professionals across disciplines are presented with attention to the applicability of methods in rural and frontier communities, and issues related to cultural sensitivity are stressed.

Successful community-level interventions rely on the efforts and commitment of the residents, effectively address legitimate community needs, involve the use of the strengths and resources of the community in a cost-effective manner, and are sustainable beyond the initial inception. Such interventions require careful planning and an in-depth understanding of the community where they will take place. This chapter is intended to serve as a tool in the planning process in addition to providing information about specific strategies for assessing need and resources and mobilizing community members to take action. The methods and procedures described are those that social scientists—representing diverse academic fields—and practicing health and mental health professionals have found to be both informative and readily implemented in rural communities.

Issues related to the assessment of need and the identification and mobilization of rural community resources can be divided into three discrete areas of concern. The first issue involves the direction of approach: assessment of needs or the identification of resources. Second, the interaction of the rural environment with the procedures must be understood. Third, regardless of the direction of approach to rural (or other) community development, interventions must be tailored to individual communities, on the basis of a clear understanding of the specific community's needs, cultural norms and values, dynamic structure, history, and available resources.

Pamela L. Mulder can be reached at 400 Hal Greer Boulevard, Huntington, WV, 25755. E-mail: mulder@marshall.edu

The activities and procedures presented in this chapter are discussed in terms of their general applicability to need or resource identification, or both, and to resource mobilization in a rural environment. Effective application of these tools is dependent on the depth of cultural awareness underlying the intervention strategy. It is not possible to cover the full scope of potential social and cultural variations, which may be encountered despite the importance of this factor. The failure of unsuccessful community interventions is frequently the result of precisely this type of ignorance, and more than one academic "expert" has struggled to establish a rural program that is based on urban (or otherwise culturally inappropriate) models only to watch this unsustainable intervention fail.

The minimum requirements, which must be met if a community intervention is to be effective and sustainable, include cultural relevance, the involvement and commitment of community residents, and a clear understanding of the community's needs and resources. Therefore, the procedures covered in this chapter can and must be modified according to the specific dynamics present in individual communities to permit effective community assessment, empowerment of community members, and management of conflict among agents of change.

Community Assessment and Mobilization

Social scientists argue the primacy of need assessment in planning, whereas community development specialists have pointed out that need assessment focuses on deficiencies and have proposed the assessment of community resources as the first step. These specialists insist that community residents must first "fall back in love with their community" if they are to have the energy and commitment needed to produce changes (Flower, 1998; Kretzmann & McKnight, 1996).

As an illustration of these differing views, consider a rural community with a large number of teenagers who lack supervised after-school activities and often get into trouble of one sort or another during the afternoon. According to a needs assessment perspective, the problem might be described in terms of a lack of extrracurricular activities for young people, a lack of adequate law enforcement, or a lack of appropriate supervision. According to an asset or resource identification perspective, the town has a sizable group of young people with energy and time to spend.

On the basis of a needs perspective, the community members might choose to establish an after-school program, try to add law enforcement personnel, or insist on a curfew of some type. On the basis of an asset or resource identification perspective, the community members might choose to find a way to motivate these young people to tackle other community problems identified during the assessment procedure.

Because these perspectives are interrelated and equally valuable, a third option becomes obvious: using both approaches to apply the resources available in the community to address the concerns and needs of the community residents. To facilitate this approach, the reader should think in terms of holistic community assessment that is based on a variety of data collection procedures.

Community Assessment Procedures

DIRECT OBSERVATION METHOD. Unbiased observers visit the community, make observations concerning the physical structures (location, condition, centrality, use, occupation, accessibility), the residents (activities, groups, emotional tones), and services (directory listings, distances, utilization) and consider the community climate likely to be associated with the observations. Carefully selected and considered observations can provide cursory but valuable information about the dynamics of community life.

The greatest advantage of direct observation is the nonintrusive nature of the procedure. Limitations, however, include a high vulnerability to observer bias and potentially inaccurate interpretation of the results by poorly trained observers. In small rural communities, observers are likely to be easily identified as outsiders, which alters the observable behavior of residents and limits the validity of the observations. Several independent observers who use planned observations minimize limitations. Observer responses should be recorded on scales that allow for an examination of interrater reliability to ensure equivalence across raters. Observations may also be made over time; this allows the presence of observers to become commonplace and minimizes some of the impact on the residents' behavior. Checking observations with several informed residents is another way of identifying the extent to which the observation itself may have contaminated the results.

ARCHIVAL DATA. Significant accumulations of previously collected data that can assist the researcher in identifying community needs, including police and emergency call rates and response times, frequency of admissions and varieties of diagnoses at local agencies, census data, community budgets, and voting records, are available in most communities. Archival data can be collected by persons not involved with the current research. Archives can be cost effective, often involving few costs beyond those directly involved with data analysis (MacCallum, 1998), although rules concerning patient confidentiality may impose restrictions on the availability of certain types of data. There are limitations to the accessibility, validity, reliability, and overall usefulness of archival data. The data may reflect changes over time, including systematic variability (i.e., mental health diagnoses that are based on different editions of manuals) and less easily identified unsystematic variability related to the training, motivation, values, and expertise of the individual data collectors.

SURVEYS AND INTERVIEWS. Questionnaires and surveys are cost effective, can be employed in a variety of contexts, and have been used frequently to collect data about communities and community residents. Issues of concern include the structure of the survey and the format of the questions asked (validity, reliability, open vs. closed and structured vs. unstructured formats, complexity and intrusiveness of items, social desirability of responses, and a tendency to obtain extreme responses under certain conditions), the context of administration (sample representativeness, degree of interaction between the researcher and respondent and among multiple respondents, confidentiality, and motivation and knowledge of the respondent), and the modality (interviews and surveys may be conducted face to face, by telephone, by mail, or online). (See Hammer & Wildavsky, 1989; Heron, 1996; Holstein & Gubrium, 1995; Kvale, 1996.)

On-site interviews. With agency permission, individuals present at preselected locations may be interviewed face to face or may complete written surveys. This procedure is particularly useful when the research objectives are site related, as when agency utilization or perceptions of service effectiveness are examined. On-site interviews frequently reach a representative sample of informed respondents. The rate of completed surveys tends to be higher for face-to-face interviews than for the complete-and-return format, and there is immediate access to the data (Rubin & Rubin, 1995; Seidman, 1991).

However, issues of confidentiality may arise. Permission to question potential respondents must be sought from the agencies involved. Responses obtained during face-to-face interviews are likely to differ from those that might have been obtained from the same sample under conditions with less researcher–respondent interaction. Individuals conducting on-site interviews must travel to the site, preferably on multiple occasions, and the results may be contaminated if the sample is composed primarily of individuals who simply happen to have the time to talk to researchers.

Mail and telephone contacts. Pen-and-paper surveys, to be completed and returned, are often mailed to respondents. Mailings can target residents in particular communities; however, confidentiality and anonymity limit the ability of the researcher to determine which recipients of the survey have responded and which individual in any given household actually completed the survey. This problem can become even more troublesome when multiple mailings are used to obtain information over a specified period of time (Brown, Cozby, Kee, & Worden, 1999; Gilbert, Fiske, & Lindzey, 1998).

Usually the number of surveys sent out must be quite large because of the poor rate of return that is a common problem associated with this technique. Some procedures have been found to increase the overall return rate for mail surveys (Brown et al., 1999; Gilbert et al., 1998; Sudau & Brown, 1984). Presurvey postcards may be sent to recipient addresses informing the residents of the forthcoming survey. Some researchers have included small gifts or payments with the surveys in an attempt to create a sense of respondent debt that could be cleared by compliance. After the survey has been mailed, follow-up postcards may be sent. Follow-up cards may include instructions for obtaining another copy of the survey if the original has been misplaced or discarded. Preaddressed, stamped return envelopes should always accompany any survey. Because the intangible costs of responding to the survey include respondent time, and because increased respondent costs are associated with lower return rates, the length and overall complexity of this type of survey should be minimized.

Telephone surveys and interviews have the advantages of producing immediate results, being somewhat more likely to obtain responses from a specified respondent (the head of the household, for example), and of making sequential surveys more feasible. Twenty minutes is probably the upper limit of what respondents will spend on a telephone survey. Respondents are sometimes particularly unwilling to speak with researchers who call them unexpectedly, and it is possible that a precall postcard, similar to those used in mail surveys, may increase compliance (Brown et al., 1999; Gilbert et al., 1998; Groves & Bieler, 1988; Thomas & Purdon, 1994). Telephone-interviewed respondents are also more likely to provide candid responses—particularly on sensitive subjects—than are those interviewed face to face. However, sample representativeness, survey completion rates, and research costs (equipment and personnel) are often problematic (Brown et al., 1999; Gilbert et al., 1998).

Not all residents are equally likely to be included in telephone surveys, because not all residents have telephones; this problem is particularly prevalent in rural and frontier regions. Of residents who do have telephones, a significant proportion (estimated at 10%–25%) have unlisted telephone numbers, and the majority of these unlisted numbers are likely to belong to younger residents, usually single women. Random number systems are of value in overcoming this problem and should be routinely employed in telephone surveys (Groves & Bieler, 1988; Thomas & Purdon, 1994).

Online surveys and interviews. This cost-effective method has become more popular as personal computer access has increased. One advantage to online interviews, as opposed to "complete and return" or "complete and submit" online surveys, is the ability to conduct these interviews in real time. Another potential advantage of online interviewing is associated with "chat room" capability, which allows the researcher a limited opportunity to observe participants interact (Chen & Hinton, 1999; Chenail, 1997; Strategic Focus Online, 1998). Disadvantages include questionable confidentiality, questionable security of data, and lack of certainty concerning the identity and demographic description of the respondent. Representativeness of the sample is also an issue because not all possible respondents have equal access to computers or the skills to express themselves in this format, and specific populations, including many rural and frontier populations, may be excluded entirely. Therefore, this method is not appropriate for research with requirements for broad or random sampling.

Individual, joint, and group interview contexts. One-on-one interviewing has been the format most commonly employed (Neuman, 1991; Rubin & Rubin, 1995; Seidman, 1991; Weiss, 1994). However, in many cases, joint or even group interviews may be the most appropriate approach; moreover, individual interviews conducted with or without an appointment can unexpectedly become joint or group interviews when other individuals in the vicinity insist on being present or participating. The quality and quantity of information obtained are likely to be affected by the context of the interview and by any actions that the researcher chooses to take after the interview has begun (Arksey, 1999).

Individual meetings give interviewers access to the opinions and reactions of one person without the interference or contamination from others. Joint interviews can be extremely effective in obtaining information from married couples, across generations in a family, and between caregiver or service provider and the individual, consumer, or client receiving the care or service (Arksey, 1999; Seymour, Dix, & Eardley, 1995). A combination of individual and joint or group interviews may allow the researcher to obtain specific types of information. It also may ensure the opportunity for expression for each participant and enable researchers to corroborate information (Arksey, 1999; Seymour et al., 1995).

Group interviews can elicit a great deal of information from a large number of respondents, are usually less costly than individual interviewing, and may help the researcher recognize a particular need or asset that would not have been so clearly identified under other conditions (Arksey, 1999). Group interviews permit interaction among interviewees, which may result in clarification of responses or the emergence of a consensus, or both, as the individuals involved consider, compare, and react to the opinions of others. Group discussion could demonstrate that seemingly different issues have the same underlying cause. Group interviews may also help determine which needs are of greatest concern to the community. When asked to identify the three most critical needs in their community, individuals interviewed alone may each mention the first three that come to mind. However, after the opportunity to interact with others, these same individuals may determine that one or another issue is actually of greatest importance to them all.

Group interaction may also result in negative reactions between individuals who unexpectedly discover that they are in disagreement. One respondent may monopolize the interview, intimidate another respondent, or foster an environment in which other participants are not comfortable. Power differences and gender role expectations can be problematic in parent–child, husband–wife, and other interview dyads or groups (Arksey, 1999; Seymour et al., 1995). The characteristics and behavior of the interviewer or, in the case of the focus groups described next, the group facilitator are important factors in determining the final outcome of group interactions.

Focus groups and town hall meetings. Focus groups usually consist of 6–10 individuals from the local community, preferably strangers, who meet with a trained facilitator for the purpose of discussing one or a very few issues (Gibbs, 1997). This process has the advantages of obtaining the opinions of several people simultaneously in an interactive setting (Kitzinger, 1994, 1995; Morgan, 1997; Morgan & Kreuger, 1993), facilitating clarification of vaguely described concerns, and broader discussion of needs and resources. It can be difficult to schedule these groups, and a well-trained facilitator must be available to maintain the group's focus on the topic, to ensure that all members are heard, and to prevent dissension that may arise in the interactive process. Significant care must be taken to ensure that the sample, both within and across groups, is representative of the community. The initial contact with potential members is most likely to be via mail or telephone, and the representativeness of the sample is likely to be affected by the factors that limit these procedures.

This process can be costly, and multiple groups are usually required, but the advantages often outweigh the costs.

Numerous resources are available to the novice researcher who would like to use this method (Powell & Single, 1996; Powell, Single, & Lloyd, 1996; Smith, Scammon, & Beck, 1995; Stewart & Shamdasani, 1992; White & Thomson, 1995). This method is also useful for mobilizing community action, as is discussed in a later section (Race, Hotch, & Parker, 1994).

The town hall process involves scheduling and publicizing an open meeting for local citizens (Brown et al., 1999; Gilbert et al., 1998) and is not a useful means of gathering initial information. The individuals who attend the meeting may represent only the most highly motivated members of the community and are not likely to be a representative sample. Participants may have agendas, which make it difficult to maintain focus, achieve consensus, and avoid negative interactions.

LEADERSHIP ANALYSIS AND KEY INFORMANTS. There are two types of leaders in communities: those who hold a formal office or position (mayor, police chief, or fire chief) and those who may have no official role but are identified by residents as informed individuals whose opinions are valued (Brown et al., 1999; Gilbert et al., 1998). These community leaders who hold informed opinions concerning community needs are valuable *key informants* whose participation should be actively solicited (Garkrovich, 1989).

Regardless of the survey or interview process used, the validity of the community assessment is likely to be improved by including a significant number of key informants and by continuing the data collection process until a high degree of consistency is identified. When key informants are carefully chosen, relatively few—perhaps four to eight—interviews are usually sufficient to gather consensual information related to a specified need in a given community (Garkrovich, 1989).

Mobilizing Community Residents

Community resources are varied, and money is not necessarily the most valuable asset. The people in the community and their talent, the buildings, and even geographical features can be community assets. Opportunities for involvement, such as organized charitable events, a school carnival, or a church social represent opportunities to inform, motivate, and mobilize residents of the community. Respondent participation can be empowering, producing an increased awareness of need, a sense of personal involvement, and motivation to take action. Group discussion and interaction, sometimes assuming the characteristics of "brainstorming" sessions, reveal valuable community assets and strategies (Kitzinger, 1994, 1995; Maxwell, 1997; Morgan, 1997; Morgan & Kreuger, 1993).

COMMON MOTIVATION TECHNIQUES. Effective sustainable community interventions require the active involvement of many residents and agencies in the community. Unfortunately, the lay population sometimes avoids techniques that are effective in securing active participation because they involve elements of manipulation and coercion, even though these elements are commonly accepted as a part of their daily lives. People are manipulated by television advertisements, by news broadcasts, by teachers, by family members, by employers, even by friends. People generally do not like to feel that they have been manipulated, but most are willing to be persuaded, motivated, recognized, and rewarded.

The "door-in-the-face" and "foot-in-the-door" techniques. Either increasing or decreasing the cost of involvement in a systematic manner can increase compliance. The "door-in-the-face" procedure involves making a request that is absurdly costly and then following the expected refusal with a more reasonable request. For example, a local merchant might first be asked to donate a large sum of money to a particular cause; then, when the merchant denies the request, the requester asks the merchant to donate an item or a gift certificate for a raffle to benefit that same cause. The merchant is not only very likely to comply with the second, more reasonable request but is also actually more likely to donate an item to the raffle because the initial request was refused.

The "foot-in-the-door" procedure works in the opposite direction, with the use of carefully escalated requests. The merchant is asked to hang a small sign advertising a meeting of concerned citizens in the storefront window. This is a small request, and many local business people commonly allow this type of advertising. Later, the merchant is asked to hang a larger sign or to make literature available at the cashier's station. Little cost to the merchant is involved, and once again, it often produces compliance. Later still, the merchant is asked to send a representative to the meetings, to make a monetary donation, or to contribute raffle items. Each act of compliance increases the probability that the merchant will respond favorably to the next request (Brown et al., 1999; Gilbert et al., 1998).

Social reinforcement. Rewards for participation can also help to increase involvement and motivation. The hypothetical merchant described previously becomes more likely to comply with future requests and even to value involvement with the group when social reinforcements are judiciously applied (Brown et al., 1999; Gilbert et al., 1998). Examples of appropriate social reinforcement would be those that increase patronization of the merchant's business and publicly praise involvement. Framed certificates of appreciation are readily and inexpensively prepared, and the recipient is likely to display the recognition publicly. A large, easily noticed item in a religious bulletin, group newsletter, or community newspaper publicly identifying and thanking the hypothetical merchant (or similar others in the community) for involvement is an effective social reinforcement, which increases future compliance. Because these rewards were not expected, the merchant is unlikely to attribute previous compliance to *payment* for involvement.

Group identity as a motivator. As the costs of involvement increase, such merchant may begin to wonder why they have become so involved. To explain their own behavior, these people will probably arrive at two common reasons: Either they have allowed others to manipulate them into taking actions that they did not wish to take or they have become involved because of their own interest and concern about the issue. People are most likely to attribute their actions to their own personal characteristics. Therefore, when the involvement has been generally pleasurable and rewarding and the issue is unlikely to arouse significant opposition (such as collections for the needy or projects to prevent teenage smoking, child abuse, or domestic violence), the merchants are most likely to decide that they have become involved by choice. They may even come to view themselves as quasi-members of the group (perhaps leading to full membership in the future) who are deeply committed to the group's goals. Identification with the group, in turn, increases motivation, involvement, and compliance further still (Brown et al., 1999; Gilbert et al., 1998; Maxwell, 1997).

CONFLICT MANAGEMENT. To implement effective community change, the efforts of many agencies must be combined in planned intervention. Many discrete systems within the community may be affected by a community intervention, the causes and effects of an identified problem may be very widespread, and it is unlikely that members of any one group will be aware of the entire situation. Potential contributors may vary significantly in terms of their missions, goals, methods, perspectives, and management styles. "Turf wars" and competition between community agencies and professionals in related fields may arise when resources are perceived as limited or boundaries (implicit or explicit) are threatened. The potential for conflict should be acknowledged forthrightly, and agreement to apply conflict management principles in their interactions should be secured from all group members. Although conflict resolution techniques, including mediation and negotiation, are valuable tools, conflict management procedures that prevent the escalation of conflict are preferable (Maxwell, 1997; see also Kozan, 1997; Secemsky, Ahlman, & Robbins, 1999; Slaikeu, 1996; Van de Viert, Nauta, Giebles, & Janssen, 1999).

In most instances, the group's ultimate success is dependent on adopting an informed and creative perspective that facilitates the search for innovative solutions to community concerns through the use of existing or obtainable resources. The interdependence that is required for success should be emphasized; group members must learn to protect the self-esteem of their colleagues and respect one another as equals who have agreed to cooperate for the sake of their community.

Members must allow themselves and others to start fresh at every meeting. The "new start" principle allows members to "cool down" after disagreements, to change their minds about issues between meetings without recrimination or derision, to learn from one another and incorporate new information without embarrassment, and to present new information without bias. When members change and develop over time, the group interaction is a dynamic process, and conflict is redefined as educational opportunity. The value of an open, creative, future-oriented perspective should be emphasized, whereas clinging to the solutions and processes of the past should be discouraged.

Group members must agree to keep any conflict within the meetings, thereby avoiding interactions outside the group, which might be viewed as exclusionary. Members must also agree that personal opinions expressed during meetings will be treated confidentially and are not to be discussed outside the group without the speaker's permission. Members should refrain from attempts to speak for one another, and no member should attempt to explain or describe the position of another without permission.

Honesty and openness should be encouraged when members describe their needs, their goals, and their most fundamental principles. Areas of agreement should be emphasized, and areas of disagreement should be brought forth for discussion. Members must demonstrate respect for diversity and for the right of each individual to have an opinion. Members must be allowed to speak openly and to be heard without undue interruptions. Attacks on character, motivations, and intentions should be avoided and, although the expression of strong feelings and reactions may be appropriate, the manner of expression need not be negative. Accusations, threats, force, coercion, stonewalling, blaming, and contempt have no place in the group process and are likely to escalate conflict.

Group members should not approach the largest or most controversial concerns first, and they should "table" issues that cannot be resolved during the meeting or that seem to defy solution, agreeing to return to these issues in the future. Working together to solve smaller, less threatening problems provides practice and experience, allowing the group members to employ conflict management procedures more effectively when larger, more controversial issues are tackled. Small successes help to build group cohesion and increase the group's perceived efficacy. Group members should focus on only one issue at a time, and each member should be invested in maintaining that focus.

Escalation of conflict is usually associated with increased physiological arousal, and members can learn to recognize these reactions in themselves and take steps to inhibit the escalation. Unscheduled breaks can be taken if needed, and relaxation techniques can be taught and employed.

Conclusions and Recommendations

Utilize the Assistance of Community Leaders

A leader who will aid in establishing the needs-assessment procedures appropriate for a given community should be selected. To effect meaningful, sustainable change in a given community, the procedures to be employed must be tailored by an informed and culturally sensitive researcher, activist, or community leader to match the values, dynamics, and historical experiences of the community residents. As residents become more aware of unmet needs and begin to explore the potential for applying existing resources to meet these needs, the community becomes empowered to make changes.

Base Interventions on Accurate Needs and Resources

Interventions must be based on accurate assessment of the needs and the assets present. This requires selection of the method or methods, sources of information, and procedures that are most appropriate for the community.

Interventions must then be tailored to address the actual needs of the community, through the use of resources that have been identified and that are available. After implementation, the effectiveness of an intervention, including both process and outcome, must be objectively evaluated.

Use Culturally Adapted Methods, Including Adaptations for Rural and Frontier Culture

The methods and procedures that will enable researchers to appropriately assess the needs of a rural or frontier community should be established. In many educational programs designed to prepare students for professional work, the curriculum includes courses covering research methods and statistical analyses. Few of these programs, however, emphasize the need for methods and procedures that are uniquely appropriate and useful in rural and frontier communities.

Ascertain the Costs and Ensuring that the Cost-to-Benefit Ratio Is Acceptable

The cost of such training and, eventually, the cost of conducting appropriate assessments and evaluations are minimal in comparison with the potential costs of a program that is unsustainable, which fails to address actual needs or is maintained without evidence of a measurable and beneficial outcome.

In the preceding sections, we have presented a number of specific data collection methods designed to identify community needs and resources, procedures that can be applied to motivate and empower community residents to take action, and guidelines for facilitating positive interactions among change agents. However, we have presented only an initial framework for community action. The reader is encouraged to explore additional resources that may be applicable to specific populations or situations and that can be used to evaluate the impact and efficacy of changes that have been implemented. For example, Wadsworth (1997) discussed the modifications needed when community members conduct their own assessment as participant–researchers, and Miller (1991) provided a comprehensive guide to survey design and outcome evaluation measures.

References

Arksey, H. (1999). Collecting data through joint interviews. *Social Research Update, 15,* Paper 4. Retrieved November 28, 2000, from http://www.soc.surrey.ac.uk/sru/SRU15.html

Brown, K. W., Cozby, P. C., Kee, D. W., & Worden, P. E. (1999). *Research methods in human development* (2nd ed.). Mountain View, CA: Mayfield.

Chen, P., & Hinton, S. M. (1999). Realtime interviewing using the World Wide Web. *Sociological Research Online, 4*(3). Retrieved November 28, 2000, from http://www.socresonline.org.uk /socresonline/4/3/chen.html

Chenail, R. J. (1997). Interviewing exercises: Lessons from family therapy. *The Qualitative Report, 3*(2). Retrieved November 28, 2000, from http://www.nova.edu/sss/QR/QR3-2 /chenail.html

Flower, J. (1998). A tool kit for building a healthy city. *National Civic Review, 87,* 293–310.

Garkrovich, L. E. (1989). Local organizations and leadership in community development. In J. A. Christenson & J. W. Robinson, Jr. (Eds.), *Community development in perspective* (pp. 196–218). Ames, IA: Iowa State University Press.

Gibbs, A. (1997). Focus groups. *Social Research Update, 19,* Paper 2. Retrieved November 28, 2000, from http://www.scu.edu.au/schools/sawd/ari/ari-wadsworth.html

Gilbert, D. T., Fiske, S. T., & Lindzey, G. (Eds.). (1998). *The handbook of social psychology* (4th ed.). New York: McGraw-Hill.

Groves, R. M., & Bieler, P. P. (Eds.). (1988). *Telephone survey methodology.* New York: Wiley.

Hammer, D., & Wildavsky, A. (1989). The open-ended, semi-structured interview: An (almost) operational guide. *Craftways: On the organization of scholarly work.* Piscataway, NJ: Transaction Publishers.

Heron, J. (1996). *Co-operative inquiry: Research into the human condition.* London: Sage.

Holstein, J. A., & Gubrium, J. F. (1995). *The active interview.* Thousand Oaks, CA: Sage.

Kitzinger, J. (1994). The methodology of focus groups: The importance of interaction between research participants. *Sociology of Health, 16*(1), 103–121.

Kitzinger, J. (1995). Introducing focus groups. *British Medical Journal, 311,* 299–302.

Kozan, M. K. (1997). Culture and conflict management: A theoretical framework. *International Journal of Conflict Management, 8,* 338–360.

Kretzmann, J., & McKnight, J. P. (1996). Assets-based community development. *National Civic Review, 85,* 23–29.

Kvale, S. (1996). *Interviews: An introduction to qualitative research interviewing.* Thousand Oaks, CA: Sage.

MacCallum, R. (1998). Commentary on quantitative methods in I-O research. *The Industrial/Organizational Psychologist, 35*(4), 38–43.

Maxwell, J. P. (1997). Conflict management and mediation training: A vehicle for community empowerment? *Mediation Quarterly, 15*(2), 83–96.

Miller, D. C. (1991). *Handbook of research design and social measurement* (5th ed.). Thousand Oaks, CA: Sage.

Morgan, D. L. (1997). *Focus groups as qualitative research.* London: Sage.

Morgan, D. L., & Kreuger, R. A. (1993). When to use focus groups and why. In D. L. Morgan (Ed.), *Successful focus groups: Advancing the state of the art* (pp. 5–13). London: Sage.

Neuman, W. (1991). *Social research methods: Qualitative and quantitative approaches.* Boston: Allyn & Bacon.

Powell, R. A., & Single, H. M. (1996). Focus groups. *International Journal of Quality in Health Care, 8,* 499–504.

Powell, R. A., Single H. M., & Lloyd, K. R. (1996). Focus groups in mental health research: Enhancing the validity of user and provider questionnaires. *International Journal of Social Psychology, 42,* 193–206.

Race, K. E., Hotch, D. F., & Parker, T. (1994). Rehabilitation program evaluation: Use of focus groups to empower clients. *Evaluation Review, 18,* 730–740.

Rubin, H. J., & Rubin, I. S. (1995). *Qualitative interviewing: The art of hearing data.* Thousand Oaks, CA: Sage.

Secemsky, V. O., Ahlman, C., & Robbins, J. (1999). Managing group conflict: The development of comfort among social group workers. *Social Work with Groups, 21*(4), 35–48.

Seidman, I. E. (1991). *Interviewing as qualitative research: A guide for researchers in education and the social sciences.* New York: Teachers College Press.

Seymour, J., Dix, G., & Eardley, T. (1995). *Joint accounts: Methodology and practice in research interviews with couples* (Social Policy Reports No. 4). York, England: Social Policy Research Unit, University of York.

Slaikeu, K. A. (1996). *When push comes to shove: A practical guide to mediating disputes.* San Francisco: Jossey-Bass.

Smith, J. A., Scammon, D. L., & Beck, S. L. (1995). Using patient focus groups for new patient services. *Joint Commission Journal on Quality Improvement, 21*(1), 22–31.

Stewart, D. W., & Shamdasani, P. N. (1992). *Focus groups: Theory and practice.* London: Sage.

Strategic Focus Online. (1998). *Strategic focus online? Information about online focus groups.* Retrieved November 28, 2000, from http://www.sfionline.com

Sudau, S., & Brown, N. (1984). Improving mailed questionnaire design. In J. Lockhart (Ed.), *Making effective use of mailed questionnaires* (pp. 33–47). San Francisco: Jossey-Bass.

Thomas, R., & Purdon, S. (1994). Telephone methods for social surveys. *Social Research Update, 8,* 3–8.

Van de Viert, E., Nauta, A., Giebles, E., & Janssen, O. (1999). Constructive conflict at work. *Journal of Organizational Behavior, 20,* 475–491.

Wadsworth, Y. (1997). *Do it yourself social research* (2nd ed.). Sydney, Australia: Allen & Unwin.

Weiss, R. S. (1994). *Learning from strangers: The art and method of qualitative interview studies.* New York: Free Press.

White, G. E., & Thomson, A. N. (1995). Anonymized focus groups as a research tool for health professionals. *Qualitative Health Research 5,* 256–261.

6

Health Planning for Rural and Frontier Mental and Behavioral Health Care

Gil Hill, Alison Howard, Donald L. Weaver, and B. Hudnall Stamm

In this chapter, we present information for health planning and funding. The first section encompasses identifying and selecting target areas and robust models for designing service delivery systems that incorporate the formal and informal health resources and allow for the incorporation of new health needs or resources. The second portion of the chapter provides information about locating and securing funds for building and sustaining health systems.

The difference between having health care services and having a delivery system can be understood in the historical origin of the services within a community. Fractionated, underfunded services typical in many rural communities may have grown topsy-turvy, without system or fiscal planning. The best and most sustainable systems are judiciously planned and funded. The information in other chapters in this book, particularly chapters 5 and 8, combined with public health approaches (see chapter 7), can enable health planners to be proactive in designing or mending gaps in health care systems.

Health Planning

Healthy People

The definitive health planning document for the U. S. government is *Healthy People,* which is revised each decade. The document is developed with input from health providers, planners, researchers, and communities throughout the United States. Each decade, there are overarching, aspirational goals that coordinate with topically arranged goals. The 28 topical goals are organized by (a) the aspirational goal, (b) an overview, (c) issues, (d) trends, and (e) disparities (often related to rural status). The goals include information about the

Mr. Hill can be reached at 1910 S Street NW, Washington, DC 20009. E-mail: gilhill1910@aol.com. Dr. Weaver can be reached at National Health Service Corps, 8th Floor, 4350 East-West Highway, Bethesda MD 20814. E-mail: DWeaver@HRSA.GOV

prevalence, when data are available, or indicate that data should be collected or exist but are unreliable.

Healthy People 2010 (U.S. Department of Health and Human Services, 2000; www.healthypeople.gov), was released in November 2000. The two main goals described in *Healthy People 2010* were to increase quality and years of healthy life and to eliminate health disparities. *Healthy People 2010* also introduced the concept of health indicators, a concept analogous to economic indicators. The 10 health indicators, which represent the overall health of the nation and focus on healthy people living in healthy communities, are (a) physical activity, (b) overweight and obesity, (c) tobacco use, (d) substance abuse, (e) responsible sexual behavior, (f) mental health, (g) injury and violence, (h) environmental quality, (i) immunization, and (j) access to health care.

Nearly all the goals of *Healthy People 2010* have some behavioral aspects. However, some specifically concern behavioral health and mental illnesses, whereas other sections are closely related to but not categorized as mental or behavioral health. The section that addresses mental health and mental disorders is Goal 18. Goal 26 addresses substance abuse, and Goal 27 addresses tobacco use. Some of the goals that are closely tied to behavioral health include cancer (Goal 3), diabetes (Goal 5), heart disease and stroke (Goal 12), human immunodeficiency virus (HIV) infection (Goal 13), injury and violence prevention (Goal 15), nutrition and overweight (Goal 19), physical activity and fitness (Goal 22), and sexually transmitted diseases (Goal 25). Goal 1, access to quality health services, applies to nearly all planning endeavors but particularly to underserved areas, most of which are rural. *Healthy People 2010* assists planners in identifying areas to target for improvement. However, like other taxonomies, the *Healthy People* series does not contain definitions for how the targets should be addressed. Planners can use the *Healthy People* series to meet the needs and resources of their communities and to establish a model of care that suits the temperament and culture of their communities.

Developing a Model Health Service Delivery System

A case can be made that the health care system in the United States is really not a system at all. Health care professionals know that there are health care disparities. The system is like a patchwork quilt that is warm and secure for many and threadbare, worn, or nonexistent for far too many others. However, all communities have the potential to craft their own "patches" to ensure that everyone in the community has access to primary health care—physical, oral, and mental or behavioral health—the ultimate outcome, as specified by the *Healthy People* series, being the increased quality and years of healthy life and the elimination of health disparities. This pattern for improving health accounts for the fact that each community needs a systematic approach to health improvement and that, although rural and frontier areas suffer from chronic health care underservice, there are options.

"If you've seen one rural health care model, you've seen one model" is a true statement, but there are similarities across successful models. First, they are grounded in guiding principles; second, they go through a series of steps to achieve their success; and, third, they continue to evolve into effective, high-quality, integrated primary care community health systems.

GUIDING PRINCIPLES. There are four guiding principles: (a) community responsiveness, (b) cultural competence, (c) interdisciplinary efforts, and (d) life cycle sensitivity. Successful communities have a system of care that addresses individual and community needs. They ensure collaboration between the primary care and public health. Successful systems also account for the richness of diversity. Designers of such systems realize that each person is guided by a cultural foundation of values, traditions, beliefs, and perceptions of health care. They use this richness to develop and improve their systems to ensure that care is of the highest quality. In successful communities, the interdisciplinary team, with emphasis on each person's strengths, is used. Finally, successful programs are based on a systematic view, accounting for all aspects of the life cycle. Prenatal, pediatric, adolescent, adult, and geriatric populations are to ensure that they are included. There is continuous monitoring to ensure that communities within a community are not left out.

Although every community is unique, and the model that each community builds reflects that uniqueness, the components are similar, regardless of how they are put together. Figure 6.1 shows an organizational schema that incorporates a variety of types of formal and informal resources. The potential members of the "egg" (right side of figure) are nearly unlimited, but anyone can take part in the process. Some members are pivotal to the plan, whereas others take a supporting or ancillary role. The next section provides a step-by-step process for determining how the "egg" will look for a particular community. The model is dynamic, and pieces can be added or subtracted without losing the vision of the whole as the needs and resources of the community change.

STEPS TO SUCCESS. For a community to improve its health care system, one or more persons must take a leadership role. This individual or individuals may come from any of a variety of backgrounds, which may or may not be in the formal health delivery realm, but they must be willing to serve as catalysts to help a community ready to transform.

Next, the individual or group that has assumed the leadership role must enlist other leaders to create a coalition to guide the effort. The decision of who becomes a member of the guiding coalition is community specific. Coalition members *talk* about increasing access and eliminating disparities, using *Healthy People* and their local needs and resource assessment. Together they identify the disparity or disparities that they believe their community can address, and they build a plan to reduce the disparities, using their combined skills.

After the identification of health targets, the coalition, composed of community champions from diverse backgrounds, makes a *commitment* to meet for the purpose of increasing access and eliminating disparities. There are always available seats at the coalition table; new leaders with fresh perspectives are always welcome, as is represented by the empty spaces attached to the "egg."

Representing the commandment made by the leadership, the coalition will *declare* its desired goal. Many goals could be selected. For example, one

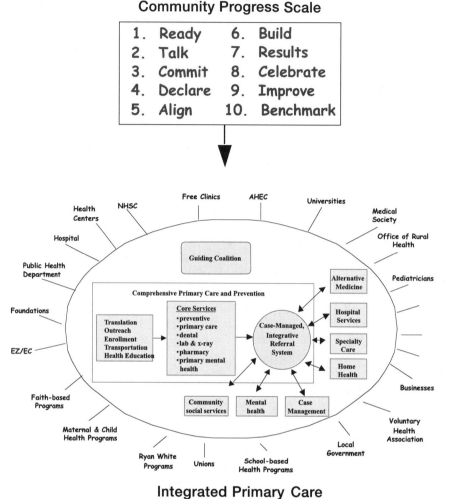

Community Progress Scale

1. Ready	6. Build
2. Talk	7. Results
3. Commit	8. Celebrate
4. Declare	9. Improve
5. Align	10. Benchmark

**Integrated Primary Care
Community Based Health System**

Figure 6.1. Celebrate, improve, and benchmark community progress.

goal, concerning access, may be that every uninsured person who is 150% or below the federal poverty level will have access to services. Another goal, concerning a disparity, is that all women will be screened and appropriately treated for depression. Regardless of what is selected, declaring a goal is a key step, because clearly stated goals attract resources both inside and outside the community. These are the goals around which to structure funding selection and requests, as well as an evaluation plan.

The community's assets are inventoried and *aligned* so that coalition members can pursue the shared goal of increasing access and eliminating disparities. The systems that evolve are centered on primary care and prevention. Collaboration with secondary and tertiary care fills out the picture but does not dominate the system. With common goals and an alignment of assets, the community is now ready to add elements to achieve its goals. This can take the form of strengthening existing partners, bringing on new partners, soliciting new resources through grants, or a combination of these. The result is to *build* a dynamic system to meet the defined needs of a community now and incorporate new needs and resources as the community's health needs and resources change over time.

Securing Funding

Once a model incorporating community responsiveness, cultural competence, interdisciplinary efforts, and life cycle sensitivity has been defined for a specific community, it serves as the blueprint for identifying sources of funding. Although there is a rich history of funding programs for rural health care (e.g., Ricketts, 1999), successfully securing funds depends on understanding the funding process. There are various *types* of funding, including gifts, grants, appropriations (funds mandated in legislation at the local, state, or federal level), and contracts. The *sources* of funding can be classified by their level (national, state, and local) and source (public and private). A new strategy termed *blended funding* (Dunbar, 1999) can be used to link multiple funding streams into a unified administrative or service delivery project.

Funding is partly a reflection of the policy trends in health care; therefore, a planner who is knowledgeable about policy trends is more likely to know what type of money is available and how to present ideas so those ideas are attractive to various funding agencies (see www.nrharural.org and www.gmu.edu/departments/chpre/ruralhealth for information on policy). Members of government and nongovernment organizations are willing to support the development of new knowledge (research), the operation of health services, assistance in training, and support of infrastructure (e.g., telehealth networks). In general, different organizations specialize in different types of funding; therefore, it is important to understand the mission and scope of the agency from which money is sought. For example, the goals of a rural community seeking service funding to reduce health disparities would be at odds with the requirements of research funding, in which the goal is the production of new knowledge.

It is important to seek funding in an ongoing way, using the master plan developed in the planning process. Trying to find a source only when the need arises may introduce frustrating elements such as rushing to meet deadlines or delays due to the review process. A potential applicant needs ongoing contact with organizations (both governmental and nongovernmental) that award grant funds. In addition, it is a good idea to learn as much as possible about likely funding sources through an understanding of their rules, guidelines, and funding limitations as well as of their mission and how it might complement an applicant's plan.

In organizations, various solicitations are used for applications. These solicitations share common elements in their structure. Most begin with a précis of the project; continue with a brief review of background information (which may include a literature review), the specific goals and objectives to be met by applicants, and information about the required format; and end with contact information. Although the definitions are not strictly adhered to, some generalizations can be made. A *request for proposal* (RFP) is probably the most common and most generic mechanism. An RFA, or request for application, is also commonly used. Some agencies use a program announcement (PA), and others use an RFI (request for interest). The latter is more commonly used to solicit participants into multisite studies or cooperative agreements that share a common methodology or data collection system.

Where to Find Funding

There are many directories of funding agencies, but the World Wide Web is generally the fastest and most up-to-date source of funding information. For readers who do not have access to the Web, reference volumes such as the *Federal Yellow Book* (Leadership Directories, Inc., 1999) or the *Foundation Directory* (http://fconline.fdncenter.org) contains addresses and telephone numbers from which information can be obtained. A general source of information is The Grantsmanship Center (www.tgci.com). In addition to providing valuable links to sites containing requests, the Center conducts training, provides technical assistance, and operates an online forum. Some of the key links to pursue are listed as follows:

1. Daily *Federal Register* and *Federal Register* archives for federal regulations and proposed actions, including the establishment of new funding streams.
2. *Catalog of Federal Domestic Assistance* (grants and contracts).
3. *Commerce Business Daily* (federal procurement actions for contract proposals).

The Foundation Center is another source of information (www.fdncenter.org); it is a clearinghouse that fosters public understanding of foundations by collecting, analyzing, and disseminating information on foundations, corporate giving, and related subjects. It covers activity on national, state, and local levels. Links to individual foundations with detailed information on foundation interests and application procedures are also provided. The Foundation Center's Web site, with entries for all 50 states and the District of Columbia, contains information on state and local funding directories.

The lead federal agency for rural health is the Office of Rural Health Policy (ORHP), of the Health Resources and Services Administration. This agency has federal governmentwide responsibility for rural health and the grant programs that are announced on their Web site (www.hrsa.gov /orhpgrant.html) and it is housed within the administration of the Department of Health and Human Services. Another important agency, the Office for the Advancement of Telehealth (OAT), is also located in the Health Resources and Services Administration. This new agency has responsibility for the administration of an important grant program relating to the rural behavioral health care infrastructure. Information on this and other responsibilities of

OAT can be found on their Web site (telehealth.hrsa.gov). An additional general site is the "Federal Support for Rural Health" (www.nal.usda.gov /ric/richs).

Specific information on other rural health programs is available from many federal agencies such as the Department of Health and Human Services (www.dhhs.gov), the Department of Agriculture (www.usda.gov), the Department of Commerce (www.commerce.gov), the Department of Defense (www.defenselink.mil); the Department of Education (www.ed.gov), the Department of Justice (www.usdoj.gov), the Department of Labor (www.dol.gov), and the Department of Veterans Affairs (www.va.gov).

Writing the Proposal

Proposal writing is arduous. Each organization has a unique proposal format, but there are similarities across formats. A good proposal specifies the problem, offers a solution, specifies a method for documenting the outcomes, and shows that the requesting organization has appropriate technical, management, and budget competency. Proposal writing can be eased with planning and careful organization. The previous section offered suggestions about planning, and the following section provides step-by-step suggestions for proposal writing.

STEP 1. Once the planner has a model and targets for change (goals), he or she should begin by contacting the funding source via telephone, e-mail, or letter of inquiry or intent (most private foundations require this). The most effective way to develop a relationship with a funding source is to visit in person. If possible, the planner should schedule an appointment with the responsible official to learn about funding priorities and the official's reaction to the planner's model and goals. In many cases, the program officer will work with the planner to develop a fundable proposal. If the interest of the funding organization will be enhanced by a site visit to the planner's facility, it may be possible to arrange for such a visit.

STEP 2. The second step in the application process is the development of the proposal. As mentioned earlier, successful rural proposal development often involves collaboration. In the fields of rural health (in which the few providers present in a rural area must work together) and substance abuse (in which treatment is best provided in a community context), proposals are strengthened by evidence of collaboration. A successful application involves matching the interests of the funding organization with the goals of the applicant.

The written funding solicitation is the most important source of guidance. It should be read and outlined with great care by the writer to ensure that all *mandatory* and *desirable* requirements are understood and addressed in the application. The writer should not hesitate to use services of the program officer, even to the extent of asking the officer to review and comment on a draft application.

General rules to follow in proposal development include the following:

- Achieve excellence in all areas (treat all aspects of the proposal with respect).
- Develop the proposal as a logical whole (seamless presentation).

- Construct the proposal to present a positive outcome, but be realistic and factual.
- Check the details (facts, spelling, grammar, and so forth).

STEP 3. The details of the proposal should be conveyed carefully to the granting organization. The elements of a good (successful) proposal include a variety of topics:

1. *Background:* Orient the reader (reviewer) to the problem in a relevant and concise manner. Include a literature review, data, and a needs assessment (when appropriate).
2. *Rationale:* Describe the principles, practices, or observations that underlie the project, as well as the model (conceptual framework) of the request. Whenever possible, build credibility by relating this proposal to other efforts being conducted by the applicant.
3. *Objectives:* Use the model and health targets to guide the objectives. The objectives should be *appropriate* (linked to the problem statement in the rationale and addressing the purposes of the proposal request). They should identify what is to be *accomplished,* be written in *measurable terms,* and be *realistic* in view of the time and money requested.
4. *Project methods:* Describe the *process* for achieving objectives—who, what, when, where, and how for each objective. Describe *activities* to be completed for each objective (be concrete, avoid vagueness, be realistic, and do not overpromise). Describe *organizational and administrative* arrangements. It helps to work closely with the business orgrants office to capture accounting controls, purchasing procedures, and other financial aspects. Also, describe a management plan that establishes the qualifications of your organization.
5. *Evaluation:* The evaluation section of an application can be only as good as the objectives. The evaluation should address both process (formative evaluation) and outcomes (summative evaluation). Quantitative and qualitative measures should be specified, and when possible, instrumentation should be specified. Care should be taken to demonstrate the evaluation expertise and commitment of project personnel.
6. *Applicant summary and resources:* In addition to demonstrating the project director's expertise, it is important to establish the credibility and record of accomplishment of the applicant institution, specifying institutional support, participation, and cooperation with other institutions. Letters of support and participation should also be included.
7. *Budget:* In accordance with the format prescribed by the funding organization, the budget should be developed through the expertise of both the funding organization and the applicant organization's finance or grants offices. It is extremely important for the budget to match and support the project objectives. If the applicant organization plans to match or provide "in-kind" resources, this should be specified, because it shows organizational investment in the project.

STEP 4. Be sure to include all requested *supplemental information.* One such portion of information is the biographical information on the project director and other project personnel. A curriculum vita, in the form specified by the funding agency, should show a focus that relates to the project. A comprehensive bibliography demonstrates that a thorough literature search has been conducted and that all sources of relevant data have been examined.

STEP 5. Finally, *never be late with an application.* It is easy for a funding organization to assume that an applicant is inept because the proposal is late. It is often policy to reject a late application. It is also useful to have your application read by a fresh set of eyes—a person not involved in the application preparation but informed on the subject matter—before it is submitted. Often, errors are missed by those overly familiar with the document.

Barriers in Seeking Funding

Knowing about the difficulties and barriers to funding can help planners work to overcome them. Barriers include lack of a track record (no history of successful grant awards), absence of adequate administrative support, absence of on-site expertise, and lack of organizational commitment. The lack of a track record can be overcome by collaborating with experienced grantees or by building a detailed, well-documented proposal that is based on the latest knowledge (research). Reviewers are usually content experts, and when they read applications that are based on research sources they know to be current and on the cutting edge of the field, they are more inclined to place less importance on the relative inexperience of the applicant. If the applicant recognizes an absence of on-site expertise, this can sometimes be corrected by including expert consultants in the proposal. This is a judgment call in which the importance of expertise to the core of the proposal must be weighed.

Conclusions and Recommendations

After designing and building a community-based, culturally competent, interdisciplinary system that addresses health care across the life cycle, it is important to *celebrate* success, whether funding has been obtained or not. When a community has learned how to become more successful in one aspect of health care, it is poised to be successful in a variety of ways. Recommendations to assist communities in building and funding health care systems are listed as follows.

Show How Quality Health Care Benefits the Community as a Whole

Help to create an awareness of the impact that quality health care can have on a rural community, as a way to ensure continuing communal support. Gaining the resources to provide interdisciplinary care for rural and frontier communities not only adds to the quality of life of rural residents but also makes major contributions to rural community development. Local rural economies depend on rural residents to purchase locally produced goods and services, including health care. When people living in rural areas go elsewhere to obtain health services the infrastructure of the community is damaged, health care providers are negatively affected, and the attractiveness of the rural community to businesses and other organizations who might locate there is decreased.

Build Local Leadership to Monitor Funding Opportunities

Establishing a leader willing to monitor the national and international funding opportunities is a critical step toward obtaining funding. This person or a second person must have the ability to successfully write grants. The take-home message of this chapter is that the interdisciplinary program developer and manager (as well as any providers who participate) must assume the function of resolutely seeking and monitoring sources of support. Opportunities can arise as aresult of public acknowledgment and awareness of a health problem (e.g., the sequelae of male adolescent violence), natural disasters (e.g., the forest fires of summer 2000), economic conditions (e.g., the persistent problem of family farm survival), and other circumstances.

Support Interagency Information Sharing

Creating a network of communication and organizations helps keep the fundraiser apprised of available funding and ensures the continued success of the community's health care model. In order to provide the highest level of access and quality of care to rural patients, planners must be vigilant for every possible source of funding. As the dot-com world continues to evolve, the World Wide Web will be an even more important source of information support. "Federal Support for Rural Health" (http:www.nal.gov/ric/richs/), mentioned previously, is an excellent place to begin. Planners should learn how to surf the Web and develop opportunities to bolster their programs.

Improve the System

After one success, planners should move on to the next task. If access continues to be an issue, they should "raise the bar." If the community has achieved the access goal, which health disparities are they now willing to tackle? This is continuous quality improvement at its best.

Benchmark the Project

When a community declares victory over its barriers to access and its disparities, it becomes a benchmark for others. Successful communities are willing to share their models. The same communities are always learning new and improved ways to deliver care from others. It really is like a quilt, beautiful in its diverse components and sewn together with love to serve a meaningful purpose. The answer to a community's health model lies within the community. The challenge is to acquire the skills to turn barriers into opportunities.

References

Dunbar, E. R. (1999). Strengthening services in rural communities through blended funding. In I. B. Carlton-LaNey, R. L. Edwards, & P. N. Reid (Eds.), *Preserving and strengthening small towns and rural communities* (pp. 15–26). Washington, DC: National Association of Social Workers Press.

Leadership Directories, Inc. (1999). *Federal yellow book.* Washington, DC: Author.

Ricketts, T. C. (Ed.). (1999). *Rural health in the United States.* New York: Oxford University Press.

U.S. Department of Health and Human Services. (2000, November). *Healthy people 2010* (2nd ed., 2 vols.). Washington, DC: U.S. Government Printing Office. Retrieved March 16, 2001, from http://www.health.gov/healthypeople/Document/tableofcontents.htm

Part II

Service Delivery in Rural Communities

7

A Public Health Approach to the Challenges of Rural Mental Health Service Integration

John A. Gale and Ronald D. Deprez

Discussions of the delivery of mental health care in rural areas tend to focus on system-level issues, including parity, historic barriers between physical and mental health systems, the growing role of managed care, the traditional separation of funding streams, and the shortage of qualified mental health providers willing to practice in rural areas. Although these public policy issues deserve attention, they are not particularly amenable to local solutions. In these system-level discussions, the needs of rural consumers and providers are often overlooked, and attention is diverted from the development of local-level solutions to the problems of rural mental health delivery systems.

In this chapter, we suggest an alternative perspective, that of the public health model, to inform the discussion of delivering mental health services in rural areas. Within the context of the public health model, we take a broad view of mental health services that includes both a mental health orientation and a mental illness orientation. We describe the *de facto rural mental health system,* discuss the populations served by the existing systems and their service needs, identify access issues and barriers for these populations, and provide a series of tools with which stakeholders can begin to analyze their local delivery system. By doing so, stakeholders will develop a context for understanding how the various components of the system fit together. These tools will enable stakeholders to identify the multiple points of access within their community, to categorize those access points according to a logical framework, and to identify the clinical roles and functions of the various providers, agencies, and organizations that constitute their local mental health system. Within this context, we suggest opportunities to improve and integrate existing components of local mental health delivery systems in rural areas to better meet the needs of the people served by them.

Elements of the Public Health Approach

Public health focuses on the diagnosis, treatment, and etiology of disease; epidemiological surveillance of the health of the population at large; health pro-

Mr. Gale can be reached at the Edmund S. Muskie School of Public Service, 96 Falmouth Street, P.O. Box 9300, Portland, ME 04104-9300. E-mail: jgale@usm.maine.edu

motion; disease prevention; and access to and the evaluation of services (Last & Wallace, 1992). Although the public health model overall is concerned with the health of a population (U.S. Department of Health and Human Services, 1999, p. 3), its core is concerned with the health of at-risk populations. The application of a public health approach to mental health and mental illness is one of the overarching themes of the Surgeon General's Report on Mental Health (U.S. Department of Health and Human Services, 1999, pp. 3–4), in which it was argued that a population-based focus on mental health treatment and promotion is needed.

In this chapter, we adapt and expand on the public health approach identifying and addressing local mental health delivery system problems. This method has two parts. One is to understand the mental health epidemiological features of the population (see Deprez, 1994–1995, 1995; Deprez & Horton, 1996). The second is to understand the specific (private and public) components of the local delivery system that address the populations at risk. From these perspectives, policymakers, mental health professionals, and other mental health stakeholders can determine how to use available local resources to attend to the population's mental health needs.

More specifically, this approach enables a population's mental health needs to be addressed through the mobilization of local community partnerships with specialty mental health providers, primary care providers, community agencies, school systems, clergy, consumers, and other key stakeholders. Partners help identify and solve access problems; expand and coordinate acute, preventive, and crisis mental health services at the community level; promote the integration of mental health, general medical, and substance abuse services; and develop outreach efforts to ensure that all members of the community are able to obtain needed mental health services.

Mental Health and Mental Illness: Points on a Continuum

Central to the public health model is the recognition that health promotion and disease prevention are, in many ways, as important as the diagnosis and treatment. The Surgeon General's Report on Mental Health (U.S. Department of Health and Human Services, 1999) suggests that "mental health and mental illness are not polar opposites but may be thought of as points on a continuum" (pp. 4–5). All too often, mental health systems focus on the treatment of disease at the expense of prevention and health promotion. This is particularly true in rural areas, in which a limited mental health infrastructure is insufficient to deal with the community's acute care needs.

Mental health, according to the Surgeon General's Report on Mental Health (U.S. Department of Health and Human Services, 1999), "is a state of successful performance of mental function, resulting in productive activities, fulfilling relationships with other people, and the ability to adapt to change and adversity" (p. 4). Because the conceptualization of mental health is culturally based and therefore grounded in the values of the individual's culture, the definition of mental health as defined by the Surgeon General's Report on Mental Health varies among all individuals. Although rural populations are often treated in the literature as a relatively homogeneous group, there are in reality likely to be more differences between rural populations in various communities than there are between the broader categories of urban and rural populations (Cordes, 1990). Rural communities are diverse both geographically and in the composition of the cultural background of their populations. This presents a challenge for rural mental health providers, who may be called upon to work with a variety of cultural and ethnic groups.

Mental illness, at the other extreme, is defined as a clinically significant behavior or psychological syndrome or pattern that is associated with present distress (e.g., painful syndrome), disability (e.g., impairment in one or more important areas of functioning), or a significantly increased risk of suffering death, pain, disability, or an important loss of freedom (American Psychiatric Association, 1994). *Mental illness* refers collectively to a broad range of diagnosable mental disorders that are characterized by alterations in thinking, mood, or behavior (or some combination thereof) in association with distress, impaired functioning, or both.

Somewhere in between these two points are mental health problems that, according to the Surgeon General's Report on Mental Health (U.S. Department of Health and Human Services, 1999), "are signs and symptoms of insufficient intensity or duration to meet the criteria for any mental disorder" (p. 5). Commonly experienced by most individuals at some point in their lives, these behavioral health problems may necessitate active intervention to ameliorate symptoms and to prevent further deterioration. Mental health problems can be precipitated by individual difficulties or communitywide economic changes. Examples at an individual level include grief caused by bereavement, feelings of powerlessness caused by the loss of a job, and depression caused by divorce. Examples at a community level include the loss of a major employer or the farm crises of the 1980s and 1990s that triggered economic hardship and rapid social change, which adversely affected the mental health of many rural residents (Beeson, 1999; Hoyt, O'Donnell, & Mack, 1995; Ortega, Johnson, Beeson, & Craft, 1994; Williams, 1996). For farm families, these stresses affect those who choose to remain on the farm (Bultena, Lasley, & Geller, 1986; Walker & Walker, 1988; Williams, 1996), as well as those who were forced out of farming (Heffernan & Heffernan, 1986).

Prevalence of Mental Health Disorders in Rural Populations

Equally central to the public health model is an understanding of the incidence of mental and behavioral health disease within a given community's populations. Although national incidence rates provide a good starting point for this process, the smallness of the population in rural areas precludes reliance solely on nationally derived rates. It is essential that these rates be supplemented with community- and population-specific data on the incidence and types of mental and behavioral health disorders in order to effectively maximize the use of scarce resources.

Findings from the National Comorbidity Survey and the National Household Survey on Drug Abuse suggest that the prevalence of clinically defined mental health problems among rural adult populations is similar to that among urban adult populations (Hartley, Bird, & Dempsey, 1999; Kessler et al., 1994). The survey also revealed comparable 12-month and lifetime rates for any substance abuse disorders across residential settings (National Rural Health Association, 1999). Approximately 28%–30% of the overall adult population has either a mental or an addictive disorder (Kessler et al., 1994; Regier et al., 1993). A subset of this group (5.4%) comprises those who have a serious mental illness (SMI) that interferes with social functioning (Kessler et al., 1996). Half of those (2.6% of the total) have severe and persistent mental illness (SPMI; Kessler et al., 1996; National Advisory Mental Health Council, 1993). The prevalence of SMI and SPMI is consistent across residence (Greenley et al., 1992).

Nationally, 20% of children and adolescents experience the symptoms of a disorder listed in the *Diagnostic and Statistical Manual of Mental Disorders, 4th Edition* (*DSM–IV;* American Psychiatric Association, 1994) during the course of a year (U.S. Department of Health and Human Services, 1999, p. 193). Approximately 5%–13% of all children suffer from serious emotional disturbances (Friedman, Katz-Leavy, Manderscheid, & Sondheimer, 1998). Although national data do not reflect a comparison of rural and urban populations, most mental health experts believe that factors other than residence are more likely to be predictive of mental health or substance abuse issues among children and adolescents (Oetting, Edwards, Kelly, & Beauvais, 1997). Similarly, the prevalence of mental disorders is not well documented among adults 55 years of age and older. Although urban–rural comparisons are not possible at this time, it is estimated that approximately 19.8% of all older adults have a diagnosable mental disorder during a 1-year period (U.S. Department of Health and Human Services, 1999, p. 336). Almost 4% have SMI and another 1% have SPMI (Kessler et al., 1996; Regier et al., 1993).

Rural Mental Health Infrastructure Issues

These studies demonstrate the generally equal prevalences of mental health problems in America. Although equal prevalence requires equal levels of resources, rural areas generally have fewer resources than do urban settings. This statement, however, is an oversimplification of the issue because the vast differences in mental health problems among populations and geographic areas of the country are underrecognized (American Psychological Association, Office of Rural Health, 1995; Deprez, 1995). Different arrays of problems necessitate different types of resources. This fact exacerbates the resource disparities between rural and urban areas because rural areas do not have the same complement of resources. Thus, the lack of both resource strength (numbers) and provider diversity in rural areas mandates an approach to solving delivery system problems that is different from those typically employed in urban areas.

The total number of individuals suffering from mental disorders is comparatively small in rural areas and spread across wider geographic regions. These differences have important implications for rural mental health infrastructure development. These factors, in combination with the weak economic bases of many rural areas, suggest that the development of specialty mental health services may not be economically feasible (Geller, Beeson, & Roden-hiser, 2000).

The constraints of rural practice make it difficult to recruit and retain specialty mental health providers, even if the local population is of sufficient size to support their practice. Rural mental health providers must treat patients outside of their expertise, make complex decisions without advice from other professionals, and interact with patients in a variety of nonclinical roles (Roberts, Battaglia, & Epstein, 1999). They are often subject to professional isolation and have a high potential for burnout (Beeson, 1991; Stamm, 1999).

Not surprisingly, rural areas have a smaller supply of specialty mental health providers than urban areas, both in the percentage of counties with any mental health services and in specialty mental health organizations (Hartley et al., 1999; Human & Wasem, 1991). This lower level of availability translates directly into access disparities between rural and urban residents (Lambert & Agger, 1995). Overall, residents of rural areas utilize behavioral health services at significantly lower rates than do residents of urban areas (Cohen & Hesselbart, 1993; Goldsmith, Wagenfeld, Manderscheid, & Stiles, 1997). When rural residents are able to gain access to services, they often are required to accept compromises that include long-distance travel to receive care, limited choices of providers, loss of confidentiality as a result of the visibility of mental health services in small communities, and a heightened sense of personal stigma (Calloway, Fried, Johnsen, & Morrissey, 1999).

Because of the shortage of specialty mental health services, primary care practices and emergency rooms are key settings for the early identification of mental health problems. Ideally, medical and mental health care would intersect during the primary care visit (Cunningham, 1997). In practice, they often intersect in the emergency room, usually in relation to drug and alcohol problems.

The De Facto Mental Health System in Rural Areas

Mental health systems in most rural communities are anything but a coordinated system of specialty mental health. Instead, there is a fragmented assortment of service venues and providers, collectively referred to as the *de facto mental health system* (Regier, Goldberg, & Taube, 1978; Regier et al., 1993). The term *system,* in this context, conveys an understanding of where persons with mental disorders or problems receive services. The characteristics and composition of the mental health system in any community are determined by a variety of heterogeneous factors rather than a single guiding set of organizing principles. Regier et al. identified four major sectors in which mental health services may be provided.

The specialty mental health sector is composed of psychiatrists, psychologists, psychiatric nurses, and social workers practicing in community mental health centers; public and private agencies; state, county, private, nonprofit psychiatric and substance abuse treatment hospitals or treatment units of general hospitals; residential treatment centers; freestanding outpatient, public, and multiservice clinics; halfway houses; and private practices. This is the sector most commonly thought of in discussions of the mental health system. Providers deliver various specialty mental health services to patients with acute, chronic, and preventive needs. As stated, the primary access issue related to this sector is the relative dearth of specialty mental health providers in rural areas.

The general medical or primary care sector is composed of family physicians, pediatricians, internists, nurse practitioners, and physician's assistants practicing in rural health clinics, private practices, community health centers, general hospitals, and nursing homes. Providers in this sector render a full range of health services, including but not limited to mental health services. Unfortunately, these providers often do not have the training to recognize early warning signals. Even if they do, opportunities to refer patients to specialty care are limited, and such care is often poorly accessible.

Social welfare, criminal justice, education, and religious and charitable organizations form the human services sector. As in the general medical sector, members of agencies and providers are unlikely to be adequately trained to recognize mental health issues and so are faced with the same limited opportunities. It is useful to discuss the role of clergy and religious organizations within the mental health system. Members of the clergy hold a position of respect and trust in rural communities and, as such, are often the first caregivers to notice that an individual or family needs special help, especially with mental health (Heffernan, 1999). They constitute an important, although frequently overlooked, resource.

The voluntary support network sector encompasses self-help groups; family members; social groups; and organizations committed to education, communication, and support. Examples of these groups are 12-step and other programs for addictive disorders and an array of family management programs and strategies. The National Institute of Mental Health has also been involved in supporting this sector with public education directed toward improving early detection of mental disorders by patients, family members, and professional caregivers (Regier et al., 1988).

Because of the nature of rural areas and the lower supply of specialized mental health providers, rural mental health systems are even more de facto than mental health systems in urban areas (Calloway et al., 1999). Rural practice is characterized by a lack of available services, a scarcity of resources, severe shortages of specialized mental health practitioners and providers, the underuse of services, the impracticality of specialization, and a recognition that clients must be supported beyond the narrow range of medically critical services (Beeson, Britain, Howell, Kirwan, & Sawyer, 1998).

In the presence of these realities, it is important to view the various sectors of the de facto system not as substitutes for one another but as different points of access and levels of care that complement one another. In the context of the public health model, policymakers, mental health professionals, and other mental health stakeholders should be concerned with more than the individuals who "show up at the front door" of specialty mental health facilities. Rather, they should also be concerned with the mental health needs of the entire at-risk population. The broader view acknowledges that there are multiple "doors" through which individuals with behavioral health needs might enter the system. The challenge becomes coordinating and facilitating their movement across the various sectors and ensuring that their needs are met at the most appropriate level.

The Needs of the Various Populations in Rural Areas

Understanding the pathological features of diagnosed and undiagnosed conditions experienced by a given area's populations is a prerequisite to understanding the area's service needs (Deprez, 1994–1995). Because both pathological conditions and services (as well as access points) differ by age and gender, policymakers, mental health professionals, and other mental health stakeholders must examine clinical and access issues of children, adolescents, and older adults apart from those of the general adult population. Before an examination of the differences in the clinical and access issues of each population is undertaken, it is important to understand the common issues that they share. Within each group, individuals may have mental health needs that include primary and secondary preventive care, acute intervention, and long-term management of chronic conditions. Any individual may have needs that span these three areas.

An individual's point of access to the system will depend on whether he or she has a mental health issue that has caused him or her to previously interact with the specialty mental health sector. For individuals without identified mental health problems, the primary point of access is likely to be either the general medical or primary care or human services sectors. For those with identified mental health issues, the point of contact is frequently the specialty mental health sector. For individuals in crisis, it may be the general medical sector (particularly the local emergency room), the human services sector (including the criminal justice system), or the voluntary support network sector (such as a minister or local support group). During these periods, individuals frequently enter the system through whichever sector offers the most rapid response.

Once in the system, their needs may be met in any one of the four sectors. Acute treatment may be provided in either the specialty medical, general medical, or primary care sectors. Also, an individual might be enrolled in a 12-step program in the voluntary support network sector, interact with the human services sector around housing or support issues, receive specialty mental health services from a psychologist or social worker, and receive medication management services as well as routine primary care services from a primary care physician. The challenges are to identify mental health needs at any of the four points, facilitate the movement of patients to the appropriate sector, manage the flow of information, and coordinate the delivery of services across the sectors.

CHILDREN AND ADOLESCENTS. The key challenge is to identify children and adolescents with mental health needs as early as possible and to engage them at the appropriate level within the de facto system. Children living in rural and urban areas are almost equally likely to use mental health services in any sector; however, rural children are less likely to have used services in the specialty mental health sector than are urban children (Burns et al., 1995). Consistent with this observation is the reality that primary care practices and schools are key settings for the early recognition of mental health problems and disorders for this population. Children and adolescents diagnosed with serious emotional disturbances exhibit multiple problems that necessitate treatment across service sectors.

OLDER ADULTS. Mental health problems are often underrecognized in older adults. Symptoms that would be recognized as warning signals in other populations are frequently attributed to the aging process. However, mental and cognitive disorders are not part of the normal aging process and should not be treated as such. By virtue of their age, older adults are frequently subject to a larger number of stressful life events, such as deteriorating health, loss of friends and family members, and declining levels of independence. Not surprisingly, older adults are subject to a variety of mental disorders (such as depression and anxiety) and mental health problems (such as bereavement issues) related to these stresses. Fortunately, many of these conditions are amenable to treatment.

The Surgeon General's Report on Mental Health (U.S. Department of Health and Human Services, 1999, p. 19) identified three problems that are particularly troublesome for this group. Dementia and other cognitive disorders reduce levels of independence among older adults and are leading contributors to the need for expensive long-term care in the last years of life. Depression contributes to a reduced ability of individuals to remain independent and the rate of suicide is high among men in this population. Schizophrenia continues to be a disabling and expensive illness among older adults, despite the recovery of function by some individuals in middle to late life.

Primary care practitioners are a key source of medical services and, as such, can serve to identify mental health issues in older adults, distinguish between physical and mental health problems, and direct patients to appropriate specialty mental health services. Of particular concern among older adults is the increased isolation that results from the loss of friends and reduced physical mobility. This source can be easily overlooked at earlier, more treatable stages.

Barriers to Access and Care

Rural residents suffer from a variety of system-level problems that negatively affect their ability to gain access to needed mental health services. These system-level problems include lower numbers of specialty mental health providers; the inability of many rural areas to support specialty mental health services; limited funding for public services; disproportionately high populations of uninsured and underinsured residents; widely dispersed and culturally diverse populations; limited supportive resources such as public transportation, housing, and vocational assistance; long travel times to available services; and the lack of provider coordination within and among the four sectors of the de facto system. Along with these problems, the stigma associated with psychiatric disorders is an important barrier to access of care in rural communities, in which it is difficult to maintain anonymity (Hoyt, Conger, Valde, & Weihs, 1997; Hoyt, O'Donnell, & Mack, 1995; and Rost, Smith, & Taylor, 1993.)

Local Solutions to Community-Level Problems and Access Issues

In discussions of the weaknesses of rural mental health systems, the focus is too often on problems external to the community, such as the shortage of qualified providers, the lack of parity between mental and physical health, the growth of managed behavioral health care, and inadequate funding levels. Amundson (1993) referred to this tendency as the "ain't it awful what they are doing to us" theme (p. 177). This focus diverts attention from the issues that are within the control of the community, such as better integration of available services or the transfer of patients among sectors. Local-level interventions alone will not solve the problems of rural mental health delivery systems; both public policy and local-level solutions are necessary and important.

Because many external problems are beyond the capacity of most communities to control, we focus on internal problems amenable to local solutions. Our intent is to suggest strategies to make the best possible use of existing resources, improving service capacity of rural systems in the short run, and to build a foundation for broader, system-level changes in the long run. Rural communities, because of their smaller size and smaller number of stakeholders, have an opportunity to develop and maintain collaborative relationships, not only among specialty mental health providers, but also across the community's spectrum of health and human services. Rural specialty mental health providers, because of their central role in the provision of services, are positioned to assume leadership roles in the development of local systems. In the absence of specialty mental health providers or because of the unwillingness of local specialty mental health providers to assume this role, other community leaders from one of the four sectors, especially primary care providers, may provide the necessary leadership as long as they are positioned to influence the participation of relevant providers and agencies. Regardless of who provides the leadership for this effort, it is crucial that that person solicits and secures the participation of all relevant providers and organizations within the four sectors of the de facto system as well as the participation of consumers.

After suitable leadership is established and broad-based participation is secured, the first task is to understand and document the various points of access to the community's mental health system. Identifying both potential and actual points of access (Aday & Anderson, 1974) in a given community provides the framework within which to focus efforts for improvement and coordination of patients' actions across the four sectors. These different points of access in a given community probably include but may not be limited to specialty mental health providers, primary care providers, school systems, clergy, the criminal justice system, social service agencies, and, when appropriate, lay providers. It is entirely likely that additional organizations and individuals that should be brought into the group will also be identified. Finally, this exercise will help the group to develop outreach strategies to "draw in" individuals who are not part of the system.

Once all points of access are established and categorized according to their positions in the sectors, it is necessary to understand ways in which the various sectors can work together. At the beginning of the process, participants should agree on a common clinical language. Either the *DSM–IV*

(American Psychiatric Association, 1994) or the *International Classification of Diseases, Ninth Revision, Clinical Modifications* (*ICD–9–CM*; Practice Management Information Corporation, 2000) is appropriate for coding as long as all participants are in agreement about which coding system to use. At the very least, information should be requested according to the coding system (either *DSM–IV* or *ICD–9–CM*) most commonly used by the sector from which the information is to originate.

The level of diagnostic specificity should be appropriate to the specialization of the referring sectors. For example, official psychiatric diagnostic categories are often unsuitable for use with patients seen in a general medical practice because these categories are based on the assumption that patients have passed through a series of diagnostic screenings before arriving at the psychiatric clinic (Eisenberg, 1992). Many of the patients seen in a general practice office simply do not fit neatly into the mental health's nomenclature; mixed states of depression and anxiety are common (Barrett, Barrett, Oxman, & Gerber, 1988). In addition, many primary care physicians are not conversant with the multiaxial evaluation system inherent in the *DSM–IV*. Asking them to provide "Axes 1 through 5" diagnoses on a patient referral form may not be appropriate or necessary. Agreeing to a common language and the type of required information (e.g., a description of the problems affecting the patient's functioning rather than a formal diagnosis) simplifies transfer of the patient across the sectors.

Another important task is to develop a group understanding of the role that each type of provider and agency can play in the provision of mental health services to rural clients. The intent is not to carve out territory, but rather to determine what is provided in the community and how the various pieces fit within the existing system. By analyzing the various functions and services performed by each participant, the group can build a base upon which to facilitate the transfer and care of patients across the sectors. The system members can also begin to develop a better understanding of the various gaps in the local system and develop strategies to fill those gaps.

Once points of access are identified, a common language is agreed upon, and the roles and functions of each system participant are understood, the group members should turn their attention to improving the functioning of the system from the patient's perspective. Clinical *vignettes* are useful tools for facilitating this discussion. For purposes of confidentiality, the group members should not use the examples of specific patients; rather, they should develop a series of vignettes that represent amalgams of a variety of patients. These vignettes can be used as part of a mental health "grand rounds" to highlight access issues, coordination difficulty, and gaps in the system's capacity. Used in this way, vignettes provide a focused opportunity to discuss issues in the context of specific patient problems and needs.

Conclusions and Recommendations

The provision of rural mental health services has always been and will probably remain a challenge. This challenge is complicated by a variety of issues whose resolution is beyond the capacity of many communities. Members of the health care industry should continue to advocate for better reimbursement and funding levels, parity with physical health benefits, programs to improve the supply of providers in rural areas, and other public policy solutions. At the same time, they should not neglect the fact that many mental health systems are not functioning optimally. Benefits can be gained at the local level through a focus on the needs of patients and at-risk populations. This focus includes developing prevention and treatment programs to improve access to services, expanding outreach efforts, identifying and addressing gaps in the local mental health infrastructure, improving coordination between existing services and providers, providing opportunities to gain a better understanding of the contributions made by members of the de facto system's four sectors, and building in opportunities to interact with one another. By creating a solid local foundation, rural communities will be better able to cope with local and system-level opportunities as they arise.

To effectively maximize the use of existing resources and to plan for the effective integration, we recommend that each community undertake the following three initiatives.

Use Community-Level Prevalence and Incidence Data

A thorough understanding of the rates and types of mental and behavioral health problems by a community's population is essential to the development of an effective and integrated local delivery system. It is vital that communities develop effective baseline and follow-up surveillance systems. These systems can enable providers to determine the combination of mental and behavioral health problems in the community by population (including but not limited to age, gender, and ethnicity) and to measure outcomes related to improvements in the local delivery system.

Develop an Understanding of the Community's Service and Workforce Needs

This process should involve the development of an inventory of existing community-level resources across the de facto mental health system. It is important to be as inclusive as possible in order to develop the contacts that will support efforts to integrate the system as a whole. Once the inventory of resources is complete, these data should be combined with the data collected on the incidence rates in the community in order to begin to identify gaps in the local service delivery system and in the mental health workforce. This information can also be used to target education efforts to upgrade the skills of existing providers. For example, if one of the major gaps in the local delivery system is a lack of medication management services, educational programs can be developed to increase the skills of primary care physicians to prescribe appropriately. This information can also be used to develop telephone consultation support for physicians. The mix and range of services and educational support will vary by community according to the unique needs of their populations and the availability of existing services.

Link Primary Care and Mental Health Providers With the De Facto Mental Health System

The various sectors of the local delivery system, including specialty mental health services, general medical or primary care services, human service providers, and voluntary support networks, must be effectively integrated. In view of the shortage of specialty mental health services (as well as most other services), it becomes vital to minimize waste in the system. Providers must know what services are available in the community and how patients can make the transition from one level of service to another with minimal effort. This is necessary not only to prevent patients from "falling through the system's cracks" but also to allow providers to focus their efforts on the patient's treatment needs. As discussed earlier, this involves identifying the system's providers, the system's points of access, and the ways in which patients move across the system. To achieve these goals, providers must agree to a common clinical language and clearly identify the level of information needed for the various components of the system to work together.

Three primary obstacles will hinder the ability of providers to conduct these community-level, small-area analyses: time, money, and expertise. We recommend that appropriate federal agencies such as the Office of Rural Health Policy and the Substance Abuse and Mental Health Services Administration provide funding to communities to conduct these activities. At the same time, simply providing funding at the community level is not sufficient. It is also important to fund the development of templates and training materials to assist communities. *Caring for the Rural Community: An Interdisciplinary Curriculum,* prepared by the American Psychological Association's Office of Rural Health (1995), is an example of an existing document that could be readily adopted by rural communities. These agencies could sponsor local or regional training seminars to train rural providers and community leaders in conducting the community assessments (including the identification of necessary data sources) without requiring undue travel time and expense. Finally, these agencies could identify appropriate individuals to assist communities in conducting these assessments.

Although it may not be possible to immediately address all the behavioral health resource needs of local communities in the short run, it is possible to assist communities in maximizing the functioning and integration of existing resources. This assistance will enable mental health professionals and stakeholders to strengthen the foundation of the rural mental health infrastructure to better meet the needs of their rural citizens and provide a base upon which to support the development of longer term, system-level changes.

References

Aday, L., & Anderson, R. (1974). A framework for the study of access to medical care. *Health Services Research, 9,* 209–220.

American Psychiatric Association. (1994). *Diagnostic and statistical manual of mental disorders* (4th ed.). Washington, DC: Author.

American Psychological Association, Office of Rural Health. (1995). *Caring for the rural community: An interdisciplinary curriculum.* Washington, DC: Author.

Amundson, B. (1993). Myth and reality in the rural health service crisis: Facing up to community responsibilities. *Journal of Rural Health, 9,* 176–187.

Barrett, J., Barrett, J., Oxman, T., & Gerber, P. (1988). The prevalence of psychiatric disorders in a primary care practice. *Archives of General Psychiatry, 45,* 1100–1106.

Beeson, P. (1991). The successful rural mental health practitioner: Dimensions of success, challenges, and opportunities. *Rural Community Mental Health, 18*(4), 4–7.

Beeson, P. (1999, Winter). Farm crisis and mental summit: A summary of findings. *National Rural Health Association Party-Line, 7*(4), 21–32. Retrieved November 1, 2000, from http://www.narmh.org/facrfrtn.htm

Beeson, P., Britain, C., Howell, M., Kirwan, A., & Sawyer, D. (1998). Rural mental health at the millennium. In R. W. Manderscheid & M. J. Henderson (Eds.), *Mental health, United States* (8th ed., pp. 82–97). Washington, DC: U.S. Government Printing Office.

Bultena, G., Lasley, P., & Geller, J. (1986). The farm crisis: Patterns and impact of financial distress among Iowa farm families. *Rural Sociology, 51,* 436–448.

Burns, B., Costello, E., Angold, A., Tweed, D., Stangl, D., Farmer, E., et al. (1995). Children's mental health use across service sectors. *Health Affairs, 14,* 147–159.

Calloway, M., Fried, B., Johnsen, M., & Morrissey, J. (1999). Characterizations of rural mental health service systems. *Journal of Rural Health, 15,* 296–307.

Cohen, R., & Hesselbart, C. S. (1993). Demographic factors in the use of children's mental health services. *American Journal of Public Health, 83*(1), 49–52.

Cordes, S. M. (1990). Come on in, the water's just fine. *Academic Medicine: Journal of the Association of American Medical Colleges, 65*(Suppl. 3), S1–S9.

Cunningham, R. (1997). Long road ahead to integration of primary and behavioral care. *Medicine and Health Perspectives, 51*(16), 1–4.

Deprez, R. D. (1994–1995, Winter). Using epidemiology methods in community needs assessments. *Fellowship Alumni Network Newsletter, 1.* San Francisco: The Healthcare Forum.

Deprez, R. D. (1995). Comparison of mental health factors for Las Vegas, New Mexico; Jackson, Wyoming; and Lame Deer, Montana. In American Psychological Association Office of Rural Health, *Caring for the rural community: An interdisciplinary curriculum* (pp. 55–69). Washington, DC: American Psychological Association.

Deprez, R. D., & Horton, S. (1996). Community health status and service needs assessment: An analytic tool for the changing health care delivery system. *Journal of Hospital Marketing, 10*(2),117–128.

Eisenberg, L. (1992). Treating depression and anxiety in the primary care setting. *Health Affairs, 11*(3), 149–156.

Friedman, R. M., Katz-Leavy, J. W., Manderscheid, R. W., & Sondheimer, D. L. (1998). Prevalence of serious emotional disturbances in children and adolescents. An update. In R. W. Manderscheid & M. J. Henderson (Eds.), *Mental health, United States* (8th ed., pp. 110–112). Washington, DC: U.S. Government Printing Office.

Geller, J., Beeson, P., & Rodenhiser, R. (2000). Frontier mental health strategies: Integrating, reaching out, building up, and connecting: *Letter to the field No. 6.* Frontier Mental Health Services Resource Network, Western Interstate Commission for Higher Education, Denver, CO. Retrieved August 11, 2000, from http://www.wiche.edu/mentalhealth/frontier/letter6.html

Goldsmith, H. F., Wagenfeld, M. O., Manderscheid, R. W., & Stiles, D. (1997). Specialty mental health services in metropolitan and non-metropolitan areas: 1983 and 1990. *Administration and Policy in Mental Health, 24,* 475–488.

Greenley, J., Barry, K., Fleming, M., Greenberg, J., Hollingsworth, E., McKee, D., et al. (1992). Rural mental health services: Research at the mental health research center, University of Wisconsin. *Outlook, 2*(3), 24–25.

Hartley, D., Bird, D., & Dempsey, P. (1999). Rural mental health and substance abuse. In T. Ricketts (Ed.), *Rural health in the United States* (pp. 159–178). New York: Oxford University Press.

Heffernan, J. (1999, Winter). Mental health and ministry: The vital connection. *National Rural Health Association Party-Line, 7*(4), 16–18 Retrieved August 11, 2000, from http://www.narmh.org/facrtwel.htm

Heffernan, J., & Heffernan, W. (1986). Impact of the farm crisis on rural families and communities. *The Rural Sociologist, 6*(3), 160–170.

Hoyt, D. R., Conger, R. D., Valde, J. G., & Weihs, K. (1997). Psychological distress and help-seeking in rural America. *American Journal of Community Psychology, 25,* 449–470.

Hoyt, D., O'Donnell, D., & Mack, K. (1995). Psychological distress and size of place: The epidemiology of rural economic stress. *Rural Sociology, 60,* 707–720.

Human, J., & Wasem, C. (1991). Rural mental health in America. *American Psychologist, 46,* 232–239.

Kessler, R., Berglund, P., Zhao, S., Leaf, P., Kouzis, A., Bruce, M., et al. (1996). The 12-month prevalence and correlates of serious mental illness. In R. W. Manderscheid & M. A. Sonnenschein (Eds.), *Mental health, United States* (7th ed., pp. 59–70). Washington, DC: U.S. Government Printing Office.

Kessler, R., McGonagle, K., Zhao, S., Nelson, C., Hughes, M., Eshleman, S., et al. (1994). Lifetime and 12-month prevalence of *DSM–III–R* psychiatric disorders: Results from the National Comorbidity Study. *Archives of General Psychiatry, 51,* 8–19.

Lambert, D., & Agger, M. S. (1995). Access of rural AFDC Medicaid beneficiaries to mental health services. *Health Care Financing Review, 17*(1), 133–145.

Last, J. M., & Wallace, R. B. (Eds.). (1992). *Maxcy-Rosenau-Last public health and preventive medicine* (13th ed.). Norwalk, CT: Appleton & Lange.

National Rural Health Association. (1999). *Mental health in rural America.* Retrieved August 11, 2000, from http:/www.nrharural.org/dc/issuepapers/ipaper14.html

National Advisory Mental Health Council. (1993). Health care reform for Americans with severe mental illness: Report for the National Advisory Mental Health Council. *American Journal of Psychiatry, 150,* 1447–1465.

Oetting, E. R., Edwards, R. W., Kelly, K., & Beauvais, F. (1997). Risk and protective factors for drug use among rural American youth. In E. B. Robertson, Z. Sloboda, G. M. Boyd, L. Beatty, & N. Kozel (Eds.), *Rural substance abuse: State of knowledge and issues* (National Institute on Drug Abuse Research Monograph No. 16, National Institutes of Health Publication No. 97-4177, pp. 90–130). Washington, DC: U.S. Government Printing Office.

Ortega, S., Johnson, D., Beeson, P., & Craft, B. (1994). The farm crisis and mental health: A longitudinal study of the 1980s. *Rural Sociology, 59,* 598–619.

Practice Management Information Corporation. (2000). *International classification of diseases, ninth revision, clinical modifications* (6th ed.). Los Angeles: Author.

Regier, D., Goldberg, I., & Taube, C. (1978). The de facto U. S. mental health services system. *Archives of General Psychiatry, 35,* 685–693.

Regier, D., Hirschfeld, R., Goodwin, F., Burke, J., Lazar, J., & Judd, L. (1988). The NIMH Depression Awareness, Recognition, and Treatment Program: Structure, aims, and scientific basis. *American Journal of Psychiatry, 145,* 1351–1357.

Regier, D., Narrow, W., Rae, D., Manderscheid, R., Locke, B., & Goodwin, F. (1993). The de facto U.S. mental health and addictive disorders service system: Epidemiologic Catchment Area prospective 1-year prevalence rates. *Archives of General Psychiatry, 50,* 85–94.

Roberts, L., Battaglia, J., & Epstein, R. (1999). Frontier ethics: Mental health care needs and ethical dilemmas in rural communities. *Psychiatric Services, 50,* 497–503.

Rost, K., Smith, G., & Taylor, J. (1993). Rural-urban differences in stigma and the use of care for depressive disorders. *Journal of Rural Health, 9,* 57–62.

Stamm, B. H. (1999). Creating virtual community: Telehealth and self-care updated. In B. H. Stamm (Ed.), *Secondary traumatic stress: Self-care issues for clinicians, researchers and educators* (2nd ed., pp. 179–210). Lutherville, MD: Sidran Press.

U.S. Department of Health and Human Services. (1999). *Mental health: A report of the Surgeon General.* Rockville, MD: U.S. Department of Health and Human Services, Substance Abuse and Mental Health Services Administration, Center for Mental Health Services, National Institutes of Health, National Institute of Mental Health. Retrieved August 11, 2000, from http://www.surgeongeneral.gov/library

Walker, J., & Walker, L. (1988). Self reported stress symptoms in farmers. *Journal of Clinical Psychology, 44*(1), 10–16.

Williams, R., (1996). The on-going farm crisis: Extension leadership in rural communities. *Journal of Extension, 34*(1). Retrieved August 11, 2000, from http://www.joe.org/1996february/a3.html

8

Rural Social Service Systems As Behavioral Health Delivery Systems

Samuel F. Sears, Jr., Garret D. Evans, and Bradley D. Kuper

Rural areas are often characterized by population scarcity, but this does not necessarily imply a scarcity of social service systems. In fact, social service systems may be of greater importance in rural areas because they serve as a congregation point for individuals and families. The social service systems of education, health, and religion serve the needs of rural residents but often work independently of one another. Nonetheless, established social service systems in rural communities are potential partners for the ambitious, committed rural behavioral health provider.

The collaboration between a behavioral health provider and a social service system requires a framework for the partnership. Franklin and Streeter (1995) developed a taxonomy in which they distinguished levels of school-based health and social service collaboration as follows: *informal, coordinated, partnerships, collaborative,* and *integrated.* Although developed for school-based collaborative health services, the definitions are useful guides for all social service systems. We have adapted these definitions for the purposes of this chapter but have retained the labels for illustration. In Table 8.1, we define each of the degrees of social service system collaboration.

The purpose of this chapter is to review four systems spanning education, health, and religious systems that could accommodate the provision of behavioral services and to examine the assets and barriers to such collaboration. In the final section of the chapter, we provide recommendations for collaborations.

The four delivery systems presented here have been explored as conduits for rural behavioral health to some degree, but no universally accepted model has yet been derived. Thus, they are presented as possibilities that possess inherent strengths and weaknesses.

Dr. Sears can be reached at National Rural Behavioral Health Center, University of Florida, P.O. Box 100165, Gainesville, FL 32610-0165. E-mail: ssears@hp.ufl.edu

Table 8.1. Collaboration With Social Service Agencies

Type of collaboration	Description of collaboration
Informal	A common arrangement in which the social service agency is aware and in contact with the agency on an as-needed basis.
Coordinated	A social service agency member develops links with community agencies, which enables the appropriate referral of persons to health resources external to the social service system.
Partnerships	Networks of contracted employees remain independent of the social service agency while simultaneously contracted for on-site social service or health services.
Collaborative	This relationship requires a merging of resources and responsibilities between a social service agency and health providers.
Integrated	The social service agency and health provider are considered full partners who work together, share responsibilities, resources, personnel, and a complementary vision for the development of a reformed system of care and service delivery in a particular setting.

Behavioral Health Delivery Systems

Education Systems

COOPERATIVE EXTENSION SERVICE. The United States Department of Agriculture actively maintains a cooperative model of education that is among the most important sources of community education support in rural areas of the United States: the Cooperative Extension Service (CES). However, the potential of this vast network of educators has not traditionally been harnessed for behavioral health. This may be explained partially by its historical foundations in agricultural and natural resource education. The roots of the CES were set with the passage of the Morrill Act in 1862, which established the Department of Agriculture and granted land to state governments to develop colleges for teaching farmers the science of agriculture. The passage of the Smith-Lever Act of 1914 formally established the CES. The extension service program funded the establishment of education extension offices in every county in the Union and charged local educators with *extending* the knowledge gained through research and scholarly efforts at the land grant institution to solving local problems. During the twentieth century, the CES education programs expanded to address the problems of impoverished rural families (e.g., malnutrition, insufficiency, and poor money management).

Despite the growing emphasis on socially relevant programs, the presence of CES-based mental health education and service was rare until the farm crisis of the mid-1980s, when rural communities experienced a dramatic rise in rates of depression, anxiety, family conflict, cognitive impairment, and other stress-related symptoms (Beeson, Johnson, & Ortega, 1991; Beltane, Lasley, & Geller, 1986; Heffernan & Heffernan, 1985; Walker & Walker, 1988). County CES professionals saw a growing pattern of emotional distress.

In what catalyzed an already evolving menu of social science programs, the farm crisis prompted CES officials to quickly expand their efforts in creating programs in stress management, family communication, coping with economic loss, preventing depression and suicide, and similar issues (Molgaard, 1997). Many of these programs were developed with the understanding that rural residents perceived traditional mental health providers and agencies as offering far less help than other institutionalized sources of support in their community (e.g., churches, CES; Williams, 1996).

The momentum of the farm crisis has not subsided. Virtually every state CES in the nation has active programming in mental health issues. Many of these efforts are preventive in nature. Education classes on parenting (Evans, Ross, & Mixon, 1999), 4-H programs designed specifically to build self-esteem and promote good decision making by children (Hobbs, 1994), and depression and suicide prevention programs (Walker, 1992) are common examples.

Two programs that feature collaborative efforts between mental health professionals and CES professionals have gained attention for their ability to use the CES platform for mental health service delivery. The Institute for Social and Behavioral Research at Iowa State University has collaborated with Iowa State University Extension Services since the early 1990s in the creation and delivery of the Strengthening Families Program, a parenting skills and substance use prevention program that has shown promising results (Molgaard, 1997; Spoth, Redmond, & Lepper, 1999). The CES network again proved to be a valuable asset to service delivery efforts: Officials assembled teams of local social service agencies in 30 separate counties for training and dissemination of the Strengthening Families Program after its worth had been proven in validation trials. The success of the Strengthening Families Program has allowed for its dissemination across the country (Center for the Study and Prevention of Violence, 1999).

A second collaborative model of mental health service delivery is found in the University of Florida (UF) Rural Psychology Program. In response to the psychological effects of Hurricane Andrew in 1992, the UF CES officials teamed with officials from the Department of Clinical and Health Psychology and the North Florida Area Health Education Center to improve access to mental health education and services. The program was established to accomplish three primary objectives: (a) to provide consultative and supervisory services for health programs offered through the UF CES, (b) to improve access to behavioral and mental health services through direct care services to rural Floridians, and (c) to provide training and methods of rural and behavioral health practice to future health practitioners. Since its inception, the program has developed mental health service initiatives and educational curricula for coping with postdisaster stress (Evans, Sears, and Williamson, 1999), self-care for better health, teenage parents (Evans et al., 1997), and improving fathers' positive impact on their children (Evans & Williamson, 1999). There is considerable empirical evidence emerging from the UF Rural Psychology Program to support the use of a collaborative model of mental health service delivery that involves CES (Evans, Ross, & Mixon, 1999).

Perhaps the CES's greatest assets for providing services of any kind are the extensiveness of its network and its relationship to a major university. With offices in virtually every county in the nation, the CES network affords an opportunity to implement education programs and large-scale mental health service delivery with minimal organizational obstacles and startup costs. Furthermore, with its connection to at least one land-grant university in each state, CES places a premium on delivering services that are connected to recent research efforts and built on empirically validated principles. In addition, CES has long been recognized as one of the most important and credible service agencies in rural areas of the United States. Through the organization of county fairs, in-school home economics courses, 4-H programs, agriculture and natural resource community education, and mental and behavioral health programs, CES serves most rural residents in one way or another. By collaborating with CES professionals, mental health professionals engage the familiarity and credibility of the CES (Sears, Evans, & Perry, 1998).

Unfortunately, although the CES offers many advantages as a partner, there are limitations. Just as CES staff can be viewed as vital collaborators in a mental health service program, they are viewed as equally vital to other programs as well. County agents often have numerous obligations across content areas and events. County agents may wish to collaborate but simply do not have the resources to participate. Second, as Molgaard (1997) astutely noted, county CES staff are typically charged with responding to pressing community issues that tend to shift from one year to the next. Thus, they may be unable to commit to a multiyear mental health program. Third, the CES is dedicated to serving community residents with education programs that address local problems. There are certain to be exceptions across state CES programs and situations, but to a large extent, CES is best used as a partner in programs designed to prevent mental disorders through education in areas such as family relations, stress management, parenting, symptom vigilance, and management.

SCHOOL-BASED SERVICES. Although the integration of health services in school settings has a long history in the United States, the movement has gained increased attention since the early 1990s. This trend is attributed to research findings, and subsequent media attention, that focus on the high rates of violence, substance abuse, and symptoms of mental disorders reported by students.

Confronted with social, emotional, health, and behavioral problems among students, school administrators and policymakers have begun to embrace in-school health care and social service programs. Many of the most sophisticated models of school-based health service delivery have occurred in urban areas. These include alcohol and drug prevention (Zavela et al., 1997), sex education and the prevention of sexually transmitted diseases (Hacker, 1989), and the prevention and treatment of mental disorders (Farie, Cowen, & Smith, 1986; King & Kirschenbaum, 1990). Less attention has been paid to school-based health services as part of a national strategy for minimizing barriers to receiving health services in rural areas of the United States.

School-based service delivery models account for the fact that school officials may have the will but rarely the necessary resources to meet the health and social service needs of their students. However, these models do have three critical assets to contribute to an effective rural health service delivery program: (a) almost constant access to the targeted population, (b) space that is geographically close to this population in which to provide services, and (c) connections with local policymakers and health professionals who can assist in putting the needed pieces in place. Community practitioners and members of other agencies often collaborate with school officials to provide skilled personnel and health services that can be focused on specific health issues.

Access to the target population is increased by the frequent contact offered in the school setting. Also, the school staff is often an excellent source of surveillance for child and adolescent health problems that may go unnoticed or unreported by parents (e.g., poor hygiene, substance use or other high-risk behavior, signs of physical or emotional abuse). S. W. Evans (1999) summarized research that suggested that school-based behavioral health services may be particularly effective in increasing service utilization rates and in improving treatment effectiveness and generalization. The stigma of seeking treatment may be lessened through the integration of treatment into a school-based service (Dryfoos, 1997; Rost, Smith, & Taylor, 1993).

There are also obstacles to effective school-based health service delivery. The support for school involvement in health service delivery has varied across generations and continues to vary across individual communities. The use of school settings for improving health service delivery in rural communities may conflict with the need to increase class size, limit special education services, and eliminate school arts, sports, and other activity programs to meet budgetary constraints. Claims that effective, school-based health service delivery is a fiscally sound decision—which are based on the model's ability to improve educational efficiency by lowering relative costs associated with truancy; with student conduct problems; and with the misdiagnosis or underdiagnosis of health, behavior, and learning problems—may have some validity. However, this research has yet to be done. Thus, political issues continue to play a pivotal role in any community's efforts to improve school-based health services.

Professional turf issues may be obstacles to school-based health service delivery (Dryfoos, 1997). Role expectations, differing policies and procedures, and relative responsibilities of school and other agency personnel are only some of the challenges in such a collaborative effort. Rural school districts are often severely underfunded, and school administrators and teachers may express concern about school and community resources devoted to expanding services or hiring professionals not formally employed by the school. Finally, special attention must be paid to developing working agreements between school staff and health professionals with regard to accepted policies and procedures for referring students and families, delivering services, and exchanging information. Specifically, parental consent for receiving health care services and the confidentiality of the student's participation and records related to such services have been pointed out as significant concerns among parents and children when school-based health services, particularly behavioral health services, are considered (Evans, 1999).

Health Systems

Primary care is *primary* for both physical and mental health needs of rural residents. In most cases, this is because of the lack of specialty mental health services in many rural areas. Rural residents depend on primary care providers for health care, including mental health care. Therefore, rural behavioral health providers trained in traditional mental health settings should recognize their colleagues in medicine and nursing and their respective clinical practices as key components of a rural delivery system. Primary care providers generally embrace a definition of primary care that emphasizes accessible, comprehensive, continuous care in which the importance of family and community in an individual's health is recognized (Institute of Medicine, Committee on the Future of Primary Care, 1995). This definition remains consistent with the prevailing conceptualizations of some behavioral health providers, such as health psychologists, consultation-liaison psychiatrists, and social workers, who embrace the biopsychosocial model of health (Engel, 1977). The biopsychosocial model emphasizes systems around an individual that affect health, such as the biological, psychological, and social domains.

Rural behavioral health care providers are needed in primary care because of the high demand for services placed on rural primary care providers. Philbrick, Connelly, and Wofford (1996) used a primary care screening, administered by trained medical students, and found a 34% prevalence rate of mental disorders in a rural primary care setting in Virginia. Hauenstein and Boyd (1994) found that approximately 41% of young, rural, predominantly low-income, and poorly educated of the women in their sample self-reported significant depression. Similarly, Sears, Danda, and Evans (1999) employed nurses to administer a psychiatric screening to consecutive rural primary care patients and found that 40% of the sample was classified as depressed.

A prominent issue for quality of care and behavioral health collaboration concerns the underdetection of mental disorders. Contributing factors include the variable presentations of the disorders, physician time constraints, lack of continued training for physicians in mental health, lack of expertise in asking appropriate questions, and patients' nonrecognition of their own mental health needs (Badger et al., 1994; Docherty, 1997; Hartley, Korsen, Bird, & Agger, 1998; Rost, Humphrey, & Kelleher, 1994). Rost et al. (1998) monitored a group of 98 depressed primary care patients and as shown by a self-report instrument found that in 32%, their depression was still not detected over the course of a year and that almost half had developed suicidal ideation.

Behavioral health providers in primary care must strive for absolute utility with practical patient benefits. Behavioral health professionals can achieve maximal utility if they are able to provide general care within at least two major dimensions: mental health and behavioral health. Mental health encompasses the diagnosis and treatment of psychological difficulties manifested in affective, behavioral, and cognitive domains of functioning. In the strictest sense, behavioral health is the recognition and modification of risk factors and high-risk behaviors (e.g., smoking, obesity, and sedentary lifestyle) and maintenance of behaviors that promote health or prevent disease. The generalist model is consistent with an emerging role for psychologists that involves emphasizing the idea of being a "health provider" rather than a mental health specialist (Belar, 1995). Primary care providers do not limit themselves to physical medicine and ignore mental health; nor should behavioral health providers limit their practices to health behavior modification, neglecting other aspects of mental health.

Rural primary care practices provide the most helpful access point to the behavioral health care provider. Therefore, mental and behavioral heath services can be efficiently delivered as part of a health care team. Rural residents may view their health in a monistic manner that includes health as the sum of physical, mental, and social functioning. Thus, they are likely to appreciate the "one-stop health care shopping" provided through integrated primary care. With proper modification of typical practice patterns, both providers and patients can appreciate the effectiveness of behavioral health systems.

In contrast, some weaknesses span both *provider-based* limitations and *practice-based* limitations. Provider-based limitations include a more limited exposure to rural primary care. Few training programs for rural behavioral health care exist. Therefore, few behavioral health providers have a comprehensive understanding of the ambitious mission of rural primary care providers (Haley et al., 1998). Some mental health training even encourages the separation of mind and body, a concept that is reinforced by managed care carve-outs that attempt to isolate mental health problems as independent of more broadly defined health concerns. Practice-based limitations include differences between mental and behavioral health practitioners in terms of the settings and manner in which they typically provide care. The majority of mental health professionals practice in relatively isolated, "mental health only" settings and typically see their patients in 1-hour segments; interprofessional communication is often limited by confidentiality concerns. In contrast, behavioral health providers tend to be trained in medical settings as part of multidisciplinary teams, and they use comprehensive, biopsychosocial treatment approaches to achieve optimal health. These professionals, therefore, may find the "fit" for rural primary care more suitable (Haley et al., 1998).

Religious Systems

Local churches and other small religious meeting places have traditionally assumed a central role in providing psychosocial and spiritual support within rural communities and are well established and accepted by many rural residents. Rural clergy members assume a major role in providing behavioral health care to rural residents and serve as a natural link in the delivery of mental health services to rural residents (Voss, 1996). The ability of religious leaders to make appropriate referrals to mental health care professionals is often compromised by the combination of a lack of resources and a lack of knowledge of available resources (Clinebell, 1984). Establishing a referral system in which religious leaders can identify congregation members in need of behavioral heath services and refer them to the most appropriate professional provides a mutually enhancing relationship that benefits the community. Behavioral health professionals can facilitate such a network by cooperating with a number of local rural religious institutions (Voss, 1996). This approach provides an avenue for behavioral health professionals to receive referrals for patients in need, while at the same time providing religious leaders peace of mind in knowing they are providing congregation members the most appropriate referral available.

A network of religious institutions can also form an alliance, and their officials can contract with a behavioral health professional as a method of establishing a viable referral system (Voss, 1996). Collaborating institutions can benefit from such arrangements in a number of ways. First, in establishing a contract with the behavioral health professional, religious leaders would probably feel more comfortable referring their congregation members. Second, because the alliance of local institutions supports the behavioral health professional, congregation members can use services regardless of socioeconomic status, increasing institution leaders' ability to engage in outreach. Despite these advantages, it may be unrealistic to presume that an alliance of rural religious institutions would be able to support a licensed behavioral health professional. Consequently, it may be more realistic for urban behavioral health professionals to establish rural satellite offices (Voss, 1996).

Rural religious institutions can also sponsor psychoeducational sessions conducted by behavioral health clinicians. The content of these presentations could vary, depending on the needs of the community, but may include behavioral health topics such as parent training, stress management, depression management, or smoking cessation. These activities could also be offered in the evening or as part of weekend retreats or ongoing education programs. Leaders of progressive institutions may even want to offer these workshops to entire rural communities in buildings separate from the institutions in order to create an outreach ministry to citizens who do not normally attend religious services.

Religious institutions in rural communities may have facilities, such as fellowship halls, that are suitable for hosting support group meetings, which is consistent with their goals of optimal health. Members of groups in which 12-step programs are used, such as Alcoholics Anonymous, often meet in church buildings. Rural behavioral health providers may be able to extend these activities by offering support groups to congregation members with special needs, such as those who have experienced a traumatic event, those who are experiencing grief, or even those who have special medical problems such as chronic pain or medical disability. Again, officials of several rural religious institutions may be willing to establish an alliance in order to support the behavioral health professional who would facilitate these activities.

Perhaps the greatest advantage of integrating behavioral health services with religious communities is the fact that religious institutions in rural areas are intrinsically linked to the regions in which they are found. Many rural churches, for example, have been in existence for decades and have served as places of worship and refuge for generations. Rural religious institutions are often viewed as "natural helpers" for people in crisis. Moreover, leaders and elders within individual institutions are typically viewed as influential in the community. As the behavioral health professional gains the trust of these individuals, it is likely that the community as a whole will begin to accept and trust the behavioral health professional as a person who can provide treatment and comfort during times of need. Consequently, effective collaboration with the religious community has the potential to increase the likelihood that the behavioral health professional will be viewed as a trusted member of the community rather than as an unfamiliar and mysterious outsider.

Despite the potential advantages of integrating the services of a behavioral health provider with rural religious institutions, there are barriers that may impede the realization of these advantages. First, many rural religious institutions lack financial resources. It may be very difficult for a rural church or a group of rural churches to contract with a behavioral health professional. Thus, the institution may serve simply as a referral source. Second, a perceived conflict may exist between behavioral health services and spiritual beliefs. Some religious leaders and congregation members may view behavioral health professions such as psychology and psychiatry as being antithetical or even hostile to specific religious teachings. Rural behavioral health providers may need to spend time with religious leaders and congregation members to help them understand that behavioral health services have the potential to provide relief to those in need without challenging or interfering with the practice of religious beliefs.

Conclusions and Recommendations

Be Aware That Members of Communities Learn

Recognizing the "learning history" of a community in its collaboration efforts can be critical in understanding sources of possible resistance to plans that appear to be "win–win" for all parties. It is sometimes true that collaborations such as those proposed here have been tried and have failed and that this failure limits the interest of potential partners in seeking further collaborations. However, even under these circumstances, the lessons learned, combined with a strong commitment by the rural behavioral health provider, can serve as the needed ingredients for success. Initial meetings with community leaders that allow for the discussion of previously successful collaborations, along with identification of ongoing health needs, help those leaders acknowledge the existing efforts and commitment of potential partners. It is important to recognize that these potential partners have attempted to address the specific health needs being discussed and that the new behavioral health provider may represent an additional resource that simply needs to be connected to the established plan. The strategies that emerge from these meetings with community leaders ideally reflect a shared vision that creates the best chances of success. In addition, the criteria for success and the outcomes of interest and how to measure them may be key skills that the behavioral health provider contributes. The academic background of both science and practitioner training may prove crucial. Finally, ongoing assessment and troubleshooting must be expected and completed for long-term collaboration between a behavioral health provider and social service agency to be attained.

Table 8.2.   Summary of Presented Social Service System Collaboration
Considerations

Social service agency	Populations within reach	Behavioral health problems they address	Barriers to implementation
County extension agencies	Broad population of adults and children	Limited	Education-focused
Primary care	Broad population of adults and children	Broad	Broad-based biopsychosocial emphasis of all partners
Local school districts	School-aged children	Broad	Bureaucracy
Local churches	Church-attending families	Life adjustment difficulties	Perceived conflict between mental health treatment and spiritual beliefs

Collaborate With Established Agencies for Early Success

Collaboration with established social service agencies by the rural behavioral
health provider may represent a key strategy for successful rural practice. Our
review of education, health, and religious collaborators revealed that each may
be particularly well positioned to serve as a conduit for behavioral health that
can provide a desirable solution to multiple parties (Table 8.2). The potential
rural behavioral health provider must determine the degree of integration
from a selected social service agency that is needed or desired for success. As
with any collaboration, each of the social service agencies has specific
strengths and weaknesses from the perspective of behavioral health collaboration and strategic planning. Finally, a specific plan of collaboration involving a systematic approach to engaging a rural community and a social service
system is presented; a combined strategic and sensitive approach may be most
effective for initiating collaboration.

References

Badger, L. W., de Gruy, F. V., Hartman, K., Plant, M. A., Leeper, J., Ficken, R., et al. (1994). Psychosocial interest, medical interviews, and the recognition of depression. *Archives of Family
Medicine, 3,* 899–907.

Beeson, P. G., Johnson, D. R., & Ortega, S. T. (1991). *The farm crisis and mental health: A longitudinal (1981, 1986, 1989) and comparative study of the economy and mental health status.*
Unpublished manuscript.

Belar, C. D. (1995). Collaboration in capitated care: Challenges for psychology. *Professional Psychology: Research and Practice, 26,* 139–146.

Center for the Study and Prevention of Violence (1999). *Blueprints for violence prevention: Promising programs? Iowa strengthening families.* Retrieved December 15, 1999, from http://www.colorado.edu/cspv/blueprints/promise/index.html

Clinebell, H. (1984). Referral counseling. In H. Clinebell (Ed.), *Basic types of pastoral care and counseling: Resources for the ministry of healing and growth* (pp. 310–322). Nashville, TN: Abingdon Press.

Docherty, J. P. (1997). Barriers to the diagnosis of depression in primary care. *Journal of Clinical Psychiatry, 58*(1), 5–10.

Dryfoos, J. G. (1997). School-based youth programs: Exemplary models and emerging opportunities. In R. Illback, C. Cobb, & H. Joseph, Jr. (Eds.), *Integrated services for children and families* (pp. 23–52). Washington, DC: American Psychological Association.

Engel, G. (1977). The need for a new medical model: A challenge for biomedicine. *Science, 196,* 129–136.

Evans, G. D. (Ed.), Perkins, D., Smith, S., Pergola, J., Allen, B., Rutledge, J., et al. (1997). *"Teening-up" with your adolescent: Parenting children ages 10–16* [Videorecording]. (Available from the University of Florida Cooperative Extension, Gainesville, FL 32611.)

Evans, G. D., Ross, M., & Mixon, R. (1999, October). *Teening-up with your adolescent. Results for an extension parenting education program.* Paper presented at the Annual Meeting of the Florida Associations of Extension Professionals, Kissimmee, FL.

Evans, G. D. (Writer and Co-Executive Producer), Sears, S. F. (Writer and Co-Executive Producer), & Williamson, A. (Producer and Director). (1999). *Triumph over tragedy: A community response to post-disaster stress* [Videorecording]. (Available from University of Florida, Institute of Food and Agricultural Sciences, Educational and Media Services, P.O. Box 110190, Gainesville FL 32611).

Evans, G. D. (Writer and Producer), & Williamson, A. (Director). (1999). *What a difference a dad makes: A father involvement program* [Videorecording]. (Available from University of Florida, Institute of Food and Agricultural Sciences, Educational and Media Services, P.O. Box 110190, Gainesville, FL 32611).

Evans, S. W. (1999). Mental health services in schools: Utilization, effectiveness, and consent. *Clinical Psychology Review, 19,* 165–178.

Farie, A. M., Cowen, E. L., & Smith, M. (1986). The development and implementation of a rural consortium program to provide early, preventive school mental health services. *Community Mental Health Journal, 22,* 94–103.

Franklin, C., & Streeter, C. L. (1995). School reform: Linking public schools with human services. *Social Work, 40,* 773–782.

Hacker, S. S. (1989). AIDS education is sex education: Rural and urban challenges. *Journal of Social Work and Human Sexuality, 8,* 155–170.

Haley, W. E., McDaniel, S. H., Bray, J. H., Frank, R. G., Heldring, M., Johnson, S. B., et al. (1998). Psychological practice in primary care settings: Practical tips for clinicians. *Professional Psychology: Research and Practice, 29,* 237–244.

Hartley, D., Korsen, H., Bird, D., & Agger, M. (1998). Management of patients with depression by rural primary care practitioners. *Archives of Family Medicine, 7,* 139–145.

Hauenstein, E. J., & Boyd, M. R. (1994). Depressive symptoms in young women of the Piedmont: Prevalence in rural women. *Women and Health, 21*(2/3), 105–123.

Heffernan, J. B., & Heffernan, W. D. (1985). *The effects of the agricultural crisis on the health and lives of farm families* (Statements prepared for a hearing of the Committee on Agriculture, U.S. House of Representatives, Washington, DC; available from William Heffernan, Rural Sociology Department, University of Missouri–Columbia, 102 Sociology Building, Columbia, MO 65211).

Hobbs, A. C. (1994, Fall). A nation at risk: Extension responds. In *Children, youth & families at risk reporter* (A publication of the Cooperative Extension System, USDA, p. 1). Washington, DC: Government Printing Office.

Institute of Medicine, Committee on the Future of Primary Care. (1995). *Defining primary care: An interim report.* Washington, DC: Division of Health Care Services, Institute of Medicine.

King, C. A., & Kirschenbaum, D. S. (1990). An experimental evaluation of a school-based program for children at risk: Wisconsin early intervention. *Journal of Community Psychology, 18*(2), 67–177.

Molgaard, V. K. (1997). The extension service as key mechanism for research and services delivery for prevention of mental health disorders in rural areas. *American Journal of Community Psychology, 25,* 515–544.

Philbrick, J. T., Connelly, J. E., & Wofford, A. B. (1996). The prevalence of mental disorders in rural office practice. *Journal of General Internal Medicine, 11,* 9–15.

Rost, K., Humphrey, J., & Kelleher, K. (1994). Physician management preferences and barriers to care for rural patients with depression. *Archives of Family Medicine 3,* 409–414.

Rost, K., Smith, G. R., & Taylor, J. L. (1993). Rural-urban differences in stigma and the use of care for depressive disorders. *Journal of Rural Health, 9,* 57–62.

Rost, K., Zhang, M., Fortney, J., Smith, J., Coyne, J., & Smith, G. (1998). Persistently poor outcomes of undetected major depression in primary care. *General Hospital Psychiatry, 20,* 12–20.

Sears, S. F., Danda, C. E., & Evans, G. D. (1999). PRIME-MD and rural primary care: Detecting depression in a low-income rural population. *Professional Psychology: Research and Practice, 30,* 357–360.

Sears, S. F., Evans, G. D., & Perry, N. W. (1998). Innovations in training: The UF rural psychology program. *Professional Psychology: Research and Practice, 29,* 504–507.

Spoth, R., Redmond, C., & Lepper, H. (1999). Alcohol initiation outcomes of universal family-focused preventive interventions: One- and two-year follow-ups of a controlled study. *Journal of Studies on Alcohol, 13,* 103–111.

Voss, S. V. (1996). The church as an agent in rural mental health. *Journal of Psychology and Theology, 24,* 114–123.

Walker, J. A. (1992). *Tackling tough stuff: Adolescent skills to understand depression (4-H youth development)* [Brochure]. St. Paul, MN: Minnesota Extension Service.

Walker, J. L., & Walker, L. J. S. (1988). Self-reported stress symptoms in farmers. *Journal of Clinical Psychology, 44,* 10–16.

Williams, R. T. (1996). The on-going farm crisis: Extension leadership in rural communities. *Journal of Extension, 34*(1). Retrieved March 17, 2001, from http://www.joe.org/jpe/1996february/a3.html

Zavela, K. J., Battistich, V., Dean, B. J., Flores, R., Barton, R., & Delaney, R. J. (1997). Say yes first: A longitudinal, school-based alcohol and drug prevention project for rural youth and families. *Journal of Early Adolescence, 17,* 67–96.

9

Nonphysician Prescribers in Rural Settings: Unique Roles and Opportunities for Enhanced Mental Health Care

Morgan T. Sammons

A defining feature of health care in the United States is the rapidly expanding scope of practice of nonphysician health care providers. Advanced practice nurses, pharmacists, psychologists, and providers in other specialties are increasingly employing treatments once considered the exclusive purview of physicians. Two such areas of expanded practice are the acquisition of independent prescriptive authority and, in some instances, collaborative drug therapy management. These trends are analyzed in light of long-extant shortcomings in the provision of rural mental health services. The positive implications of expanded nonphysician scopes of practice for rural residents in need of mental health services are discussed, and recommendations are made for instituting changes in training programs and scope of practice to the benefit of rural populations.

Mental health care providers include specialists from a variety of training paths, including psychiatrists, psychologists, psychiatric nurse practitioners, clinical social workers, counselors, and paraprofessionals. Psychiatrists, who attend medical school and then complete 3 years of specialty training, have been the traditional prescribers of psychotropic medications. Psychiatric nurse practitioners, who generally have mental health master's degrees in addition to their general nursing training, are increasingly prescribing medications for psychiatric patients. Some doctorally prepared psychologists, who have additional training in psychopharmacology, are seeking prescription privileges. In 1999, psychologists in the territory of Guam were included as health professionals who had attained the statutory right to prescribe medication (Rabasca, 1999). In 2002, New Mexico granted prescription privileges to psychologists (Daw, 2002).

The acquisition of prescription privileges by nonphysician providers brings not only a new skill but also an entirely different philosophy to patient

Dr. Sammons can be reached at Mental Health Department, Naval Medical Clinic, Annapolis, MD 21402. E-mail: MTSammons@US.MED.NAVY.MIL. Please note that the opinions presented in this chapter are solely those of the author and do not reflect the official views of the U.S. Navy or Department of Defense.

care and medication use. Many nonphysician providers (e.g., those with specialty training other than a doctor of medicine degree) approach medication as part of an overall health plan based on prevention and intervention. For example, nurses are trained in a model of health promotion in contrast to one of medical intervention. Extraordinary reliance on psychotropic drugs characterizes modern medical and psychiatric treatment of mental disorders (Pincus et al., 1998, 1999; Zarin, et al., 1998); however, nonmedical prescribers are expected to lessen the emphasis on pharmacotherapy by deploying the behavioral, psychotherapeutic, or patient management skills that are the traditional purviews of those fields. Because psychologists and psychiatric nurse practitioners undergo lengthy training in assessment, behavioral and social interventions, and psychotherapy before acquiring skills as prescribers, it is anticipated that they will prescribe medication more sparingly than do their medical confreres (Sammons, 1994, 1998). This hypothesis has yet to be tested because the number of psychologists who possess prescriptive authority is small, but some data suggest that psychologists will be more abstemious in their prescriptions of medications than are allopathically trained mental health providers (Sammons, 1999). Skills in holistic assessment, behavioral observation, psychometrics, and a variety of specific psychotherapeutic modalities will continue to be features distinguishing psychologists and nonphysician specialists with prescriptive authority from medically trained mental health providers.

The preceding discussion provides the intellectual underpinning for the argument that prescriptive authority is a legitimate and valuable extension of mental health practice by nonphysician providers. It is hoped that by achieving such authority, those who are trained in both psychological and psychotropic means will expand the range of disorders and patient populations they can successfully treat. These observations apply in any setting, but the notion of nonphysician mental health prescribers acquires particular salience in rural areas. Because access to full-spectrum mental health services is often limited in rural areas, some sectors of the population, especially those with serious and persistent forms of mental distress, are poorly served by existing health care structures. In this chapter, I examine differences in patient demographics, provider characteristics, and geographic and cultural peculiarities that distinguish rural mental health care from that provided in more populated areas, in the hope of demonstrating that the skills of prescribing psychologists can be uniquely valuable in rural environments.

Nonphysician Prescribing in Rural Areas

Characteristics, Distribution, and Practice Patterns of Health Care Providers in Rural Settings

The apportionment of care in rural settings may lead to the excessive prescription of medication and underuse of behavioral interventions in treating mental disorders, in that specialty mental health providers are underrepresented in the rural setting. Traditional practice standards in primary care, a history of underdetection of depression, and absence of behavioral training in the medical curriculum are all predictive of an excessive reliance on pharmacological inter-ventions for depression and other common forms of mental distress.

Because most treatment of mental disorders in rural areas is rendered by medical providers, often primary care providers (who have to address, on average, six problems in an appointment lasting an average of 13 min; Bryant & Shimizu, 1998; Schappert, 1994; Williams et al., 1999), rural patients probably do not receive an optimal mix of psychotherapy and pharmacological interventions. The severe time constraints under which these physicians operate, combined with their lack of training in behavioral treatments, render pharmacotherapy the mainstay of therapy, even for disorders that have been shown to respond better to nonpharmacological treatments.

In a survey of more than 75,000 patients seeking primary care, Zung, Broadhead, and Roth (1993) reported the prevalence of clinically significant depressive symptoms as 20.9%. They cited data demonstrating that primary care physicians fail to diagnose major depression in up to 50% of affected patients. These data echo earlier figures, which suggested that over 25% of all nonpsychiatric physician visits were for psychological problems and that more than 80% of all psychoactive medications are prescribed by physicians other than psychiatrists (U.S. Department of Health and Human Services [DHHS], 1984, cited in Zimmerman & Wienckowski, 1991). The DHHS study also revealed that physicians who are not psychiatrists make almost half of all primary and sec-ondary diagnoses of mental problems. These results and those of Zung et al. suggest that significant numbers of patients with mental disorders continue to be underdiagnosed in the primary care system. In addition, it follows that a number of medications are employed without the benefit of diagnostic precision.

Since the mid-1990s, enhanced physician education and the promulgation of national guidelines for the detection and management of depression have resulted in greater attention to depression in the primary care setting (see Williams et al., 1999). Nonetheless, rates of detection of mental disorders in general medical practice are relatively low, and standardized screening instru-ments have had only modest success in improving physicians' recognition of depression and other mental disorders (Gonzales, Magruder, & Keith, 1994). The results of the study by Williams et al. (1999) indicated that depression remains unrecognized in large numbers of primary care patients and that depression continues to be diagnosed on the basis of clinical impressions rather than formal diagnostic criteria. Williams et al. (1999) also examined depression diagnosis and treatment practice patterns among family practi-tioners, internists, and obstetricians. Results from the 1,350 people complet-ing the survey indicated that 72.5% of depressed patients were prescribed an antidepressant and 38.4% of those prescribed an antidepressant were also referred to a mental health specialist (primarily psychologists or social workers). Of patients in whom a major depressive episode was diagnosed, 76.9% were treated with antidepressants and 47.3% of those 76.9% were referred to mental health specialty care (Williams et al., 1999). Primary care physicians tended to be more satisfied with consultation performed by psy-chologists or social workers than with that performed by psychiatrists, and they referred more patients to nonpsychiatrists, although levels of satisfaction with mental health service provision overall were lower than those for other medical specialties. These results suggest that although drug therapy is the most common form of management of depression in primary care, a fairly large percentage of depressed patients is simultaneously referred to nonprescribing mental health specialists.

Because these researchers did not examine rural status as a covariate, it is uncertain whether the patterns just described reflect rural primary care. Ganguli, Mulsant, Richards, Stoehr, and Mendelsohn (1997) found similar rates of prescription of antidepressants for a rural Pennsylvania population and for an urban comparison group. In the rural group, however, primary care managers prescribed most antidepressants, and rates of referral to specialty mental health, even in the presence of numerous depressive symptoms, were remarkably low. A point of further interest in the Pennsylvania study is that psychiatrists were overrepresented among recognized mental health providers, inasmuch as they constituted more than 84% of the group; this fact is incongruent with most analyses of the distribution of rural mental health specialists.

Susman, Crabtree, and Essink (1995), studying a small sample, concluded that rural physicians employed a deliberate and organized approach to the recognition and management of depression but were reluctant to diagnose depression because of social stigma or fear of detrimental effects on employability or insurability. Practitioners in this study appeared reluctant to intervene unless the depression was severe. This, in the authors' opinion, was a factor contributing to the high rate of pharmacological versus psychosocial management of depression among family physicians, although lack of time and available mental health resources were also cited as factors.

The fear of stigmatization or iatrogenic creation of social or occupational problems by making diagnoses of mental disorders is, at least to some extent, an accurate reflection of the verities of rural life. Practitioner misperceptions, however, can also contribute to underdetection and undertreatment. Rural primary care physicians in one survey (Hartley, Korsen, Bird, & Agger, 1998) cited lack of available services, long waiting times for appointments, and patients' reluctance to seek specialty care as reasons not to make specialty referrals for their patients. Nevertheless, data analysis from that study revealed that mental health provider supply was not a significant predictor of referral, whereas physician knowledge and attitudes were.

In the era of tricyclic antidepressants, management of depression in primary care was often characterized by inadequate medication trials. The exponential rise in antidepressant prescriptions by primary care providers (Pincus et al., 1998) is in large part due to reduced concerns about the toxicity of newer antidepressants. Nevertheless, an adequate trial of medication (i.e., a sufficient dose for a sufficient period of time) is only one guarantor of appropriate treatment of depression. Many depressed patients fail to respond completely to pharmacotherapy alone; this is a major concern in rural areas, where treatment of depression is concentrated in primary care.

Nonphysician Providers in the Rural Setting

Although the number of physicians specializing in primary care fields has risen, there continue to be physician shortages in rural areas. Nonphysician specialties, represented largely by nurse practitioners and physician's assistants, have shown an explosive growth, to such an extent that the number of nurse practitioners is expected to equal the number of family physicians in practice by 2005 (Cooper, Laud, & Dietrich, 1998). Nevertheless, geographic distribution of nonphysician specialties tends to parallel that of physicians, with some variability as a result of the presence of training institutions or more permissive licensing laws in certain states (Cooper et al., 1998). As Cooper et al. commented, whether nonphysician providers will supplant the traditional role of physicians depends, to some extent, on their ability to distribute themselves across less well-served areas. However, nonphysicians may respond to the same pressures that deter physicians from rural settings, such as demanding call schedules and decreased opportunities for specialization. Larson, Hart, and Hummel (1994) reported a trend away from rural practice settings by physician's assistants, even though rural physician's assistants tend to be paid the same and have somewhat greater autonomy than their urban counterparts.

As of 1998, nurse practitioners have achieved completely independent prescriptive authority in 12 states and the District of Columbia (Pearson, 2002). The 12 states, but not the District of Columbia, have large rural populations, and well over half (including Alaska) are located in the mountain or far western regions of the United States. It is reasonable to assume that nurses serve with primary care physicians as first-line mental health providers in these rural areas and may even be the sole medical resource. Nevertheless, unless trained in psychiatric nursing, they are no more likely than physicians to have received training in treatment of mental disorders. A survey of nurse practitioners in Maine revealed that only one third had received specific training to treat depression, in comparison with two thirds of primary care physicians (Hartley et al., 1998).

Issues of training aside, the growing number of nonphysician prescribers will certainly influence rural health care. Pharmacists now have achieved limited prescriptive authority in 31 states; this reflects policies that have long been in place within the Indian Health Service and the Department of Veterans Affairs (Greene, 1999). The number of prescriptions written by nonphysicians doubled between 1992 and 1996 ("Nonphysician Prescribing Doubles," 1996) and again increased 45% for physician's assistants and 75% for nurse practitioners between 1995 and 2000 (Greene, 2000). These trends make it less likely that a physician will treat mental health patients, but primary care settings seem certain to remain the predominant locus of mental health service delivery in the future, particularly in rural areas of the United States. Because treatment in primary care predicates a strong reliance on pharmacological interventions, patients may continue to be deprived of mental health care unless more emphasis is placed on the provision of a complete spectrum of mental health services.

Access to Specialty Mental Health Care in Rural Settings

An analysis (Smyer et al., 1992) of the U.S. population percentage served by psychologists or psychiatrists indicated that 83.8% of all Americans had access to both specialties, 7.3% had access only to psychologists, and 1.4% had access only to psychiatrists. When population samples were restricted to rural areas, psychologists were found to be considerably more accessible than were psychiatrists. Of the rural populations, 57.7% had access to both specialties, but 18% had access only to psychologists and 3.5% had access only to psychiatrists (Smyer et al., 1992). Results of a California survey indicated that there was a paucity of both psychologists and psychiatrists in rural California counties, but psychologists were considerably more common in those counties than were psychiatrists (California Board of Examiners of Psychologists, 1998).

Other states with large rural populations have experienced increased shortages of psychiatric care. More than two thirds of Iowa counties lack a psychiatrist, and efforts to lure psychiatrists through forgiveness of school loans have failed. Patients in such areas are likely to be treated by a *circuit-riding* psychiatrist, who visits infrequently and may not be acquainted with the problems of rural areas ("Rural Health," 1999). Because it is difficult to provide ongoing psychotherapeutic services under such circumstances, it is probable that psychotropic medication represents the mainstay of mental health service in areas so served.

Underrecognition and undertreatment are not limited to the outpatient setting. Rural nursing homes in a Maine study were less likely to employ mental health specialists than were those in urban settings (40% vs. 62%), were unlikely to routinely screen for depression, and were unlikely to have a formal protocol for the treatment of depressed patients (Bolda, Dushuttle, Keith, Coburn, & Bridges, 1998). A national analysis of care in nursing facilities revealed that mental health issues tended to be widely undertreated, especially in rural areas (Burns et al., 1993).

Characteristics of Mental Health Patients in the Rural Environment

Mehl-Madrona (1998) described characteristics of a group of persons who used health care extensively ("high utilizers") in a rural primary care practice in comparison with those of a randomly selected control group. Mental health diagnoses were more common among high utilizers. Sixty-three percent of high utilizers had a diagnosed mental illness, in comparison with 14% of randomly selected patients. Multiple diagnoses were common among the high utilizers: 133 patients had 440 mental health diagnoses. Adjustment, anxiety, and depressive disorders were the most frequent diagnoses in this group. Mental health diagnoses were not among the 10 most common diagnoses of the randomly selected patients, but they ranked among the 10 most common among the high utilizers. A very high proportion (49%) of high utilizers were prescribed psychotropic medications. The medications most commonly employed were antidepressants (37%), followed by anxiolytics (22%). Of importance, only 15% of patients who were prescribed these medications reported that their symptoms had improved; more than half (51%) described problems with the medications, significant side effects, or no improvement in symptoms.

Future Role of Rural Nonphysician Prescribers

Will prescribing psychologists and other nonphysician prescribers be accepted in rural health care settings? The ability to safeguard confidential information, geographic accessibility and availability of services, integration with the existing health care system, and fee structure and reimbursement have all been identified as predictors of successful rural integration of physician's assistants and nurse practitioners (Baldwin et al., 1998). Other things being equal, it seems likely that the public will accept these new providers. Random sampling of the U.S. population suggested that the public at large has no difficulty accepting prescribing psychologists: 60% accepted the idea and 32% were opposed (Fredericks/Schneider, Inc., 1992). Acceptance by other health care providers has not been extensively studied, but the data of Williams et al. (1999), presented previously, suggest that primary care providers preferentially referred patients to psychologists and social workers over psychiatrists. In a study of Department of Defense personnel, Klusman (1998) reported high levels of acceptance for the notion of prescribing psychologists among nonpsychiatric physicians (66%), social workers (67%), and other psychologists (77%). Although one study (Bell, Digman, & McKenna, 1995) revealed that slightly fewer than half (46%) of family practitioners surveyed thought that appropriately trained psychologists should prescribe, physician acceptance is likely to increase once the contributions of prescribing psychologists are appreciated. None of these studies was performed with rural populations, but the limited data suggest that nonphysician prescribers will not experience extraordinary difficulties with acceptance by the public or other health care providers. It can be anticipated that nonmedical prescribers will be easily integrated into rural communities in which psychologists have reputations as reliable and effective providers of mental health care.

Conclusions and Recommendations

Economic and social changes are creating a true revolution in American health care (Pew Health Care Commission, 1998). Far more significant than the changes wrought by the current emphasis on managed care is the growing realization that health care providers can be trained more efficiently and economically than traditional medical education (the dominant model throughout most of the 20th century) has permitted. Nurse practitioners and physician's assistants were among the first to recognize that providers of high-quality health care could be trained in far less time and at greatly reduced cost than could physicians. The skills of well-trained physicians are unparalleled and will continue to be a fundamental component of American health care. Nevertheless, traditional medical education continues to be extraordinarily expensive, and inequities in the distribution of physicians in general, and of psychiatrists in particular, have led to problems in access to quality mental health care, problems that are especially acute in rural areas.

Because of fundamental differences in training and conceptualization of mental distress, prescribing psychologists and other nonphysician mental health prescribers are not expected to function as "junior psychiatrists" or psychiatric extenders. Instead, these practitioners have the potential to bring a unique blend of behavioral and pharmacological services to rural health care. Through the integration of these services into the primary care setting, a more complete range of services can be brought to populations that are traditionally underserved. In order for this to occur, however, nonphysician mental health prescribers must first accomplish several prerequisite tasks. Accordingly, the following recommendations are made.

Commit to Training in Psychopharmacology

Nonphysician prescribers must commit to training programs in psychopharmacology. Physician's assistants and nurse practitioners have long included training in pharmacology as a core of their curriculum. The extent of training in psychopharmacology, however, is more restricted. Even this limited amount of additional training seems sufficient to produce safe and effective prescribers. Nurse practitioners have been found to practice as safely as their physician counterparts, and patient satisfaction with nurse practitioners is also equivalent to that with physicians (Mundinger et al., 2000). Overall, patients' acceptance of nonphysician prescribers has been found to be good (Baldwin et al., 1998). Pharmacists now have the ability to prescribe either independently or under some form of collaborative practice arrangement with physicians in 31 states (S. Winckelman, personal communication, March 14, 2001). Requirements for additional training and the type of pharmacist–physician collaborative drug therapy management agreements allow pharmacists varying degrees of autonomy from state to state. As is the case with physician's assistants and advanced practice nurses, however, formal training in psychopharmacology is often not a featured component of these curricula. This is a concern not only because graduates of these programs do not possess specialist-level knowledge in psychopharmacology but also because if such practitioners are not schooled in viable alternatives to the prescription of psychotropics (e.g., psychotherapy), there may be little chance to correct the excessive reliance on pharmacological interventions for mental distress that is a hallmark of current medical treatment in rural settings.

Because their background is more exclusively in behavioral sciences, psychologists devising training programs for their colleagues who wish to prescribe have recommended a longer curriculum. The American Psychological Association (1996) recommended a 300-contact-hour curriculum encompassing studies in anatomy, physiology, neurosciences, pathophysiology, pharmacology, and psychopharmacology. Numerous programs based on these recommendations for training prescribing psychologists now exist some in states with large rural populations (including Louisiana, Georgia, Nebraska, New Mexico, Texas, and California).

Not all practitioners will seek psychopharmacology training, nor should they. Those with interests in psychopharmacology and backgrounds in health psychology or behavioral medicine will likely self-select pharmacology training programs. If various professions are to maintain the historical distinctions that allow them to bring their unique perspectives and skills to health care, formal training in psychopharmacology must largely take place after the fundamental training, which imbues a professional identity. Thus, training may be at the postlicensure level, although components of pharmacology training may be available in the graduate curriculum.

Commit to Practicing in Underserved or Rural Areas

Nonphysician prescribers must commit to practicing in rural and underserved areas. This should not pose too great a burden. Many groups of potential nonphysician prescribers, such as nurses, physician's assistants, pharmacists, and psychologists, have a history of public service, and these prescribers are better distributed in rural areas than are psychiatrists. However, they must also recognize an obligation to practice in areas where the needs are greatest, and this implies a renewed dedication to high-quality rural mental health. Other professionals seeking to expand their legal authority to prescribe might consider such stipulations, because they serve both professionals and the public in good stead.

Commit to Obtaining Prescriptive Authority

Psychologists and other nonphysician specialists must commit to the legal and political struggles necessary to obtain prescriptive authority or to expand collaborative drug therapy management. Optometrists, advanced practice nurses (including nurse midwives and nurse practitioners), physician's assistants, and pharmacists have seen significant increases in professional autonomy as a result of effective political action. Nonphysician mental health prescribers should recognize that this is the true health care revolution of today and that they participate in this revolution not only for the good of their professions but also for the good of underserved populations in rural and urban areas alike. In many instances, collaborative drug therapy management may be a viable alternative to independent prescriptive authority. Collaborative agreements between nonphysician health care providers and physicians, if reached, will reduce the necessity of a protracted legislative struggle and provide a scenario by which the professions can work together as a team to enhance the public weal. The finding that many patients in designated Health Professional Shortage Areas have poorer health status than those in areas where providers are better represented (Kohrs & Mainous, 1995) should provide impetus for all health care providers to work together to ensure that adequate services are available.

Train New Providers to Meet the Needs of Changing Health Delivery Systems

Training programs for nonphysician mental health practitioners must lead the way in producing graduates who meet health care's changing needs. Training nonphysician mental health care providers to prescribe is potentially important for providing a range of rural mental health services. In line with the recommendation made in the Pew Health Care Commission (1998) report, leaders and educators of nonphysician mental health providers must accept the charge of training practitioners to meet the needs of the health care delivery system.

References

American Psychological Association. (1996). *Prescription privileges: Model legislation and curriculum.* Washington, DC: Author.

Baldwin, K. A., Sisk, R. J., Watts, P., McCubbin, J., Brockschmidt, B., & Marion, L. N. (1998). Acceptance of nurse practitioners and physician assistants in meeting the perceived needs of rural communities. *Public Health Nursing, 15,* 389–397.

Bell, P. F., Digman, R. J., & McKenna, J. P. (1995). Should psychologists obtain prescribing privileges? A survey of family physicians. *Professional Psychology: Research and Practice, 26,* 371–376.

Bolda, E. J., Dushuttle, P., Keith, R. G., Coburn, A. F., & Bridges, K. (1998). *Does access to mental health services for rural and urban nursing home residents with depression differ* (Rural Health working paper series, No. 11). Portland, ME: Maine Rural Health Research Center.

Bryant, E., & Shimizu, I. (1998). Sample design, sampling variance, and estimation procedures for the National Ambulatory Medical Care Survey. *Vital Health Statistics, 2*(108), 1–39.

Burns, B. J., Wagner, H. R., Taube, J. E., Magaziner, J., Permutt, T., & Landerman, L. R. (1993). Mental health service use by the elderly in nursing homes. *American Journal of Public Health, 83,* 331–337.

California Board of Examiners of Psychologists. (1998). [Psychologists and psychiatrists in rural California]. Unpublished data.

Cooper, R. A., Laud, P., & Dietrich, C. L. (1998). Current and projected workforce of non-physician clinicians. *Journal of the American Medical Association, 280,* 788–794.

Daw, J. (2002). New Mexico becomes first state to gain Rx privileges. *APA Monitor, 33,* 4. Retrieved June 27, 2002, from http://www.apa.org/monitor/apr02/newmexico.html

Fredericks/Schneider, Inc. (1992). *Survey of general population of the United States on prescription privileges for psychologists.* Washington, DC: Author.

Ganguli, M., Mulsant, B. B., Richards, S., Stoehr, G., & Mendelsohn, A. (1997). Antidepressant use over time in a rural older adult population: The MoVIES project. *Journal of the American Geriatrics Society, 45,* 1501–1503.

Gonzales, J. J., Magruder, K. M., & Keith, S. J. (1994). Mental disorders in primary care services: An update. *Public Health Reports, 109,* 251–258.

Greene, J. (1999). The threat of the domino effect. *American Medical News,* June 22, 1999. Retrieved August 2, 1999, from http://www.ama-assn.org/pubs/amnews/pick_99/prfa0621.htm

Greene, J. (2000). Drug reps targeting nonphysicians. American Medical News, March 27, 2000. Retrieved October 29, 2002, from www.ama-assn.org/sci-pubs/amnews/pick_00/pr120327.htm

Hartley, D., Korsen, H., Bird, D., & Agger, M. (1998). Management of patients with depression by rural primary care practitioners. *Archives of Family Medicine, 7,* 139–145.

Kohrs, F. P., & Mainous, A. G. (1995). The relationship of Health Professional Shortage Areas to health status. *Archives of Family Medicine, 4,* 681–685.

Klusman, L. E. (1998). Military health care providers' views on prescribing privileges for psychologists. *Professional Psychology: Research and Practice, 29,* 223–229.

Larson, E. H., Hart, L. G., & Hummel, J. (1994). Rural physician assistants: A survey of graduates of MEDEX Northwest. *Public Health Reports, 109,* 266–274.

Mehl-Madrona, L. E. (1998). Frequent users of rural primary care: Comparisons with randomly selected users. *Journal of the American Board of Family Practice, 11,* 105–115.

Mundinger, M., Kane, R., Lenz, E., Totten, A., Tsai, W., Cleary, P., et al. (2000). Primary care outcomes in patients treated by nurse practitioners or physicians. *Journal of the American Medical Association, 283,* 59–68.

Non-physician prescribing doubles. (1996, June 17). *American Medical News.* Retrieved August 2, 1999, from http://www.ama-assn.org/sci-pubs/amnews/amn_96/summ0617.htm

Pearson, L. J. (2002). 14th annual legislative update. *The Nurse Practitioner, 27*(1), 10–52.

Pew Health Care Commission. (1998). *Recreating health professional practice for a new century.* San Francisco: University of California, Center for Health Professions.

Pincus, H. A., Taneilian, T. L., Marcus, S. A., Olfson, M., Zarin, D. A., Thompson, J., et al. (1998). Prescribing trends in psychotropic medications: Primary care, psychiatry, and other medical specialties. *Journal of the American Medical Association, 279,* 526–531.

Pincus, H. A., Zarin, D. A., Tanielian, T. L., Johnson, J. L., West, J. C., Pettit, A. R., et al. (1999). Psychiatric patients and treatments in 1997: Findings from the American Psychiatric Practice Research Network. *Archives of General Psychiatry, 56,* 441–449.

Rabasca, L. (1999). Guam psychologists gain right to prescribe. *APA Monitor, 30,* 2. Retrieved June 27, 2002, from http://www.apa.org/monitor/feb99/guam.html

Rural health: Profits and access on the decline. (1999, June 15). *American Health Line.* Retrieved March 13, 2001, from http://nationaljournal.com

Sammons, M. T. (1994). Prescription privileges and psychology: A reply to Adams and Bieliauskas. *Journal of Clinical Psychology in Medical Settings, 1,* 199–207.

Sammons, M. T. (1998). The case for prescription privileges for psychologists: An overview. In S. C. Hayes & E. M. Heiby (Eds.), *Prescription privileges for psychologists: A critical appraisal* (pp. 11–45). Reno, NV: Context Press.

Sammons, M. T. (1999, August). *Pills versus psychotherapy: The evidence accumulates.* Paper presented at the annual convention of the American Psychological Association, Boston, MA.

Schappert, S. M. (1994). National Ambulatory Medical Care Survey: 1991 summary. *Vital Health Statistics, 13*(116), 1–110.

Smyer, M. A., Balster, R. L., Egli, D., Johnson, D. L., Kilbey, M. M., Leith, N. J., et al. (1992). *Report of the ad hoc task force on psychopharmacology of the American Psychological Association.* Washington, DC: American Psychological Association.

Susman, J. L., Crabtree, B. F., & Essink, G. (1995). Depression in rural family practice: Easy to recognize, difficult to diagnose. *Archives of Family Medicine, 4,* 427–431.

Williams, J. W., Rost, K., Dietrich, A. J., Ciotti, M. C., Zyzanski, S. J., & Cornell, J. (1999). Primary care physicians' approach to depressive disorders: Effects of physician specialty and practice structure. *Archives of Family Medicine, 8,* 58–67.

Zarin, D. A., Pincus, H. A., Peterson, B. D., West, J. C., Suarez, A. P., Marcus, S. C., et al. (1998). Characterizing psychiatry with findings from the 1996 national survey of psychiatric practice. *American Journal of Psychiatry, 155,* 397–404.

Zimmerman, M. A., & Wienckowski, L. A. (1991). Revisiting health and mental health linkages: A policy whose time has come . . . again. *Journal of Public Health Policy, 12,* 510–524.

Zung, W. W. K., Broadhead, W. E., & Roth, M. E. (1993). Prevalence of depressive symptoms in primary care. *Journal of Family Practice, 37,* 337–344.

10

Rural Dentistry

Steven W. Friedrichsen and B. Hudnall Stamm

Of all health professionals, dentists have the most opportunity to provide services in a rural location independently of other health care services. The dental workforce is not as diverse as those of other health professions, and thus it can be relatively more available in rural locations. In this chapter, we review dental needs, including problems amenable to collaboration with behavioral health such as dental fear, as well as dental disease and special populations, such as patients infected with the human immunodeficiency virus (HIV). This chapter also addresses the availability of dental services in rural areas, considers sociodemographic and access issues, and reviews the crossover literature. The chapter concludes with recommendations for training and collaboration between dentistry and mental health.

Dentistry and mental or behavioral health have points of potential interaction. These points are diverse and range from addressing dental fears and phobias to helping dental professionals deal with personal crises of stress and isolation. Between those extremes lie multiple areas of interaction. Examples of areas of interaction include designing appropriate and effective patient compliance measures, tobacco cessation counseling, dealing with traumatic stress disorders, and helping patients cope with the chronic pain response seen in temporomandibular disorders (TMD). Dentists can also benefit from additional skills in recognizing the role that depressive disorders can play in dental care behaviors and in employing effective education and communication techniques for working with both dental staff and patients. An increasing area of interaction involves assessment of patient competence. Patient competence is a necessary aspect of understanding dental procedures and of providing informed consent.

Nearly all of these areas of potential interaction between the behavioral and dental sciences are present and, in some cases, magnified in rural areas. In all locations, particularly rural locations, the potential interaction between dental personnel and mental health professionals is rarely more than a dormant potential. There is room for significant development of professional interactions in the training of both types of professionals and in fostering practical interactions in the practice of their respective fields.

One of the most germane areas of latent interaction involves dental fears. Nearly all people experience some degree of reluctance with regard to dental

Dr. Friedrichsen can be reached at Idaho State University, Pocatello, ID 83209. E-mail: friestev@isu.edu

care. Some individuals have demonstrable phobias or serious behavioral health issues related to their beliefs and experiences surrounding dental care. In those situations, a coordinated approach between dental and mental health care can provide opportunities to understand (Liddell & Locker, 2000), prevent (Townend, Dimigen, & Fung, 2000), and reduce patient anxiety (Clay, 2000) and to facilitate provision of dental services. If dentists and mental health professionals were educated and practiced as integrated team members, many possibilities for positive changes in the care of dental patients would exist.

Rural Dentistry

Dentistry is one of the health services with the least potential to be adversely affected by location. Among health professionals, dentists have the enhanced capability of providing most services in a rural location independently of other health care services and with minimal hardship caused by infrastructure or geography. Although dentistry can be available, there are significant disparities in its availability in rural and frontier areas of the United States. The reduced availability stems from decreased numbers of dental practitioners and from deterrents to access to care, some of which are products of the rural environment.

Several characteristics of dental practice are favorable to delivery of services in rural and frontier locations. Most dental offices are stand-alone operations, not dependent on the availability of hospital or long-term care beds, medical laboratories, or diagnostic imaging services. General dentists comprise approximately 80% of the dentist workforce, and they deliver more than 80% of all dental services. Most general dentists are trained to deliver an adequate level of services with a reasonable degree of skill, so that referral to specialists is not frequently needed. In dentistry, the emergency or acute care caseload is small enough that a single practitioner can handle client needs without a burdensome rotation or call schedule. The dental workforce is not as diverse as workforces of other health professions, and the technology of care is not as onerous as that in other health care delivery systems.

Although dentistry is more readily available in rural locations than are other health care services, significant issues serve to reduce the quantity and quality of dental services available. Anderson (2000) noted that reduced access to oral health care services is associated with low-income status and location of residence. The problems of access experienced by underserved groups in general is magnified in the presence of geographic isolation, lack of transportation, diminished fiscal resources, and reduced physical presence of dentists in nonurban locations.

Dental Need

In dental literature, patient care is commonly considered to be based on a series of steps progressing from actual dental need to the provision of dental care. At each of the steps, the process may be stopped or redirected by a variety of factors. Helping patients overcome their fear of getting care can have striking psychological implications. A significant problem is dental fear, which in extreme cases qualifies as a fully developed phobia or traumatic stress reaction to a previously traumatizing dentistry-related experience. Some patients may be reluctant to seek treatment or may have cognitive impairments that make it difficult for them to understand the need for treatment. Other examples of the need for a closer alliance between dentistry and mental health professionals include working with patients toward cessation of tobacco use, restoration associated with traumatic injury such as a traumatic brain injury, the interactions of depression with TMD, and other dentally related chronic pain (Albino, 2002; Mucci & Brooks, 2001).

Dentists as a group have a low level of comfort in dealing with issues such as evaluating patients' mental health status or competency. This is most likely the result of lack of training in this area. Explaining the treatment that is needed or provided can be a difficult task if the patient is not able to comprehend or make an informed decision; this situation is exacerbated when the dentist is uncertain of the patient's level of comprehension. Dentists can benefit from additional training and from coordinating care with appropriate mental health care personnel.

Dentistry has made significant advances toward reducing the actual need for services. The use of fluorides in various forms and of dental sealants has resulted in significant reductions of dental disease. Although there have been population-wide reductions, the prevalence of dental decay is no longer evenly distributed. From 75% to 80% of the carious lesions (dental decay) occur in 20%–25% of the population (Stookey, 2000). Record numbers of elderly people have retained their teeth and represent a population increasingly affected by both dental caries and periodontal disease. The ability to develop appropriate educational and motivational methods could help reduce the ravages of disease in these highly affected populations.

Even with advances in preventative dentistry, dental disease (specifically dental caries) remains one of the most ubiquitous transmissible diseases. More than half of all children aged 6 to 8 and two thirds of all children up to the age of 15 have experienced decay (U.S. Department of Health and Human Services, 1997). Fewer than 5% of adults in the United States are completely without the effects of dental disease. Rural residents have a higher incidence and severity of dental disease and are less likely to obtain dental care (Gilbert, Duncan, Heft, & Coward, 1997). Because of the high frequency of discrete water sources and the typical infrastructure of small municipalities, residents of rural locations are less likely to have the significant benefit of water fluoridation, which is a key preventive element in dentistry (Reifel, Davidson, Rana, & Nakazono, 1997). Dental disease continues to be a significant problem (Koop, 2000) and is accelerated when fluoridation is inadequate and other preventive measures are unavailable to rural populations.

Several pockets of particular need exist. The rural population is aging faster than the population in general (Jones & Brand, 1995), which results in increased need, especially for restorative and rehabilitative dentistry. The geriatric population has a unique subset of dental needs stratified most succinctly by age. Patients who are HIV seropositive, those who have physical or intellectual disabilities, and patients who have complex medical or psychological problems that necessitate team approaches to therapy are even more likely to face significant challenges and barriers to finding adequate treatment in a rural environment.

Dentists in rural locations may have less experience with patients with a broad array of cognitive, behavioral, and physical disabilities, as well as with those who have complex medical problems. Rural dentists may see only a few people who have a particular type of disability or mental illness in their entire practice careers. The ability of a dentist to treat these patients adequately may be severely limited by experience. To complicate matters, many of these patients have a higher level of dental need than the general population because of their inability to engage in adequate self-care (Castro & Linares, 1998), accompanied by diminished capacity to determine their level of need for care (Cumella, Ransford, Lyon, & Burnham, 2000). Very often, special-needs patients' fiscal resources are drained by the higher level of nondental health care services needed.

The negative attributes of rural special-needs populations are usually counterbalanced by the dentist's willingness to attempt treatment on behalf of the patient or the patient's family. Information on various disorders and diseases and the modifications necessary for safe and efficacious treatment in the dental office is available from a variety of sources. To ensure the best outcome, however, most dentists would benefit from increased resources than are commonly available through the dental literature and database. The assembly of a team for interdisciplinary care and consultation for treatment of special-care patients can be logistically difficult in a rural environment.

Availability of Dental Services

To serve the needs of rural dental patients, dental providers must be present locally. Knapp and Hardwick (2000) studied the availability of various classes of medical personnel in rural and designated Health Professional Shortage Areas (HPSAs), using zip codes of practice locations. Comparing the national average of health care practitioners to rural locations and then to designated HPSAs, they found a decline in the numbers of all available practitioners. The two most common practitioners among all types are primary care physicians and dentists. As demonstrated by Knapp and Hardwick, dentists are more common in a rural or HPSA setting than are physicians, and dentists are the health care professionals most likely to be available in rural areas or HPSAs. The average numbers of these practitioners per population of 100,000 are 95.2 physicians and 75.9 dentists nationally, 53.6 physicians and 55 dentists in rural areas, and 4.2 physicians and 29.1 dentists in HPSAs.

From these data, it appears that because of the unique characteristics of dentistry in the health care delivery system, a higher proportion of people living in rural and HPSA areas have local access to dental services. Nationally, there is a demonstrated 27.5% decrease in dentist availability in rural locations and a 61.7% decrease in their availability in HPSAs. Although this decrease is not desirable, it is better than the 43.7% and 95.6% reductions noted for physicians. Other data indicate that dentists are 19.7%–21.2% more likely to be present in HPSAs than are physicians or registered nurses (Johnson & Spencer, 2000). Data on mental health providers are not presented to make comparisons.

Dentists seem to have a reasonable presence in rural locations, which is probably a direct reflection of the financial capacity of the "system" in a particular area. In dentistry, the financial risk for profitable operation, which is directly related to the ability to continue to provide service in a rural area, rests on the individual practitioner or owner rather than on a community clinic.

The future availability of dentists in rural locations will be influenced heavily by the workforce trends in dentistry (Mages, 2000). In 1960, there were approximately 59.5 dentists per 100,000 persons; it is projected that by 2020, there will be 52.7 dentists per 100,000 persons. In 1985, 85.8% of dental practitioners practiced full time (30 or more hours per week of patient care); in 1995, 76.2% practiced full time. The interpretation of these workforce changes are mixed. It is possible there will be an inadequate number of dentists to serve the population, or it could be postulated that the increasing productivity and changes in disease patterns are well balanced with the projected changes in the workforce.

Sociodemographics and Access

The dental literature consistently identifies significant barriers to care in the rural setting or deficiencies in the system of care (U.S. Government Accounting Office Report, 2000). Few of the factors cited are unique to the profession of dentistry, and most influence all rural health care acquisition. Primary among the negative factors is the continued relevance of economic barriers to rural care. Even though most authors identify negative factors resulting in diminished dental access, there are only occasional calls for reforms to alter the current dental care delivery system, in contrast to other sectors of the health delivery system (*Building Partnerships*, 1998; U.S. Department of Health and Human Services, 2000; U.S. Government Accounting Office Report, 2000).

Many of the most commonly cited barriers or negative factors involve or are direct outgrowths of the sociodemographics of rural living. Rural residents are more likely to depend on the economics of agriculture or of locally owned and operated businesses than on those of manufacturing industries or services, and national or regional businesses (Chollett, 1987). Rural residents have a lower per capita income; decreased availability of health insurance, especially dental insurance; and minimal public transportation (U.S. Congress, Office of Technology Assessment, 1990). Rural residents are also less likely to have preventive and health promotion programs (Bushy, 1990; Weinert & Long, 1990; see also the introduction in this book). Diminished levels of dental insurance reduce the beneficial role of preventive and routine maintenance dentistry. Preventive measures and early treatment represent the mainstays responsible for the decreasing incidence and severity of dental disease since the early 1970s. Without appropriate preventive measures, rural residents will avail themselves of dentistry primarily for acute problems and problems of great severity—problems that could have been avoided with preventive care.

Rural residents find the availability of local dentists who accept public insurance limited. Many rural and frontier locations may only have one dental provider. If that available provider is not a participant in the insurance program, residents may have to travel significant distances to obtain care from a participating dentist. Multiple sources point to the paucity of dental providers willing to accept Medicaid reimbursement (Isman & Isman, 1997; National Center for Education in Maternal and Child Health, 1988). In general, there is significant disagreement between dental providers and public insurance officials concerning how to best increase the low number of participating dental providers. Dentists identify reimbursement levels below their cost of care delivery and an inordinate administrative burden for payment mechanisms as the two most significant factors involved in not participating in public insurance programs.

Medicaid and State Children's Health Insurance Program (SCHIP) reimbursements remain the strongest impediments to dentist participation in insurance programs. A report to Congress (U.S. Government Accounting Office Report, 2000) demonstrated that only four states reimburse dental fees at 75% of the state's average fees, 13 states reimburse at approximately 67%, and the other 33 states pay at lower rates, some as low as 25% of the average fees. Most dental offices have overhead expenditures of 70%–75% of fees, and so, even under the best of circumstances, treating Medicaid and SCHIP patients results in a financial loss to the dental practice in 44 of the nation's 50 states.

Values and Perceptions

Entitlement and health care supplemental programs cover 44% of the eligible urban poor and 36% of the rural poor (U.S. Congress, Office of Technology Assessment, 1990). Thus, some differences can be explained by the availability of assistance. However, the values and perceptions common in the more close-knit environment of rural living continue to attach a stigma to enrollment in government programs, and family pride also provides another disincentive (Bushy, 1990).

A comprehensive and unique study by Strickland and Strickland (1995, 1996) demonstrated the significant interplay between poverty and health care in a rural environment. Their work demonstrated several key interactions in exquisite detail. Among the key values was the difference between actual and perceived need. In the arena of preventive services, there was at least a 50% lack of recognition of the need for services across all fields. Among all health care services, the field of dentistry had the most pronounced discrepancy between actual and perceived need, which was heightened when coupled with an inability to pay.

Strickland and Strickland (1995, 1996) further found that the social values and norms among impoverished rural residents were distinctly negative with regard to preventive health care. Among the households with very low incomes, all health care became a luxury item, unless it involved potential morbidity or mortality. A particularly astute summary of the situation is as follows:

> People with similar health status do not have similar perceptions, nor do they make similar demands for health care because of differences in health

beliefs, illness behavior, social networks, willingness or ability to pay for services, and other social, psychological, economic, and cultural processes. The assessment of need is not simply a matter of relating health status to resource availability and distribution, but also the social, economic, and political environment of individuals and populations. (Patrick, Stein, Porta, Porter, & Ricketts, 1988, p. 105)

Dentistry and Mental Health

There should be strong and significant ties between the professions of dentistry and mental health. The reality is that there is not a strong allegiance between these professions; there is little interdisciplinary education and often less interactions between practicing professionals. Because of the more abundant presence of dentists in rural locations, additional training and information in patient education techniques from psychologists might provide patients with increased levels of care (Secker-Walker, Dana, Solomon, Flynn, & Geller, 2000). Efforts directed toward altering rural patients' perceptions of need for dental care could increase the persistent and early intervention efforts and reduce the need for crisis or acute care. Cotherapeutic approaches could increase dentists' comfort level and effectiveness with patients in special-needs groups, such as those with disabilities, cognitive deficits, or extreme fear of dentistry.

Although a small but significant body of literature addresses mental health and dentistry, it has been difficult to locate because it has been spread among mental health, dental science, and medical journals (Albino, 2002). Albino reviewed nine conditions that she believed held promise for collaboration between dentistry and mental health: (a) dental caries; (b) periodontal disease; (c) dental anomalies and orthodontics; (d) birth defects; (e) edentulism, or the loss of all natural teeth; (f) head and neck cancer and treatment complications; (g) trauma such as craniofacial injury; (h) chronic orofacial pain; and (i) salivary gland dysfunction. In addition to identifying these conditions, Albino arranged them in probability across the life span. Makuch and Reschke (2001) found that using age-appropriate games to teach young children (aged 3–5) good oral health habits was a good method for teaching oral health facts.

Dental anxiety has perhaps been the condition best studied. One study revealed that both early- and late-onset dental fear were associated with conditioning. In addition, early-onset fear was characterized by stress-reactive personality and specific beliefs about health professionals, whereas late-onset fear was associated more with irregular use and an external locus of control (Poulton, Waldie, Thomson, & Locker, 2001). Fear seems to be a key factor in dental anxiety (Townend et al., 2000). People with dental anxiety report significantly greater fear of severe pain, higher levels of general anxiety and somatization symptoms, and greater health and work-related stress. This fear is related to dental fear but not to other psychological symptoms (McNeil et al., 2001). Whereas NcNeil et al. found no link to dental fear and other mental disorders, Kaakko et al. (2000) found that 68% of people with fear of dental injections also had a lifetime Axis I disorder listed in the American Psychiatric Association's *Diagnostic and Statistical Manual of Mental Disorders (DSM)*.

There is variability among people with dental fear. However, these fears can generally be classified into groups: those who are anxious avoiders of dental treatment whose anxiety subsides if they avoid dental treatment (Liddell & Locker, 2000) and those who have the ability to control negative cognitions related to dental care (Locker, Shapiro, & Liddell, 1999).

Thom, Sartory, and Joehren (2000) studied two standard treatments for anxiety: benzodiazepine and stress management. The one-session psychological intervention included stress management and imaginal exposure to phobic stimuli with homework assignments. Both treatments led to reduced anxiety during dental treatment, but the patients receiving psychological intervention continued to show improvement at the 2-month follow-up, whereas those receiving the medication intervention showed postsurgical complications. Other treatments that have been studied include hypnosis (Pinnell & Covino, 2000), ambient odor of orange (Lehrner, Eckersberger, Walla, Poetsch, & Deecke, 2000), enhanced social support (Vedhara, Addy, & Wharton, 2000), eye movement desensitization and reprocessing (De Jongh, Ten Broeke, & Renssen, 1999), and emotional disclosure (Sullivan & Neish, 1999).

Psychologists and other mental health professionals can play a role in helping dentists improve communication in dental offices through improved communication skills (Newton & Brenneman, 1999). Appropriate communication and interpersonal relationship skills would benefit the dental staff and patients alike, perhaps reducing the stress of caregiving in rural areas. In view of the significant potential for professional isolation and the high stress level, psychologists can provide dentists with avenues for reducing professional burnout (Stamm, 1999). This sharing can be mutual. Rural providers of all types are often isolated, and interdisciplinary sharing can help reduce that isolation and strengthen the provider's professional quality of life.

Conclusions and Recommendations

The presence of dental practitioners in rural areas and HPSAs represents a bright spot in the rural health services picture. The ability of dentists to locate in areas isolated from other health care services and their ability to provide an array of dental services are benefits to improving access. The roadblocks to access of the dental services are reasonably known but are not seriously addressed because of their fiscal impact. Federal and state support for dental services is minimal and declining. There are conduits of interaction between dentistry and mental health that need to be filled with two-way dialogue, information, and education of both groups.

Work for Improved Reimbursement

Dentists should continue to work for inclusion of dental services in health plans. Increasing reimbursements to a realistic level will increase the participation by practitioners. Mental health and oral health practitioners are natural alliance partners for inclusion in primary care.

Improve Rural Oral Health Provider's Health Screening Activities

Oral health providers in rural and frontier areas should recognize that they have additional responsibilities as health care providers in screening for hypertension, counseling patients on tobacco cessation, advanced recognition protocols for head and neck pathosis, referral for medical conditions, and promoting lifestyle changes for oral and general health concerns.

Increase Interprofessional Activity Between Oral and Mental or Behavioral Health

Dentistry and mental health professionals should forge stronger alliances to help foster appropriate interprofessional referrals and to help develop effective methods of increasing care-seeking behaviors and decreasing dental fears.

Increase Training and Curriculum Collaboration

Members of the American Dental Association and of mental or behavioral health organizations such as the American Psychological Association should consider common curricular elements that promote the skills and knowledge of dental professionals in such areas as dental fear, facilitation of tobacco cessation, recognizing the depressive interplay of TMD and chronic pain, and treatment of developmentally disabled and dementia patients.

Provide Professional Assistance Programs

Professionals of all types experience negative effects of providing care for their clients and patients. Because rural oral health professionals tend to be in solo practice, they may be at particular risk for experiencing isolation, burnout, and even work-related trauma. Mental health professionals should consider providing assistance programs to isolated health care professionals for improving their professional quality of life and personal mental health.

References

Albino, J. E. (2002). A psychologist's guide to oral diseases and their treatment. *Professional Psychology: Research and Practice, 33,* 176–182.

Anderson, J. R. (2000). Access to oral health care services remains challenging. *Rural Clinician Quarterly, 10*(2), 2–3.

Bushy, A. (1990). Rural US women: Traditions and transitions affecting health care. *Health Care for Women International, 11,* 503–513.

Castro, A., & Linares R. (1998). Is the oral hygiene suitable in Down syndrome people? *Italian Journal of Intellective Impairment, 11,* 147–149.

Chollett, D. (1987, March 4). *Uninsured in the United States; the non-elderly population without health insurance.* Washington, DC: Employee Benefit Research Institute.

Clay, R. A. (2000). The mental/dental connection. *Monitor on Psychology, 31*(7). Retrieved November 21, 2002, from http://www.apa.org/monitor/julaug00/dental.html

Cumella, S., Ransford, N., Lyon, J., & Burnham, H. (2000). Needs for oral care among people with intellectual disability not in contact with community dental services. *Journal of Intellectual Disability Research, 44,* 45–52.

De Jongh, A., Ten Broeke, E., & Renssen, M. R. (1999). Treatment of specific phobias with eye movement desensitization and reprocessing (EMDR): Protocol, empirical status, and conceptual issues. *Journal of Anxiety Disorders, 13,* 69–85.

Gilbert, G. H., Duncan, R. P., Heft, M. W., & Coward, R. T. (1997). Dental health attitudes among dental black and white adults. *Medical Care, 35,* 255–271.

Isman, R., & Isman, B. (1997). *Oral health America: Access to health services in the United States 1997 and beyond.* Chicago: Robert Wood Johnson Foundation.

Johnson, A. E., & Spencer, W. (2000). Registered nurses in health professional shortage areas. *Health Workforce Newslink HHS/HRSA,6*(4), 1–3. Washington, DC: Health Resources and Services Administration of the U.S. Department of Health and Human Services (HHS/HRSA).

Jones, H. P., & Brand, M. K. (1995). Providing rehabilitative services in rural communities: Report of a conference. *Journal of Rural Health, 11,* 122–127.

Kaakko, T., Coldwell, S. E., Getz, T., Milgrom, P., Roy-Byrne, P. P., & Ramsay, D. S. (2000). Psychiatric diagnoses among self-referred dental injection phobics. *Journal of Anxiety Disorders, 14,* 299–312.

Knapp, K. K., & Hardwick, K. (2000). The availability and distribution of dentists in rural ZIP codes and primary care health professional shortage areas (PC-HPSA) ZIP codes: Comparison with primary care providers. *Journal of Public Health Dentistry, 60,* 43–48.

Koop, C. E. (2000). *Improving oral health: Preventing unnecessary disease among all Americans.* Atlanta, GA: Centers for Disease Control and Prevention. Retrieved June 17, 2002, from http://www.cdc.gov/nccdphp/oh

Lehrner, J., Eckersberger, C., Walla, P., Poetsch, G., & Deecke, L. (2000). Ambient odor of orange in a dental office reduces anxiety and improves mood in female patients. *Physiology and Behavior, 71,* 83–86.

Liddell, A., & Locker, D. (2000). Changes in levels of dental anxiety as a function of dental experience. *Behavior Modification, 24,* 57–68.

Locker, D., Shapiro, D., & Liddell, A. (1999). Variations in negative cognitions concerning dental treatment among dentally anxious and nonanxious individuals. *Cognitive Therapy and Research, 23,* 93–103.

Mages, M. (2000). Workforce worries: Will there be enough dentists in the future? *AGD Impact, 28*(10), 6–11.

Makuch, A., & Reschke, K. (2001). Playing games in promoting childhood dental health. *Patient Education and Counseling, 43,* 105–110.

McNeil, D. W., Au, A. R., Zvolensky, M. J., McKee, D. R., Klineberg, I. J., & Ho, C. C. (2001). Fear of pain in orofacial pain patients. *Pain, 89,* 245–252.

Mucci, L. A., & Brooks, D. R. (2001). Lower use of dental services among long term cigarette smokers. *Journal of Epidemiology and Community Health, 55,* 389–393.

National Center for Education in Maternal and Child Health. (1988, June). Building partnerships to improve children's access to Medicaid oral health services. Paper presented at the national conference of the National Center for Education in Maternal and Child Health, Lake Tahoe, Nevada.

Newton, J. T., & Brenneman, D. L. (1999). Communications in Dental Settings Scale (CDSS): Preliminary development of a measure to assess communication in dental settings. *British Journal of Health Psychology, 4,* 277–284.

Patrick, D., Stein, J., Porta, M., Porter, C., & Ricketts, T. (1988). Poverty, health services, and health status in rural America. *Milbank Quarterly, 66,* 105–136.

Pinnell, C. M., & Covino, N. A. (2000). Empirical findings on the use of hypnosis in medicine: A critical review. *International Journal of Clinical and Experimental Hypnosis, 48,* 170–194.

Poulton, R., Waldie, K. E., Thomson, W. M., & Locker, D. (2001). Determinants of early- vs late-onset dental fear in a longitudinal-epidemiological study. *Behaviour Research and Therapy, 39,* 777–785.

Reifel, N. M., Davidson, P. L., Rana, H., & Nakazono, T. T. (1977). ICS-II USA research locations: Environmental, dental care delivery system, and population sociodemographic characteristics. *Advances in Dental Research, 11*, 210–216.

Secker-Walker, R. H., Dana, G. S., Solomon, L. J., Flynn, B. S., & Geller, B. M. (2000). The role of health professionals in a community-based program to help women quit smoking. *Preventive Medicine: An International Journal Devoted to Practice and Theory, 30*, 126–137.

Stamm, B. H. (Ed.). (1999). *Secondary traumatic stress: Self-care issues for clinicians, researchers, and educators* (2nd ed.). Lutherville, MD: Sidran Press.

Stookey, G. K. (2000). Current status of caries prevention. *Compendium of Continuing Education in Dentistry, 21*, 862–867.

Strickland, W., & Strickland, D. (1995). Coping with the cost of care: An exploratory study of lower income minorities in the rural South. *Family and Community Health, 18*(2), 37–51.

Strickland, W., & Strickland, D. (1996). Barriers to preventive health services for minority households in the rural South. *Journal of Rural Health, 12*, 206–217.

Sullivan, M. J., & Neish, N. (1999). The effects of disclosure on pain during dental hygiene treatment: The moderating role of catastrophizing. *Pain, 79*, 155 163.

Thom, A., Sartory, G., & Joehren, P. (2000). Comparison between one-session psychological treatment and benzodiazepine in dental phobia. *Journal of Consulting and Clinical Psychology, 68*, 378–387.

Townend, E., Dimigen, G., & Fung, D. (2000). A clinical study of child dental anxiety. *Behaviour Research and Therapy, 38*, 31–46.

U.S. Congress, Office of Technology Assessment. (1990). *Health care in rural America* (OTA Publication No. OTA-H-34). Washington, DC: U.S. Government Printing Office.

U.S. Department of Health and Human Services. (1997). *Healthy people 2000: Review*. Washington, DC: U.S. Government Printing Office.

U.S. Department of Health and Human Services. (2000). *Oral health in America: A report of the Surgeon General*. Rockville, MD: U.S. Department of Health and Human Services, National Institute of Dental and Craniofacial Research, and National Institutes of Health.

U.S. Government Accounting Office Report. (2000). *Oral health-factors contributing to low use of dental services by low-income populations* (Publication No. GAO/HEHS 00-149). Washington, DC: U.S. Government Printing Office.

Vedhara, K., Addy, L., & Wharton, L. (2000). The role of social support as a moderator of the acute stress response: In situ versus empirically-derived associations. *Psychology and Health, 15*, 297–307.

Weinert, C., & Long, K. (1990). Rural families and health care: Refining the knowledge base. In D. Unger & M. Sussman (Eds.), *Families in community settings: Interdisciplinary perspectives*. Binghamton, NY: Hawthorne.

11

Bridging the Rural–Urban Divide With Telehealth and Telemedicine

B. Hudnall Stamm

Telehealth and telemedicine encompass many applications useful to the field of rural health, including direct patient care; training, supervision and consultation; continuing education; and an opportunity to ameliorate the isolation that can exist in rural health systems. In this chapter, I briefly review challenges and opportunities. Four challenges are presented: establishing effectiveness, reimbursement, licensure, and the uneven distribution of access to technology, often called the *digital divide*. The chapter concludes with six recommendations to increase the opportunities provided by telehealth.

There is no universal definition of telehealth or telemedicine, but since the 1990s, most people have acquired the gist of the meaning. This growth in understanding of the concept, even if not by official definition, is reflected in the growth of the use of telehealth and telemedicine.

The activities accomplished across telehealth systems are quite varied. In fact, there are no standard definitions because technological developments are opening new avenues every year. What constitutes telehealth is unclear, as is the role of the mental health provider in this emerging market (Jerome et al., 2000; Stamm, 1998b; Stamm & Perednia, 2000). The question of the role of mental health aside, the key to defining telehealth or telemedicine seems to be the use of telecommunications between the origin and delivery of an activity or service, in which there may or may not be an actual person at either end at a particular time (Stamm, 1998b). Activities such as using Web sites, telephones, e-mail, videoconferencing, store-and-forward applications, virtual reality, and transmitting information from medical device peripherals and tests such as electroencephalography and magnetic resonance imaging all have a role in psychological and general telehealth (Jerome et al., 2000; Rothchild, 1999; Stamm, 1998b, 2000a) as well as in training (Stamm, Ax, Wiggins, & Barbanel, 2000).

Telehealth and Telemedicine

Although impossible to count in numbers, the telephone is the most common telehealth tool (VandenBos & Williams, 2000). With the growth of the

Dr. Stamm can be reached at Campus Box 8174, Institute of Rural Health, Idaho State University, Pocatello, ID 83209. E-mail: bhstamm@isu.edu

Internet, viewing Web sites is probably fast approaching the telephone as a tool of choice for acquiring health care information. Besides these two inestimable tools toward what aligns more commonly with professional health care, the majority of the contacts appear to be for medication and treatment management planning. The stereotypical telehealth consultation is that of a video teleconference between clinician and patient. One of the popular and less complex uses of teleconferenceing is for educational purposes. Educational activities include grand rounds, continuing education, distance-delivery, university coursework, and community health education.

Supervision is common and particularly important in rural areas, where there are limited numbers of specialists. Supervision is composed of a range of activities that may include specialists supervising generalists, doctoral-level providers supervising midlevel or paraprofessional caregivers, supervision for licensure, and peer-to-peer supervision to prevent burnout and vicarious or secondary trauma (Stamm, 1999). Consultations are another professional-to-professional aspect of telehealth. Although it is impossible to count the number of "long-distance" health-related encounters between clinician and patient that have occurred over the telephone since its development in 1896, telehealth has formalized this long-distance practice. Beyond the telephone, secure information networks (e.g., e-mail, patient records, specialty equipment) and real-time video consultations form the core of a telehealth system (Darkins & Cary, 2000; Stamm, 1998b).

An extension of the professional-to-professional consultation occurs when the professional at the originating end presents the patient to one or more professionals at the remote end or ends. This is perhaps the most common patient consultation format. As patients become more comfortable with the technology and particularly with the provider at the remote location, there is a decreasing need for a professional at the originating end. For example, a family practice provider in a rural clinic might initiate the relationship between his or her patient and a distant mental health professional. As the patient gains confidence in the new relationship, he or she may meet directly with the remote professional with only modest technical assistance. In other scenarios, caregivers connect directly with patients in their home. Home health is a growing application for people with disabilities, chronic illnesses, and end-of-life care.

Establishing a single, set definition of telehealth or telemedicine is not very helpful. Darkins and Cary (2000) suggested a laissez-faire approach toward definitions, pointing instead to the underlying principles of the activity. General definitions accommodate new technology and applications well and yet may be too vague and not helpful. Specific definitions have the advantage of ruling in or ruling out various activities, but they may limit creative, new applications. For simplicity, in this chapter, both the terms *telehealth* and *telemedicine* are used, but I avoid the further specialization of words into field-specific entities such as *telepsychology* and *telepsychiatry* except when I refer to another's work in which the terms were used. *Telehealth* refers to the broader collection of health-related activities, whereas *telemedicine* refers more specifically to patient care.

Challenges and Opportunities

The technology of telehealth is sufficiently developed that it is practical for use. In the early years, there were so many technological glitches that it took a great deal of interest in telehealth to be willing to use it. These glitches were amplified by working in rural areas with low technological infrastructure. There are increasing types of options, including a low-bandwidth option appropriate for many rural settings. Thus, the pressing issues relate more to the fit between technology and the human aspects of telehealth than to the technology itself (Stamm & Perednia, 2000). In fact, for caregivers, the technology of telehealth is becoming less prominent compared with the caregiving it makes possible (Whitten, Sypher, & Patterson, 2000). It is critical to remember that telehealth is a service delivery mechanism, not a treatment protocol.

Although some people, such as administrators and clinicians, still question the acceptability of telehealth, their numbers are dwindling and are more likely to reflect the percentage of people assumed to have aversions to computers or technology than those with concerns about the viability of telehealth use (Rosen & Maguire, 1990; Rosen, Sears, & Weil, 1987; Rosen & Weil, 1996). Even in this group, the literature suggests that true technology phobias are rare (Rosen & Maguire, 1990) and can be modified with experience (Wilson, 1999).

Four major challenges repeatedly appear when telehealth discussed in policy and in research (see Sandberg, 1999). Although these challenges apply to urban and nonurban areas alike, they are particularly salient in rural areas, where telehealth is seen as a significant solution to isolation. The first of these challenges is establishing evidence of effectiveness. The second is reimbursement. The third challenge relates to licensure and regulatory issues. The final and perhaps the most difficult challenge to overcome is the uneven distribution of access to technology, what is sometimes called the *digital divide*.

EVIDENCE OF EFFECTIVENESS. The traditional path to acceptance for new ideas in health care is through an efficacy study, often a clinical trial. Once efficacy has been shown, there is a period of adjustment, after implementation, through effectiveness studies that show the "real world" success of the laboratory or clinical trial projects. Breaking with tradition, telehealth emanated not from efficacy studies, or even effectiveness research, but from grassroots applications. In fact, many telehealth programs existed before, and even outside of, any research (Stamm & Perednia, 2000). Certainly there are efficacy studies and clinical trials in process, but real-world effectiveness continues to be a cornerstone of telehealth research. Darkins and Cary (2000) posited that evidence of effectiveness is key to the overall care process: "We believe telehealth has the capacity to improve the quality of health care, provide equity of access to health care services, and reduce the cost of delivering health care" (p. viii).

The door through which telehealth entered onto the health care scene was that of access. Applications of telehealth to rural and underserved communities far outnumber those of other programs. Telehealth has been a way to provide care to underserved and isolated communities (Brown, 1999; Lambert & Hartley, 1998; Magaletta, Fagan, & Peyrot, 2000). Startup for telehealth programs often exceeds the cost of usual treatment; however, when Werner and Anderson (1999) suggested that rural telepsychiatry was economically unsustainable, many people took issue, often pointing to improved access as having not been considered in the cost–benefit analysis (see, for example, Smith, 1999). Authors report that telehealth is satisfactory to providers and patients. Satisfaction has been reported by children (Dossetor, Nunn, Fairley, & Eggleton, 1999; Elford et al., 2000; Ermer, 1999), the older population (Gardner-Bonneau & Gosbee, 1997; Lee et al., 2000), corrections populations (Brodey, Claypool, Motto, Arias, & Goss, 2000; Magaletta et al., 2000), military health care professionals (Stamm, 1998a), and combat veterans (Gelsomino, Hayman, Haug, & Stamm, 1999).

REIMBURSEMENT. The Balanced Budget Act of 1997 was a major breakthrough for the reimbursement of telehealth services. As a provision of this bill, Medicare providers could be reimbursed for services delivered through telehealth if the patient (not the provider) lived in a rural, federally designated Health Professional Shortage Area (HPSA). Administrators at the Health Care Financing Administration (HCFA), now the Centers for Medicare & Medicaid Services, struggled for several years to discern how to put the law into action. When the regulations went into effect in January 1999, many people, including the author of the original bill (Senator Kent Conrad of North Dakota; 1997 Rural Telehealth Act), believed that the rules and the intention of the bill had diverged in negative ways, in particular suggesting potentially illegal fee splitting between the originating and remote sites. Nonetheless, the journey had a profoundly positive impact on the regulatory system. Rather than reject the concept of reimbursement for telehealth, subsequent Congressional activities revolved around upholding and expanding the authority of reimbursement for telehealth services.

The earliest systematic *reimbursed* use of telehealth was in federal medicine, in which caregivers were paid a salary rather than reimbursed on a case-by-case basis (Marsan & Brewin, 1993). Military telehealth surged ahead in the federal system, antedating telehealth in the private or even nonmilitary public sector (e.g., Baxter, 1996; Forkner, Reardon, & Carson, 1996; Linder, 1994). Since the emergence of telehealth in the federal system, federal telehealth has had special prominence in the telehealth world. Perhaps this is because of the salaried nature of the caregiver positions, which precludes reimbursement in a fee-for-service or managed care environment.

Following the pattern set in military medicine, some private payers and managed health care organizations do reimburse for telehealth services, but it can be difficult to understand how the billing process works (Kinsella, 1998). Viewing the problem as one with ethical and legal ramifications, Koocher and Morray (2000) suggested that when third parties are billed, use of telehealth must be clearly noted on the forms to prevent the accusation of fraud from organizations that are not supportive of telehealth.

LICENSURE AND REGULATORY ISSUES. There are a number of issues related to legal and regulatory aspects of providing care at a distance. The first and most obvious relates to licensure (Nickelson, 1996, 1998). Fundamentally, should the provider of care be licensed in the state from which he or she originates or in the state to which the care goes? A more philosophical question is whether there is a third location somewhere in cyberspace. If the patient is in state A, and the provider in state B, does the provider need a license in both states A and B, or does he or she need a license only in state A or state B? At the time of this writing, no clear precedent had arisen. There are varying legal opinions that are beyond the scope of this chapter (for more information, see, for example, Schanz, 1999; Schanz & Gordon, 1998). From a practical perspective, most providers err on the side of caution. They either restrict their telehealth consultations to one state or hold licenses in the state from which the care originates and the state or states to which the care *travels electronically* to the patient. There is discussion for credentialing work in cyberspace, but, as yet, no one has seriously suggested the need for such licensing. Special rules apply to those working in the federal health care system, which includes the Bureau of Prisons, the military, the Department of Veterans Affairs, and the Indian Health Service. Perhaps the most liberal interpretation of licensure on *federal property* is that the clinician must hold a license in *a* state, not necessarily *the* state in which the federal facility exists. These federal property "areas" have provided a ground for the concept of a federal license, and development of telehealth programs has been rapid because of fewer restrictions.

Koocher and Morray (2000) surveyed states' attorneys general with regard to the delivery of mental health services through telemetry. One of their most striking findings was that there were no established standards across states. Moreover, they found that rural states had more advanced understandings and regulations than their urban counterparts had. Koocher and Morray believed that there would be an increase in the legal and regulatory criteria for providing care through telehealth. In this volatile climate, they recommended that practitioners (a) assess their competency through the medium, (b) consult with their professional liability insurance carriers, (c) seek consultation from their colleagues, (d) provide patients written emergency procedure information, (e) inform clients of the standard limitations and cautions regarding mental health care as well as potential risks to privacy entailed by the technology used, and (f) clearly inform patients what types of services can be offered. Koocher and Morray suggested that, in the case of adverse events, the incidents be carefully documented.

THE DIGITAL DIVIDE. This last challenge presents a paradox; the very tool that should improve access is limited by the frailty of the technological infrastructure in rural areas.[1] Technology in the service of caregiving is at the core of powerful societal changes that confront providers' roles as caregivers. From its inception, telehealth has been touted as a doorway to more egalitarian access to care, superseding geographical, climatic, and social barriers. Any tool to enhance service delivery to underserved and hard-to-reach populations is

---

[1]An earlier version of this section appeared in Stamm, B. H. (2000b). Telehealth puts public service caregiving in focus. *American Psychological Association: Public Service Psychology (Div. 18), 24*(1), 1, 19.

worthy of serious consideration. However, a digital divide exists between those who may only hope to receive care and those who do.

The digital divide is the gap between those with telecommunications access and those without. Historically, there have been similar gaps emerging and closing but none with the rapidity of change associated with today's digital divide. For example, after the development of the printing press in the mid-1400s, more people had access to the printed word. As centuries passed, the literacy power gap began to close. By the year 2000, literacy rates worldwide were usually 70%–100%; only in the poorest countries did those rates fall below 60% (United Nations Population Fund, 2000). This literacy gap has lasted 650 years. The digital divide has unfolded in less than 200 hundred years, and the societal cost of not addressing this rapid change can only be imagined.

In many ways, the changes in the digital age echo the profundity of change brought about by the Industrial Revolution, which fueled urbanization. Before the Industrial Revolution, goods were made one item at a time, largely in rural settings, where the raw materials were available. The changes wrought by the introduction of machines made it possible to mass-produce goods and for people to purchase products rather than make them for themselves. The expanding availability of goods created the possibility of urbanization, which was judged by some authorities to be superior to the old ways and by others as inferior (Estabrook, 1999). Whereas goods were produced rapidly, information was still produced slowly, one document at a time. Today, the changes wrought by the Information Age have made it possible to mass-produce information. As with Industrial Revolution goods, this Information Revolution is judged by some authorities to be superior and by others to be inferior to the old ways.

The most striking characteristic of the Information Revolution is the volume of information produced. Of interest is that the Industrial Revolution's mass production of goods engendered a similar feeling of societal claustrophobia. However, from a historical view coupled with a psychological perspective, the speed of adaptation to this new Information Age is remarkably different from that of the Industrial Revolution. The nascent seeds of the Industrial Revolution were sown in England in the early 1700s and blossomed into full flower in the United States between 1870 and 1920. Over a 200-year period, Western countries changed from rural agricultural societies to urbanized, wage-earning societies. In contrast, the roots of the Information Age developed with computers in the late 1940s. Only 50 years later, 320 million people worldwide had access to the Internet, and digital technology constituted 8.2% of the U. S. gross domestic product (Meares & Sargent, 1999).

The rapid adaptation has been uneven. For example, according to New York University's Taub Urban Research Center, the 20 largest cities in the United States contain about 86% of the Internet delivery capacity, excluding most of the world (Moss & Mitra, 1998). Even in urban areas, telecommunications companies focus on the financial districts and corporate or scientific areas. The poorer and residential areas are left out; in the U.S., 95% of small businesses do not have high-speed access. Thus, in the U.S., 86% of the capacity goes to the richest 10% of the 42% of the people who have access.

Income is a major predictor of access to the Internet (Moss & Mitra, 1998; National Telecommunications and Information Administration, 1999; Public

Broadcasting Service, 1999). In the U.S., the digital divide between the highest and lowest incomes widened 29% between 1997 and 1999. Profound differences exist between races; White people are more likely to have access than are members of any other racial group. Similar differences exist between rural and urban areas: Rural residents are less likely to have access (National Telecommunications and Information Administration, 1999).

Future Directions

One of the fastest growing segments of telehealth is the home health care market. Many individuals and families can benefit from home telehealth care. With the assistance of telehealth, many older people can remain independent longer. In one project, computers with video cameras were placed in the homes of senior citizens who needed support. The seniors were very receptive to the program and used the systems well (Glueckauf, Stamm, Kwon, & Norton, 1998). Home health care is also commonly used for families struggling with chronic illnesses (Hufford, Glueckauf, & Webb, 1999). Alternatively, it may be used to support independent living for those with disabilities such as serious and persistent mental illnesses.

Outside the home setting, telehealth has been used in prisons. For inmates, receiving care through telehealth prevents the humiliation of being transported in chains to a health care facility. For prison personnel, safety is less compromised. Telehealth can also be used to link inmates with their families to improve family function and to speed reintegration into the community (Magaletta, Fagan, & Ax, 1998). Similarly, telehealth can link those in the community with family members who are hospitalized (Stamm, 1998b). Telehealth can also be used to link families together when children have moved to urban areas and parents are aging in-place. Rather than the child's traveling to accompany a parent to a health care provider, it is possible for the child to attend the parent's appointment through telehealth by using teleconferencing facilities. Veterans also report liking telehealth. They prefer travelling short distances to a videoconferencing facility over longer travel to meet in person with a mental health provider (Gelsomino et al., 1999).

Telehealth can support caregivers and their quality of life. Reducing isolation can improve recruitment and retention by increasing protective factors and reducing risk factors for burnout, secondary traumatization, and medical error (Stamm, 1998a, 1999; Terry, 1999). Along with linking specialty care with primary care, telehealth can provide types of care in cases in which none have previously been available.

Conclusions and Recommendations

Many health care professionals spend their caregiving careers crossing the divides of race, class, and gender. Telehealth as a mode of service delivery is not different in this respect from other modes they have used. Although it is equally as easy to become overly enthusiastic about the potential of technology to change the world as it is to become overwhelmed by the digital divide, a middle ground is emerging. Thoughtful connectivity is used to maximize bandwidth and minimize specialty equipment in a variety of settings. Tele-health, whether in the hands of the provider or of the consumer, can give control to those who traditionally have very little control. It can support the isolated provider. It can serve to empower members of special populations who suffer from stigmatization or are underserved. Telehealth may also offer opportunities to contain or even reduce current health care costs by reducing travel or by improving the quality of care. Telehealth can yield opportunities to improve the quality of care or provide earlier (less costly) interventions. Telehealth is also an important tool for aftercare. It can allow people to return home from tertiary care centers earlier. In some cases, telehealth may prevent costly hospitalizations by supporting local providers in complex service provi-sion. Telehealth can improve everyone's sense of self-efficacy. To meet these promises, however, changes are needed in health care system to accommodate the possibilities.

Increase All Infrastructure

For telehealth and telemedicine to reach their potential in rural areas, there must be a change in the available bandwidth. Incentives for companies to develop infrastructure in rural areas could help address the cost vs. user-density problem that drives the private sector to more affluent areas.

Increase Number of Providers With Knowledge of Telehealth

Information about telehealth must be incorporated into training programs. This has been done in some programs; others are far from ready to include telehealth and technology. Directors of some programs would like to include training in using telehealth but are prohibited by the accreditation rules of their fields. For example, many training programs prevent trainees from doing any training unless there are licensed professionals in their fields physicaly present. This prevents students from training in underserved areas where there also may be provider shortages. If accreditation- and organization-approved supervision and consultation were available through video confer-encing, for example, students could train in settings that are more diverse and would probably be more likely to select rural or underserved areas for post-graduate practice sites.

Address Issues of Licensure

Until providers and reimbursement organization officials understand the requirements of licensure, they will not be eager to incorporate telehealth into their reimbursement packages. Currently, many licensing boards are trying to resolve issues of cross-state licensure, but there is no legal or research clarity on the implications of cross-state licensing. Additional funds could be allocated toward policy and practice research that could help state licensing boards make informed decisions.

Address Reimbursement Issues

At this time, it is possible to be reimbursed for telehealth services under a number of federal and private mechanisms. However, none has emerged as the benchmark for equitable or appropriate reimbursement. Additional policy and practice research, as well as cost-offset research, should improve providers' understanding of reimbursing telehealth.

Expand Cost Research to Include the Cost to the Community

Many studies on which infrastructure upgrades, licensure, and reimbursement are based do not address the total cost associated with care. To understand this cost, cost-offset research must be community based and must include comparisons of face-to-face care with telehealth care, including averted and opportunity costs. In addition, associated costs and benefits should be considered. Some of these factors include lost work due to travel time, impact on the community's economy due to the ill person's lost work, and the lost work time of those who travel with him or her. The sustainability of a community that has telehealth as an option, in terms of recruitment and retention of providers and other businesses, is increased, and the medical cost may be potentially offset by averting illness through better access to care.

Include Professional Services to Rural Providers as Reimbursable Time

Recruitment and retention are major issues for most rural communities and are usually tied to professional quality of life. Burnout, secondary traumatization, and even medical error are possible negative outcomes of highly stressed and isolated working environments. Use of telehealth as a professional and social support to improve the provider's quality of life should reduce burnout, improve quality of care, and increase recruitment and retention and, by extension, access to care. As long as the system can generate capital only by seeing more and more patients, it will be difficult to improve the quality of the provider's ability to care. The benefit of telehealth for reducing professional isolation will be realized only when caring for the caregiver is a respected part of the health care system.

References

Baxter, C. F. (1996). Telemedicine enters the fleet. *Navy Medicine, 87*(4), 4.

Brodey, B. B., Claypoole, K. H., Motto, J., Arias, R. G., & Goss, R. (2000). Satisfaction of forensic psychiatric patients with remote telepsychiatric evaluation. *Psychiatric Services, 51,* 1305–1307.

Brown, F. W. (1998). Rural telepsychiatry. *Psychiatric Services, 49,* 963–964.

Darkins, A. W., & Carey, M. A. (2000). *Telemedicine and telehealth: Principles, policies, performance, and pitfalls.* New York: Springer.

Dossetor, D. R., Nunn, K. P., Fairley, M., & Eggleton, D. (1999). A child and adolescent psychiatric outreach service for rural New South Wales: A telemedicine pilot study. *Journal of Pediatrics and Child Health, 36,* 525–529.

Elford, R., White, H., Bowering, R., Ghandi, A., Maddiggan, B., St. John, K., et al. (2000). A randomized controlled trial of child psychiatric assessments conducted using videoconferencing. *Journal of Telemedicine and Telecare, 6,* 73–82.

Ermer, D. J. (1999). Experience with a rural telepsychiatry clinic for children and adolescents. *Psychiatric Services, 50,* 260–261.

Estabrook, C. (1999). *Urban and rustic England: Cultural ties and social spheres in the provinces, 1660–1780.* Stanford, CA: Stanford University Press.

Forkner, M. E., Reardon, T. G., & Carson, G. D. (1996). Experimenting with feasibility of telemedicine in Alaska: Success and lessons learned. *Telemedicine Journal, 2,* 223–240.

Gardner-Bonneau, D., & Gosbee, J. (1997). Health care and rehabilitation. In A. D. Fisk & W. A. Rodgers (Eds.), *Handbook of human factors and the older adult* (pp. 231–255). New York: Academic Press.

Gelsomino, J., Hayman, P. M., Haug, R. J., & Stamm, B. H. (1999, August). *Potential uses of tele-health technology: A vet center initiative.* Paper presented at the 107th Annual Convention of the American Psychological Association, Boston, MA.

Glueckauf, R., Stamm, B., Kwon, S., & Norton, J. (1998, August). *Telehealth for persons with chronic medical conditions—Program evaluation developments.* Paper presented at the 106th Annual Convention of the American Psychological Association, San Francisco, CA.

Hufford, B. J., Glueckauf, R. L., & Webb, P. M. (1999). Home-based, interactive videoconferencing for adolescents with epilepsy and their families. *Rehabilitation Psychology, 44,* 176–193.

Jerome, L. W., DeLeon, P. H., James, L. C., Folen, R., Earles, J., & Gedney, J. J. (2000). The coming age of telecommunications in psychological research and practice. *American Psychologist, 55,* 407–421.

Kinsella, A. (1998, March/April). Telemedicine: The reimbursement challenge. *Home Health Care Dealer/Supplier 10,* 96–97.

Koocher, G. P., & Morray, E. (2000, October). Regulation of telepsychology: A survey of state attorneys general. *Professional Psychology: Research and Practice, 31,* 503–508.

Lambert, D., & Hartley, D. (1998). Linking primary care and rural psychiatry. *Psychiatric Services, 49,* 965–967.

Lee, J., Kim, J., Jhoo, J. H., Lee, K. U., Kim, K. W., Lee, D. Y., et al. (2000). A telemedicine system as a care modality for dementia patients in Korea. *Alzheimer Disease and Associated Disorders, 14,* 94–101.

Linder, A. (1994). Department-wide rollout planned as U.S. Navy tests ship to shore telemedicine. *Global Telemedicine Report, 1*(2), 1–5.

Magaletta, P. R., Fagan, T. J., & Ax, R. K. (1998). Advancing psychology services through telehealth in the Federal Bureau of Prisons. *Professional Psychology: Research and Practice, 29,* 543–548.

Magaletta, P. R., Fagan, T. J., & Peyrot, M. F. (2000). Telehealth in the Federal Bureau of Prisons: Inmates' perceptions. *Professional Psychology: Research and Practice, 31,* 497–502.

Marsan C. D., & Brewin, B. (1993). DOD, VA, IHS overhaul federal health systems (Department of Defense, Veterans Administration, Indian Health Service). *Federal Computer Week 7*(35), 1–3.

Meares, C. A., & Sargent, J. F. (1999). *The digital workforce.* Washington, DC: U.S. Department of Commerce, Technology Administration, Office of Technology Policy. Retrieved March 12, 2001, from http://www.ta.doc.gov/Reports/itsw/digital.pdf

Moss, M. L., & Mitra, S. (1998). *'Net equity.* New York: New York University, Robert F. Wagner School of Public Service. Retrieved March 13, 2001, from http://urban.nyu.edu/archives/net-equity/net-equity.pdf

National Telecommunications and Information Administration. (1999). *Falling through the 'net: Defining the digital divide.* Retrieved March 11, 2001, from http://www.ntia.doc.gov/ntiahome/fttn99/contents.html

Nickelson, D. W. (1996). Behavioral telehealth: Emerging practice, research, and policy opportunities. *Behavioral Sciences and the Law, 14,* 443–457.

Nickelson, D. W. (1998). Telehealth and the evolving health care system: Strategic opportunities for professional psychology. *Professional Psychology: Research and Practice, 29,* 527–535.

Public Broadcasting Service. (1999, September 17). *The digital divide.* Retrieved March 13, 2001, from http://www.pbs.org/newshour/bb/education/july-dec99/digital_9-17.html

Rosen, L. D., & Maguire, P. (1990). Myths and realities of computerphobia: A meta-analysis. *Anxiety Research, 3,* 175–191.

Rosen, L. D., Sears, D. C., & Weil, M. M. (1987). Computerphobia. *Behavior Research Methods, Instruments, and Computers, 19,* 167–179.

Rosen, L. D., & Weil, M. M. (1996). Psychologists and technology: A look at the future. *Professional Psychology: Research and Practice, 27,* 635–638.

Rothchild, E. (1999). Telepsychiatry: Why do it? *Psychiatric Annals, 29,* 394–401.

Sandberg, L. A. (1999, February). Telemedicine continues to wrestle wicked problems: Reimbursement, licensure, and bandwidth rules (or is it compliance?). *Health Management Technology 20,* 134.

Schanz, S. J. (1999). *Compendium of telemedicine laws: Selected statute excerpts and article citations relating to telemedicine.* (Available from Legamed, Inc., P.O. Box 99526, Raleigh, NC 27624-9526.)

Schanz, S. J., & Gordon, E. L. (1998). *Compendium of telemedicine laws: Selected statute excerpts and article citations relating to telemedicine.* (Available from Legamed, Inc., P.O. Box 99526, Raleigh, NC 27624-9526.)

Smith, H. A. (1999). Rural telepsychiatry is economically unsupportable: Comment. *Psychiatric Services, 50,* 266–267.

Stamm, B. (1998a, August). Improving care with technology: Reducing military caregiver stress. In R. Ax (Chair), *Federal telehealth—issues and initiatives.* Paper presented at the 106th Annual Convention of the American Psychological Association, San Francisco, CA.

Stamm, B. H. (1998b). Clinical applications of telehealth in mental health. *Professional Psychology: Research and Practice, 29,* 536–542. Retrieved March 13, 2001, from http://www.apa.org/journals/pro/pro296536.html

Stamm, B. H. (1999). Creating virtual community: Telehealth and self-care updated. In B. H. Stamm (Ed.), *Secondary traumatic stress: Self-care issues for clinicians, researchers, and educators* (2nd ed., pp. 179–210). Lutherville, MD: Sidran Press.

Stamm, B. H. (2000a). Shifting gears: Integrating models of telehealth and telemedicine into current models of mental health care. In L. G. Lawrence (Ed.), *Innovations in clinical practice* (Vol. 18, pp. 385–400). Sarasota, FL: Professional Resource Press.

Stamm, B. H. (2000b). Telehealth puts public service care giving in focus. *American Psychological Association: Public Service Psychology (Division 18), 24*(1), 1, 19.

Stamm, B. H., Ax, R. A., Wiggins, J. G., & Barbanel, L. (2000, August). *Growing the future II—What about market forces?* Paper presented at the 108th Annual Convention of the American Psychological Association, Washington, DC.

Stamm, B. H., & Perednia, D. (2000). Evaluating psychosocial aspects of telemedicine and telehealth systems. *Professional Psychology: Research and Practice, 31,* 184–189.

Terry, M. J. (1999). *Kelengakutelleghpat:* An Arctic community-based approach to trauma. In B. H. Stamm (Ed.), *Secondary traumatic stress: Self-care issues for clinicians, researchers, and educators* (2nd ed., pp. 149–178). Lutherville, MD: Sidran Press.

United Nations Population Fund. (2000). *State of the world population 2000.* Retrieved March 4, 2001, from http://www.unfpa.org/swp/1999/Swp99_action.cfm

VandenBos, G. R., & Williams, S. (2000). The Internet versus the telephone: What is telehealth anyway? *Professional Psychology: Research and Practice, 31,* 490–492.

Werner, A., & Anderson, L. E. (1999). Rural telepsychiatry is economically unsupportable. *Psychiatric Services, 50,* 267–268.

Whitten, P., Sypher, B. D., & Patterson, J. D. (2000). Transcending the technology of telemedicine: An analysis of telemedicine in North Carolina. *Health Communication, 12*(2), 109–135.

Wilson, B. (1999). Redressing the anxiety imbalance: Computerphobia and educators. *Behaviour and Information Technology 18,* 445–454.

Part III

Special Populations in Rural Communities

12

Children and Adolescents in Rural and Frontier Areas

Katherine C. Nordal, Stuart A. Copans, and B. Hudnall Stamm

Although the majority of children younger than 21 in the United States live in urban areas, nonmetropolitan dwellers form a significant minority. Most members of this minority (16 million, or 21% of children) reside in rural areas. The majority of the rural residents live primarily in the Midwest and the South. Rural children differ in other ways from their urban counterparts. As might be expected from this geographical distribution, farm-related accidents contribute to higher rates of morbidity and mortality among rural children than among urban children. Although drug abuse rates are lower, rural teenagers drink more alcohol and engage in riskier sexual behavior and at younger ages than their urban peers. Also, in comparison with urban populations, a larger proportion of rural children are White, tend to live in larger families, have parents who are married, and their parents work. This family constellation has great potential for successful parenting and well-adjusted children, as discovered by Brody, Stoneman, Smith, and Gibson (1999) in their study of Southeastern rural Black families. However, about 23.2% of rural children live in poverty and 15% of those rural children do so without health insurance. Only 55% of the children in rural families have employer-sponsored health plans, and 23% have Medicaid (Clark, Savitz, & Randolph, 1999). Their access to health and mental health care is limited accordingly. Not only are there fewer providers in rural areas than in larger urban or suburban populations but also geography and climate restrict the ability of rural dwellers to receive timely and appropriate care. For many rural children, school-based clinics provide the most frequent contact with health and mental health care providers.

In this chapter, we discuss issues relating to children and adolescents in rural areas. We begin by considering youth mortality, health risks, and mental health issues. In the second section, we consider access to care and utilization of services. After this discussion, we consider some workforce issues specific to those who care for youths, and we proceed to an overview of clinical issues. In the final section, we provide recommendations for policy and clinical care.

Dr. Nordal can be reached at The Nordal Clinic, P.A., 1121 Grove Street, Vicksburg, MS 39180, 801-634-0118. E-mail: knordal@vicksburg.com

Rural Youth

Mortality and Health Risks

Mortality from causes other than disease among children is related to accidents, poor quality of and access to health care, and exposure to social problems such as violence and substance abuse. Access to care, given fuller treatment elsewhere in this chapter, plays an important role with regard to timely and appropriate responses of providers to children who have suffered accidental injury. The leading causes of death among all children stem from various accidents and injuries, such as motor vehicle accidents, gun accidents, drowning, burning, suffocation, and poisoning, more than from any other means, including terminal illnesses (Grossman, 2000). Among rural children, farm-related accidents (especially from tractor mishaps) can be especially dangerous. According to DeMuri and Purschwitz (1999), about 100 children die every year from farm-related accidents and another 27,000 suffer injury. Despite knowing the dangers associated with operating farm machinery, farm fathers held ingrained beliefs about the importance of work, farming traditions, and the experiences that a farm boy should have (Lee, Jenkins, & Westaby, 1997). Other researchers found that fatal injuries were 44% higher among rural children than among urban children (Clark et al., 1999).

Exposure to social problems (such as suicide, violence, acquired immunodeficiency syndrome) and involvement in risky behavior (drug abuse, alcohol consumption, sex) affect the health of all children and adolescents; these behaviors and suggestions for prevention are well known to researchers (for a summary of 137 studies, see Fahs et al., 1999). For example, suicide rates among rural boys aged 15–19 are higher than among urban boys of the same age (Clark et al., 1999).

Violence also knows no boundaries. Since the early 1980s rural adolescents have been increasingly exposed to violent crimes. Gang activity at school is still three times higher in urban schools, but a substantial number of rural youths exhibit fear about violence at school. One in five students fears being attacked at school, and 13% of rural students fear being attacked while traveling to and from school (Bastian & Taylor, 1991).

Drugs are widely available: 71% of rural students report that drugs are obtainable at their schools. The drugs of choice among rural youth, however, are alcohol and tobacco. Rural youths report using alcohol while driving, which increases their risk of motor vehicle fatalities. There is also a strong relationship between early age of initiation to use and the likelihood of subsequent misuse of alcohol and other drugs. A study of 374 rural fifth graders by Valois et al. (1998) revealed that 26% of boys and 16% of girls had tried tobacco. In sum, across race and gender, at the end of the first decade of their lives, one fifth to one quarter of youths were at least trying substances associated with some of the most negative health behaviors.

Rural adolescents also have higher rates of risky sexual behavior than do their urban counterparts (DiClemente, Brown, Beausoleil, & Lodico, 1993) and are two times as likely to be sexually active, to have an earlier first sexual encounter and report in greater numbers having alcohol-related unprotected sexual intercourse. Although these adolescents had a good knowledge of the human immunodeficiency virus (HIV) and risk-reduction strategies, this information did not necessarily translate into better practice of risk-reduction behavior. Rural teens demonstrated a weak relationship between knowledge of HIV and preventive behaviors during intercourse. In view of the generally lower prevalence rates of HIV infection in rural communities than in urban communities (Steinberg & Fleming, 2000), rural adolescents may feel less vulnerable to the threat of HIV infection.

Rural Youth and Mental Health Issues

Rural life does not earn a distinction for general psychological well-being. Simons, Johnson, Beaman, Conger, and Whitbeck (1996) found that in 207 single-parent families in 104 small Midwestern communities, community population size was not related to adolescent adjustment. These adolescents showed rates of conduct disorder and psychological distress similar to those of peers in smaller urban areas. Economic disadvantage and the proportion of single parents in the population, rather than the urban–rural dichotomy, had greater impact on adolescent problem behavior, particularly in boys (this factor did not seem to affect girls). Furthermore, the proportion of single parents within the community was related to affiliation with deviant peers and to conduct problems.

Rural ethnic populations may experience a higher prevalence of certain mental health and substance abuse problems (Neighbors et al., 1992). Studies suggest that Black adolescent girls who have experienced stressful life events in the previous 12 months are more likely to suffer from depression, conduct disorder, posttraumatic stress disorder, and somatic complaints. Black adolescent boys are more likely than their White counterparts to exhibit aggression and other forms of conduct disorder. Hispanic youth exhibit more frequent depression and suicidal behavior than either Black or White youth. Native American adolescents appear to drink more heavily and to use marijuana and readily available inhalants such as gas, spray paint, and glue at higher rates than do other American adolescents. They are also more likely to commit suicide (Hoberman, 1991).

In the absence of national epidemiological studies of the prevalence of mental disorders among children and adolescents in the United States, the national Center for Mental Health Services developed methodology based on results of eight smaller, localized studies (reported in the *Federal Register,* October 6, 1997). The data were inadequate for estimating prevalence rates of serious mental illness in children younger than 9 years, but such prevalence rates of 9%–13% were projected for the 9–17 age group (Global Assessment Scale cutoff score = 60 or lower). Imposing a cutoff score of 50 or lower projected prevalence rates of 5%–9%. These impairment levels indicate serious emotional disturbances that substantially interfere with major life activities.

Access to Care and Utilization of Services

In urban areas, numerous private practitioners and well-developed transportation options create good access to services such as inpatient hospitals, day treatment programs, outpatient clinics, social service agencies, crisis centers, crisis hotlines, youth organizations, and after-school programs. However, in rural areas, there are a number of barriers to child and adolescent mental health prevention and treatment programs. Typically, rural populations are dispersed across geographically large areas, with a paucity of qualified providers, inadequate resources, inefficient communication systems, and little public transportation other than school buses. Rural communities are tight-knit, and members are not always willing to trust outsiders. Moreover, rural residents are reluctant to accept government services or public programs and instead often seek their community's informal networks of natural helpers (ministers, school counselors, school nurses, etc.; Wagner, Menke, & Ciccone, 1995). Rural parents are also wary of services that might draw attention to their children or identify them as deficient in some way. Clients may be further deterred by the need to travel long distances, which may be accompanied by a long wait for an appointment or in-office wait times.

Even when parents are willing to seek help for their children, access is limited by the shortage of child-focused providers. Despite the consensus on the treatment of attention deficit hyperactivity disorder (ADHD; National Institutes of Health Consensus Development Panel, 2000), treatment disparity is widespread (Angold, Erkanli, Egger, & Costello, 2000). Of rural children in need of mental health services, 75% receive no care, and less than 30% of those who are treated receive adequate treatment (Cutrona, Halvorson, & Russell, 1996; S. L. Martin, Kupersmidt, & Harter, 1996).

The lack of specialty mental health professionals results in reliance on primary care practitioners (Hartley, Bird, & Dempsey, 1999). Pediatricians see more children than do members of any other professional group except teachers (Costello et al., 1988), and parents willingly talk with their pediatricians about their children's mental health problems (Tarnowski, 1991). However, even pediatric specialists are in limited supply in rural communities. Many rural hospitals have closed, causing the focus of a community's health care to shift elsewhere. Health departments provide more curative services instead of fostering prevention, and the closing of facilities has increased the difficulty of recruiting and retaining primary care providers in rural communities. Finally, high rates of underinsurance prevent access to available private care for many rural residents.

S. L. Martin et al. (1996) studied 112 farmworker families with children in North Carolina to address use of mental health services. Participants were either migratory or seasonal farmworkers. Eighty-six percent were Hispanic, and the others were Black. Fifty-one percent of the children in the study were girls and 49% were boys. Sixty-four percent of these children met criteria for one or more psychological diagnoses. Of those children, 60% had an anxiety disorder, 9% had a depressive disorder, 9% had an oppositional defiant or conduct disorder, 8% were diagnosed with ADHD, and 2% had post-traumatic stress disorder. However, fewer than 50% of children who needed services saw a health professional; instead, their parents consulted school personnel, religious leaders, and friends. The others occasionally saw psychologists or child psychiatrists, but family physicians performed most of the consultations.

Bussing, Zima, and Belin (1998) studied 143 elementary students diagnosed with ADHD. They found that girls, minorities, and rural residents had lower rates of appropriate diagnoses and treatment. Primary care physicians commonly provided services, but the disorders were undetected. Overall, ADHD was managed in the primary health care setting, with some services provided in the schools or by specialists.

Workforce Considerations Specific to Child Mental Health

Recruitment

Getting mental health professionals to work in rural areas requires rural training programs and specific support. The literature suggests that professionals trained in rural areas are somewhat more likely to remain in rural areas and that training programs that recruit from rural areas are somewhat more likely to have graduates that return to there to practice. Despite progress in developing rural-oriented training programs, there is more work to do, particularly for recruitment of child specialists and stressing the future rural provider's sense of place (Cutchin, 2000; Stearns & Stearns, 2000)

A second issue is reimbursement. Child mental health care usually requires longer and more expensive training than does adult mental health care. Because graduates have larger debt loads, many rural clinics are hard-pressed to offer salaries that allow both debt reduction and minimal living expenses. New clinicians may find that they have to work in the higher paying locations (i.e., urban areas) in order to keep from defaulting on their loans. Unless reimbursement for rural clinics takes into account travel time and "no-shows"—which must include mode of transportation, geography, and climate—rural clinics will not be able to compete with their urban counterparts. Also, practitioners in urban clinics often supplement their income with private practices; this habit may not be possible in rural areas because of client poverty and low population.

Development of peer support networks is another crucial issue. Recruitment is often most successful when the recruit is paired with a peer who works in a similar situation. The scarcity of highly trained child mental health clinicians in rural areas, however, makes face-to-face meetings difficult. Yet conference calls, listservs, or private chat rooms for rural professionals may help overcome some of the problems that stymie this form of support (Stamm, 1998, 1999).

Retention

Child mental health clinicians in rural areas leave for numerous reasons, including unhappiness with the work or the agency, familial dissatisfaction with the rural environment, or monetary issues. Others remain in the same geographic location but leave child mental health work for administrative work or for work with adult patients. In order to increase provider retention, several key changes should be made in agency policies and Medicaid reimbursement guidelines. The most crucial change is the realization that work with children is more time intensive than work with adults because of the need for collateral contacts. Caseloads for child mental health clinicians should be between two thirds and three fourths of the caseloads for adult mental health clinicians. In turn, there must be differential reimbursements for those working with children, along with reimbursement for collateral contacts, such as time spent in communication with schools, the parents, or family physicians or pediatricians.

Because familial dissatisfaction often undermines retention, it is important for agencies to help ensure that the move will be positive for both the clinicians and their families (Cook, Copans, & Schetky, 1998). There are many strategies that can enhance the chances of successful family relocation, including arranging for a peer sponsor for each relocating family member.

If an agency does not need a full-time clinician, collaboration with another agency may help meet salary requirements. A barrier to such collaboration is the expense of travel between sites, so compensation should be split by the agencies involved. Also, federal reimbursement for travel time is one option that would greatly help in the recruitment of rural clinicians.

A final and crucial part of retention of rural practitioners is mandatory reimbursed attendance at off-site professional meetings. Psychologists should be expected to attend the annual meeting of the American Psychological Association at least every other year and should be granted the time and expenses to do so. Similarly, child psychiatrists should be expected to attend the meetings of the American Academy of Child and Adolescent Psychiatry (AACAP). Such meetings provide contact with peers, support for the practitioner's professional identity, and ongoing education.

Clinical Issues

Copans and Racusin (1983) and Cook et al. (1998) explained several clinical issues that child mental health clinicians must learn about and deal with if they are to practice in rural areas. Two of these are the importance of ethnocultural and geocultural issues (see chapters 2 and 18) and the possible necessity of home visits. The latter may help a clinician better grasp family dynamics or roles and conflicts between the family and their neighborhood.

Boundaries and Collaboration

Boundary concerns are very important from both ethical and legal perspectives (Schetky, 1998). In a small town, it is inevitable that children in treatment and their parents will be in a variety of relationships with family members of their therapists: as classmates, students of the therapists' spouses, on the same baseball or soccer team, in the same book group, and so forth. Confidentiality is therefore problematic, and it is important to discuss with patients how they wish to deal with the inevitable overlaps. Copans and Racusin (1983) presented several case histories to illustrate some of these boundary problems and ways to handle them appropriately.

Community collaboration is particularly important in clinical work with children. Clinicians must collaborate with parents, school personnel, and pediatricians or family physicians. In small rural agencies, relationships between doctoral-level psychologists and child psychiatrists are vital but often far easier to achieve than in the more competitive and less collaboratively oriented urban areas. Collaborative opportunities also arise in small agencies when specific staff members develop expertise in particular areas. Working together, the various professionals can better address the needs of their shared patients. For example, a psychologist may pass information to the consulting child psychiatrist about new medications for obsessive–compulsive disorder, or the child psychiatrist may pass information about new behavioral approaches to the psychologist.

Peer support is as important for child mental health clinicians as is supervision and is equally as hard to obtain. It is vital to attend meetings of professional associations for rural practitioners to discuss common issues. The AACAP has a rural listserv for members and a rural child psychiatry committee with open meetings at each year's annual meeting. The American Psychological Association also provides listservs and maintains a Committee on Rural Health that advocates for rural practitioners and supports work in rural communities.

Sample Programs for Provision of Services

Community-Based Programs

A comprehensive, community-based child- and family-centered system of care that emphasizes access and coordination with other agencies is one way to meet mental health needs of children. Case management is key to this system and core in the Ideal System Model for the Mississippi Comprehensive Community Mental Health System for Children with Serious Emotional Disturbance (Mississippi Department of Mental Health, 2001). Built on the belief that children and families should receive services close to their homes and support systems, it depends on parents to identify and meet the needs of their children. Major service components include prevention, early intervention, diagnosis and evaluation, case management, crisis intervention, protection and advocacy, day treatment, respite services, community-based residences, outpatient settings, family education and support, inpatient services, and therapeutic support. It also employs systemwide features such as education, medical and dental care, financial assistance, certain social services, transportation, and volunteers.

Children with behavioral health problems receive care at community mental health centers, in the general health system, and through schools, child welfare agencies, and the juvenile justice system. Urban youth, who have higher rates of psychological diagnoses, are more likely than rural youth to receive care, but the Mississippi program distributes services to rural youth through a widespread network of community mental health centers. The Mississippi Department of Mental Health funds community mental health centers and nonprofit mental health programs to offer general outpatient mental health services at school-based sites. Thus, regional centers are linked to satellite centers (county mental health offices) and school-based services. School officials facilitate access to mental health services for many youths and their family members and deal with the problems of transportation. School personnel promote accessibility to mental health services at the school site. Finally, school-based community mental health therapists provide individual, group, and family counseling to intervene with students with emotional problems before their schoolwork is affected adversely.

In 1991, the University of Kansas Medical Center established a comprehensive distributed care telemedicine program for rural Kansans. The psychiatry component included consultation with child and adolescent clinics whereby the community mental health center contracted with psychiatrists at the medical center. An evaluation of that program revealed a high degree of patient satisfaction and allowed many youths at risk for hospitalization to be treated in their home communities and remain with their families (Ermer, 1999).

School-Based Programs

According to the Center for Substance Abuse Prevention (CSAP; 1999), schools are the most common places for children to receive mental health prevention and early intervention services. This is a direct result of the Department of Education's policies of educating children and youth with emotional and behavioral disorders and training school personnel to meet the needs of these children. These students fail more often and have lower grades than any other category of students with disabilities. Graduation rates for emotionally or behaviorally disordered youth is only 42% (S. M. Martin & Weinke, 1998). Forty-eight percent of the students with disabilities drop out of school. They also experience significant involvement with the juvenile justice system: 73% are arrested within 5 years of dropping out of school. Thus, the mental health needs not met in childhood are ultimately shifted to the justice system, with its concomitant costs and the loss of a potential contributor to society.

Although much progress has been made in providing public school education for students with disabilities, one significant challenge is the successful inclusion of students with emotional and behavioral disorders in the regular classroom. The 1997 Individuals with Disabilities Education Act (IDEA; http://www.ed.gov/offices/OSERS/OSEP) requires that disabled students be educated in the least restrictive environment to the fullest extent possible. This implies providing services in regular classroom settings as part of responsible inclusion for such students. Furthermore, other related and necessary services to enable students to make educational progress, are also the responsibility of the school system; these include individual and group counseling, school-based day treatment programs, and assistance from intervention specialists to students and teachers in the development of behavior management protocols. To this end, officials at West Virginia University have developed an intensive 1-year graduate program to prepare regular education teachers in rural settings to work in inclusive settings with behaviorally disordered youth. Through the use of video disk and computer technology, the program offers learning experiences not readily available in West Virginia's rural setting. Other programs use interactive theater (performer–audience interactive play) to teach children concepts of understanding and thwarting potential sexual abuse (Hayward & Pehrsson, 2000).

Child Mental Health Practitioners and Collaboration With Primary Care Practitioners

Primary care is an opportune modality for meeting the mental health needs of children and adolescents. Psychologists and psychiatrists can aid in the early identification of youth at risk for behavioral, emotional, or substance abuse problems and in subsequent development of treatment programs. One problem with a collaborative model is the reluctance of many primary care practitioners to prescribe medications for seriously mentally ill children, especially those requiring polypharmacy or medications prescribed off-label (which includes almost all psychotropic medications used with children). A solution is to have a child psychiatrist focus consultations on medication concerns for the children in need of polypharmacy. Monthly child psychiatry consultation, with ongoing phone availability, enables primary care practitioners to manage psychotropic medications and collaborate with the psychologist or therapist. Moreover, current data suggest that medication *plus* therapy is more effective than either medication or therapy alone. This argues for a collaborative model involving the primary care practitioner and the therapist and consultations with a child psychiatrist when requested by the therapist or when the therapist is faced with difficult medication questions.

Conclusions and Recommendations

It seems that the most common problem for rural children is access to behavioral health care. The majority of rural youth who need mental health treatment receive none, and few receive adequate treatment. Residents of rural areas suffer from a lack of trained mental health providers, particularly those with expertise in treating children and youth, and there are too few doctorally trained school psychologists in rural school districts. Inefficient communication systems and a lack of public transportation are also barriers to access.

Collaborate With the School Systems to Provide Quality Mental Health

Expansion of mental health services in schools (and other social service systems; see chapter 8) through arrangements between school districts and rural mental health centers is a means by which more youths and their family members can receive care in a nonstigmatizing environment. Therefore, school districts should develop incentives to attract doctorally trained psychologists and psychiatrists.

Increase Recruitment and Retention Programs for Mental Health Providers

Efforts are needed to recruit and retain psychologists and psychiatrists with special expertise in treating youth. There are increasing numbers of children who need help, and compelling data suggest that these children are not getting the help that they need. Incentive programs have been successful in recruiting primary physical health providers to rural and frontier areas and are likely to work just as well with mental health providers.

Involve National Organizations in Recruitment and Retention Issues

Active collaboration between the rural committee of the AACAP and the corresponding committee of the American Psychological Association would go far to increase support for rural psychologists and child psychiatrists and could create a stronger lobby for changes in reimbursements and support for rural child mental health clinicians. In addition to traditional mechanisms such as the National Health Service Corps or Medicare and Medicaid premium payments, school district officials can play an active role in providing or collaborating in training, recruitment, and retention programs.

Seek Legislative Support for Developing Models Based on Rural Dynamics

Legislators need to know that national policies are often based only on urban models and do not provide an accurate picture of rural areas. Although only 20% of the U.S. population lives in a rural area, 72% of the nation's counties are rural (Ricketts, 1999). Moreover, data indicate that substance abuse problems in rural areas of the United States are understudied in comparison with such problems in urban areas (Robertson, Sloboda, Boyd, Beatty, & Kozel, 1997) and may be worse than was previously assumed (Booth, Kirchner, Fortney, Ross, & Rost, 2000). The rate of fatal motor vehicle crashes in which alcohol was a factor is nearly twice as high in rural areas as in urban areas (Hartley, Bird, & Dempsey, 1999). These and other studies suggest that models of funding and care must take rural factors into account.

References

Angold, A., Erkanli, A., Egger, H. L., & Costello, E. J. (2000). Stimulant treatment for children: A community perspective. *Journal of the American Academy of Child and Adolescent Psychiatry, 39,* 975–984.

Bastian, L. D., & Taylor, L. N. (1991). *School crime: A national crime victimization survey report* (NCJ Reference Service No. 131645). Washington, DC: Office of Justice Programs, Bureau of Justice Statistics.

Booth, B. M., Kirchner, J., Fortney, J., Ross, R., & Rost, K. (2000). Rural at-risk drinkers: Correlates and one-year use of alcoholism treatment services. *Journal of Study of Alcohol, 61,* 267–277.

Brody, G. H., Stoneman, Z., Smith, T., & Gibson, N. M. (1999). Sibling relationships in rural African American families. *Journal of Marriage and the Family, 61,* 1046–1057.

Bussing, R., Zima, B. T., & Belin, T. R. (1998). Differential access to care for children with ADHD in special education programs. *Psychiatric Services, 49,* 1226–1229.

Center for Substance Abuse Prevention. (1999, December). *Findings symposium: Division of knowledge development and evaluation.* Symposium conducted at the meeting for Substance Abuse Mental Health Services Administration, Washington, DC.

Clark, S. J., Savitz, L. A., & Randolph, R. K. (1999). Rural children's health. In T. C. Ricketts (Ed.), *Rural health in the United States* (pp. 150–158). New York: Oxford University Press.

Cook, A. D., Copans, S. A., & Schetky, D. H. (1998). Psychiatric treatment of children and adolescents in rural communities: Myths and realities. *Child and Adolescent Psychiatry Clinics in North America, 7,* 673–690.

Copans, S., & Racusin, R. (1983). Rural child psychiatry. *Journal of the American Academy of Child Psychiatry, 22,* 184–190.

Costello, E. J., Costello, A. J., Edelbrock, C., Burns, B. J., Culcan, M. K., Brent, D., et al. (1988). Psychiatric disorders in pediatric primary care: Prevalence and risk factors. *Archives of General Psychiatry, 45,* 1107–1116.

Cutchin, M. P. (2000). Retention of rural physicians: Place integration and the triumph of habit. *Occupational Therapy Journal of Research, 20*(Suppl. 1), 106S–111S.

Cutrona, C. E., Halvorson, M. B. J., & Russell, D. W. (1996). Mental health services for rural children, youth, and their families. In C. A. Heflinger & C. T. Nixon (Eds.), *Families and the mental health system for children and adolescents: Policy, services, and research* (pp. 217–237). Thousand Oaks, CA: Sage.

DeMuri, G. P., & Purschwitz, M. A. (2000, December). Farm injuries in children: A review. *Wisconsin Medical Journal, 99*(9), 51–55.

DiClemente, R. J., Brown, L. K., Beausoleil, N. I., & Lodico, M. (1993). Comparison of AIDS knowledge and HIV-related sexual risk behaviors among adolescents in low and high AIDS prevalence communities. *Journal of Adolescent Health, 14,* 231–236.

Ermer, D. J. (1999). Experience with a rural telepsychiatry clinic for children and adolescents. *Psychiatric Services, 50,* 260–261.

Fahs, P. S., Smith, B. E., Atav, A. S. , Britten, M. X., Collins, M. S., Morgan, L. C., et al. (1999). Integrative research review of risk behaviors among adolescents in rural, suburban, and urban areas. *Journal of Adolescent Health, 24,* 230–243.

Grossman, D. C. (2000, Spring–Summer). The history of injury control and the epidemiology of child and adolescent injuries. *Future Child, 10*(1), 23–52.

Hartley, D., Bird, D. C., & Dempsey, P. (1999). Rural mental health and substance abuse. In T. C. Ricketts (Ed.), *Rural health in the United States* (pp. 159–178). New York: Oxford University Press.

Hayward, K. S., & Pehrsson, D. E. (2000). Interdisciplinary action supporting sexual assault prevention efforts in rural elementary schools. *Journal of Community Health Nursing, 17,* 141–150.

Hoberman, H. M. (1991) Ethnic minority status and adolescent mental health services utilization. *Journal of Mental Health Administration, 19,* 246–267.

Lee, B. C., Jenkins, L. S., & Westaby, J. D. (1997). Factors influencing exposure of children to major hazards on family farms. *Journal of Rural Health, 13,* 206–215.

Martin, S. L., Kupersmidt, J. B., & Harter, K. S. M. (1996). Children of farm laborers: Utilization of services for mental health problems. *Community Mental Health Journal, 32,* 327–340.

Martin, S. M., & Weinke, W. W. (1998). Using cutting edge technology to prepare teachers to work with children and youth who have emotional/behavioral disorders. *Education and Treatment of Children, 21,* 385–395.

Mississippi Department of Mental Health. (2001). *Mississippi Department of Mental Health state plan for community mental health services: Children with severe emotional disturbance and adults with serious emotional disturbances.* Jackson, MS: Mississippi Department of Mental Health, Division of Planning and Public Information.

National Institutes of Health Consensus Development Panel. (2000). National Institutes of Health Consensus Development Conference statement: Diagnosis and treatment of attention-deficit/hyperactivity disorder (ADHD). *Journal of the American Academy of Child & Adolescent Psychiatry, 39,* 182–193.

Neighbors, H. W., Bashur, R., Price, R., Selig, S., Donabedian, A., & Shannon, G. (1992). Ethnic minority mental health service delivery: A review of the literature. *Research in Community and Mental Health, 7,* 55–71.

Ricketts, T. C. (Ed.). (1999). *Rural health in the United States.* New York: Oxford University Press.

Robertson, E., Sloboda, Z., Boyd, G. M., Beatty, L., & Kozel, N. (Eds.). (1997). *Rural substance abuse: State of knowledge and issues* (National Institute on Drug Abuse Research Monograph No. 168, National Institutes of Health Publication No. 97-4177). Washington, DC: U.S. Government Printing Office.

Schetky, D. H. (1998). Ethics and the clinician in custody disputes. *Child and Adolescent Psychiatric Clinics of North America, 7,* 454–463.

Simons, R. L., Johnson, C., Beaman, J., Conger, R. D., & Whitbeck, L. B. (1996). Parents and peer group as mediators of the effect of community structure on adolescent problem behavior. *American Journal of Community Psychology, 24,* 145–171.

Stamm, B. H. (1998). Clinical applications of telehealth in mental health. *Professional Psychology: Research and Practice, 29,* 536–542. Retrieved March 13, 2001, from http://www.apa.org /journals/pro/pro296536.html

Stamm, B. H. (1999). Creating virtual community: Telehealth and self care updated. In B. H. Stamm (Ed.), *Secondary traumatic stress: Self-care issues for clinicians, researchers and educators* (2nd ed., pp. 178–210). Lutherville, MD: Sidran Press.

Stearns, J. A., & Stearns, M. A. (2000). Graduate medical education for rural physicians: Curriculum and retention. *Journal of Rural Health, 16,* 273–277.

Steinberg, S., & Fleming, P. (2000, Winter). The geographic distribution of AIDS in the United States: Is there a rural epidemic? *Journal of Rural Health, 16*(1), 11–19.

Tarnowski, K. J. (1991). Disadvantaged children and families in pediatric primary care settings: I. Broadening the scope of integrated mental health services. *Journal of Clinical Child Psychology, 20,* 351–359.

Valois, R. F., Dowda, M., Trost, S., Weinrich, M., Felton, G., & Pate, R. R. (1998). Cigarette smoking experimentation among rural fifth grade students. *American Journal of Health Behavior, 22,* 101–107.

Wagner, J. D., Menke, E. M., & Ciccone, J. K. (1995). What is known about the health of rural homeless families? *Public Health Nursing, 12,* 400–408.

13

The New Psychology of Men: Application to Rural Men

Ronald F. Levant and Corey Habben

Those not familiar with the new psychology of men sometimes ask, "Why do we need a psychology of men? Isn't all psychology the psychology of men?" The answer is yes, men have been the focal point of most psychological research, but only in studies that viewed men as representative of humanity as a whole. Feminist scholars challenged this traditional viewpoint by arguing for a gender-specific approach and have rewritten the canon on the psychology of women. In the same spirit, since the mid-1980s, men's studies scholars have examined masculinity not as a normative referent but rather as a complex and problematic construct. In so doing, they have provided a framework for a psychological approach to men in which they question traditional norms, such as the emphasis on competition, status, toughness, and emotional stoicism. Within this framework, certain male problems, such as aggression and violence, devaluation of women, fear and hatred of homosexual people, detached fathering, and neglect of health needs, are viewed as unfortunate but predictable results of the male role socialization process (Brod, 1987; Levant & Pollack, 1995; O'Neil, Good, & Holmes, 1995; Pleck, 1981, 1995). Men's studies scholars have also provided a framework for creating positive new definitions of masculinity that support optimal development of men, women, and children.

In this chapter, we provide a brief introduction to the new psychology of men, covering, in turn, the gender role strain paradigm, masculinity ideology, and types of male gender role strain. We continue with an application of this new work to rural men and end the chapter with a series of recommendations for behavioral health care work with rural men.

This new psychology of men is both overdue and urgently needed. Men are disproportionately represented among many problem populations: substance abusers; the homeless; perpetrators of family and interpersonal violence; parents estranged from their children; sex addicts and sex offenders; victims of homicide, suicide, and fatal automobile accidents; and victims of lifestyle- and stress-related fatal illnesses (Brooks & Silverstein, 1995; Eisler, 1995). A new psychology of men may contribute to the understanding and solution of

Dr. Levant can be reached at Nova Southeastern University, 3301 College Avenue, Ft. Lauderdale, FL 33314. E-mail: levantr@nova.edu.

Several sections in this chapter are reprinted from "The New Psychology of Men" by R. Levant, 1996, *Professional Psychology: Research and Practice, 27,* 259–265. Copyright 1996 by the American Psychological Association. Adapted with permission.

some of the male problems that have long affected women, men, children, and society in negative ways.

Moreover, because of long delays in dealing with many of these problems, there currently exists a "crisis of connection" between men and women (Levant, 1996). As a result, the pressures on men to behave in ways that conflict with various aspects of traditional masculinity ideology have never been greater. These new pressures—pressures to commit to relationships, to communicate their innermost feelings, to nurture children, to share in housework, to integrate sexuality with love, and to curb aggression and violence— have shaken traditional masculinity ideology to such an extent that there is now a "masculinity crisis" in which many feel bewildered and confused, and the pride associated with being a man is lower than at any time (Levant, 1997a). Many such men are gravitating to organizations such as Promise Keepers (Promise Keepers, 1994) and the Fatherhood Initiative (Blankenhorn, 1995), which propose to return the man to his "rightful place" as the "leader of his family"; some critics of such organizations say that these groups are reversing the gains of the women's movement. A new psychology of men might help men find solutions to the masculinity crisis and the crisis of connection, solutions that enhance rather than inflame gender relations, and provide men with tools for a reconstruction of the traditional male code (Levant & Kopecky, 1995). Indeed, there is some indication that this new psychology is becoming an important part of gender studies (see Cohen, 2001, Kimmel, 2000; Kimmel & Messner, 2001).

The purpose of this chapter is to introduce this new field and sketch out its potential to rural men. We cover the *gender role strain paradigm,* masculinity ideology, and the three varieties of male gender role strain: (a) discrepancy strain, (b) dysfunction strain, and (c) trauma strain.

The New Psychology of Men and Its Implications for Rural Mental Health Care

The Gender Role Strain Paradigm

According to the new psychology of men, gender roles are viewed not as biological or even social givens but rather as psychologically and socially constructed entities that bring advantages and disadvantages and, of more importance, can change. In this perspective, biological differences are acknowledged, but the biological differences of sex do not make for *masculinity* and *femininity*. These notions are socially constructed from bits and pieces of biological, psychological, and social experience. Traditional constructions of gender serve patriarchal purposes; nontraditional constructions, such as those that Gilmore (1990) described among the Tahitians and the Semai, serve more egalitarian purposes.

The gender role strain paradigm, originally formulated by Pleck (1981), is the forerunner of social constructionism in the new psychology of men, of social constructionism, and of modern critical thinking about masculinity. It spawned a number of major research programs that produced important data, which deepened the understanding of the emotional strain that men experience when they attempt to live up to the traditional, yet impossible, male role.

Pleck demonstrated that the paradigm that dominated the research on masculinity for 50 years (1930–1980), the *gender role identity paradigm,* not only poorly accounted for the observed data but also promoted the patriarchal bifurcation of society on the basis of stereotyped gender roles. In its place, Pleck proposed the gender role strain paradigm.

According to the older gender role identity paradigm, people have a psychological need to have a gender role identity, and optimal personality development hinges on its formation. The extent to which this *inherent* need is met is determined by how completely people embrace traditional gender roles. The development of appropriate gender role identity is viewed as a failure-prone process; and failure for men to achieve a masculine gender role identity is thought to result in homosexuality, negative attitudes towards women, or defensive hypermasculinity. The gender role identity paradigm springs from the same philosophical roots as the *essentialist* or *nativist* view of sex roles: the notion that there is a clear masculine *essence* that is historically invariant.

In contrast, according to the gender role strain paradigm, contemporary gender roles are contradictory and inconsistent; the proportion of people who violate gender roles is high; violation of gender roles leads to condemnation and negative psychological consequences; actual or imagined violation of gender roles leads people to overconform to them; violating gender roles has more severe consequences for men and boys than for women and girls; and certain prescribed gender role traits (such as male aggression) are often dysfunctional. In this paradigm, appropriate gender roles are determined by the prevailing gender ideology (which is operationally defined by gender role stereotypes and norms) and are imposed on the developing child by parents, teachers, and peers—the cultural transmitters who subscribe to the prevailing gender ideology. As noted previously, this paradigm springs from the same philosophical roots as social constructionism, which is the perspective that notions of masculinity and femininity are relational, socially constructed, and subject to change.

Masculinity Ideology

Thompson and Pleck (1995) proposed the term *masculinity ideology* to characterize the core construct in the research assessing attitudes toward men and male roles. Masculinity, or gender ideology, is a construct very different from the older notion of gender orientation. Gender orientation arises out of the identity paradigm and "presumes that masculinity is rooted in actual differences between men and women" (p. 130). This approach has attempted to assess the personality traits associated more often with men than with women. In contrast, studies of masculinity ideology have been conducted according to a normative approach, in which masculinity is viewed as a socially constructed gender ideal for men. Whereas the masculine man in the orientation or trait approach is one who possesses particular personality traits, the traditional man in the ideology or normative approach "is one who endorses the ideology that men *should* have sex-specific characteristics" (p. 131). Thompson and

Pleck adduced evidence to support the idea that gender orientation and gender ideologies are independent and have different correlates.

MASCULINITY IDEOLOGIES. According to the strain paradigm, there is no single standard for masculinity, nor is there an unvarying masculinity ideology. Rather, because masculinity is a social construction, ideals of manhood may differ for men of different social classes, races, ethnic groups, sexual orientations, life stages, and historical eras. Following the example of Brod (1987), we therefore prefer to speak of masculinity *ideologies*. To illustrate, consider these descriptions of male codes among four ethnic groups in the United States:

> African-American males have adopted distinctive actions and attitudes known as *cool pose*. . . . Emphasizing honor, virility, and physical strength, the Latino male adheres to a code of *machismo*. . . . The American-Indian male struggles to maintain contact with a way of life and the traditions of elders while faced with economic castration and political trauma. . . . Asian-American men resolve uncertainty privately in order to save face and surrender personal autonomy to family obligations and needs. (Lazur & Majors, 1995, p. 338)

TRADITIONAL MASCULINITY IDEOLOGY. Despite the diversity in the contemporary United States, Pleck (1995) pointed out that "there is a *particular* constellation of standards and expectations that individually and jointly have various kinds of negative concomitants" (p. 20). It is common to refer to this as *traditional* masculinity ideology, because it was the dominant view before the deconstruction of gender that began in the 1970s.

Traditional masculinity ideology is thought to be a multidimensional construct. David and Brannon (1976) identified four components of the traditional ideology: Men should not be feminine (labeled by David & Brannon as "no sissy stuff"); men should strive to be respected for successful achievement ("the big wheel"); men should never show weakness ("the sturdy oak"); and men should seek adventure and risk, even accepting violence if necessary ("give 'em hell"). More recently, Levant et al. (1992) defined the traditional ideology in terms of seven dimensions: the requirement to avoid all things feminine; the injunction to restrict one's emotional life; the emphasis on toughness and aggression; the injunction to be self-reliant; the emphasis on achieving status above all else; nonrelational, objectifying attitudes toward sexuality; and fear and hatred of homosexual people.

Types of Male Gender Role Strain

Pleck (1995), in an update on the gender role strain paradigm, pointed out that his original formulation of the paradigm stimulated research on three varieties of male gender role strain, which he termed *discrepancy strain, dysfunction strain,* and *trauma strain* (p. 12). Discrepancy strain results when a man fails to live up to his internalized manhood ideal, which is often a close approximation of the traditional code. Dysfunction strain results when a man fulfills the requirements of the male code, because many of the characteristics viewed as desirable in men can have negative side effects on the men themselves and on those close to them. Trauma strain results from the ordeal of the male role socialization process, which is now recognized as inherently traumatic.

DISCREPANCY STRAIN. One approach to investigating discrepancy strain used a version of the time-honored self/ideal-self research paradigm (e.g., Deutsch & Gilbert, 1976), in which participants were asked first to describe the ideal man and then to describe themselves, both times using adjectival rating scales. The discrepancy between the two ratings was used as an index of discrepancy strain, which was then studied in terms of its correlations with other variables such as self-esteem. This line of research has not been particularly productive.

Another method has been more fruitful. This approach involves not asking participants whether discrepancy strain exists for them but, rather, inquiring whether they would experience particular gender discrepancies as conflictual or stressful if they did exist. Investigators in two major research programs have used this approach: O'Neil et al. (1995), in their work on male gender role conflict, and Eisler and Skidmore (1995), in their work on masculine gender role stress.

DYSFUNCTION STRAIN. The second type of gender role strain is dysfunction strain. The notion behind dysfunction strain is that fulfillment of the male code requirements can be dysfunctional because many of the characteristics viewed as desirable in men can have negative side effects on both the men and those close to them. Pleck (1995) reviewed some of the research that documents the existence of dysfunction strain, including studies that revealed negative outcomes associated with masculine gender-related personality traits on the one hand and lack of involvement in family roles on the other hand.

Brooks and Silverstein (1995), in a far-reaching discussion of the "dark side" of masculinity, provided a taxonomy of the problems that result from dysfunction strain. These are significant social and public health problems that, Brooks and Silverstein argued, result from adherence to traditional masculinity ideology. These problems include (a) violence, including male violence against women in the family, rape and sexual assault, and sexual harassment; (b) sexual excess, including promiscuity, involvement with pornography, and sexual addiction; (c) socially irresponsible behaviors, including chemical dependence, risk-seeking behavior, physical self-abuse, absent fathering, and homelessness and vagrancy; and (d) relationship dysfunctions, including inadequate emotional partnering, nonnurturing fathering, and nonparticipative household partnering.

TRAUMA STRAIN. The concept of trauma strain has been applied to groups of men whose experiences with gender role strain were thought to be particularly harsh. This includes professional athletes (Messner, 1992), war veterans (Brooks, 1990), and survivors of child abuse, including sexual abuse (Lisak, 1995). It is also recognized that gay and bisexual men are traumatized by male gender role strain by growing up in a heterosexist society (Harrison, 1995). Beyond this recognition, there has emerged a perspective on the male role socialization process in which socialization under traditional masculinity ideology is viewed as *inherently* traumatic (Levant & Kopecky, 1995; Levant & Pollack, 1995).

Application to Rural Men

In view of the assumptions underlying the social construction of masculinity (that is, that masculinity is socially constructed from a combination of biological factors, psychological variables, and social experience), the rules of masculinity that are internalized by men rely rather significantly on the environment. As boys learn the masculine code from fathers, mothers, peers, teachers, neighbors, coaches, and countless others, the rules that are passed on to them represent the doctrine of generations past; these are the lessons learned from necessary adaptations to an environment. The ethic of hard and dangerous work, for example, did not emerge spontaneously; it emerged out of necessity from a combination of factors such as time, place, and available resources.

As environments vary, so do the subsequent "rules" (i.e., ideologies) that emerge from them. A relatively stable, isolated environment can be thought of as a precursor to a culture. As we have noted, masculinity ideologies can vary from culture to culture. Furthermore, it appears that masculinity ideologies also vary *within* cultures. For example, it may be cumbersome to determine what is considered traditional African American masculinity ideology, inasmuch as there are certainly many "masculinities" within African American subcultures. What can be presumed in this observation is that various cultures socially construct masculinity somewhat differently.

Cultures need not be thought of as only a collection of similar ethnicities or races. Various collections of people have unique cultures. Military culture, Appalachian culture, academic culture, and gay culture are some examples of cultures in which gender ideologies or socially constructed rules can help define an identity. Rural lifestyle is another of these so-called cultures. Rural masculinity ideology may be just as different as it is similar to what is often referred to as traditional masculinity ideology. However, both share the same elements of male gender role strain (condemnation and negative psychological consequences for violation of gender roles and a resulting pressure to over-conform to them). Just as in other cultures, there is probably more diversity *within* rural male culture than there is between rural male culture and other cultures. The masculinity code for a man raised on a Hopi Indian reservation in northeastern Arizona may be different from that of a Norwegian man raised in a rural Minnesota town.

The psychological study of masculinity and that of rural health are relatively young fields. As a result, little has been written about rural men from the perspective of the new psychology of men. How then, does a clinician practice with a full understanding of the culture of rural men? Sue (1998) identified three elements of the culturally competent counselor: *scientific mindedness* in forming hypotheses about a culturally-different client; *dynamic sizing,* or the ability to know when to generalize and when to individualize; and *culture-specific expertise* in understanding and obtaining specific knowledge about the cultures of a client as well as culture-appropriate interventions.

These elements are important to consider in working with rural men. The characteristics of a rural area (e.g., less crowding, less access to a variety of services, more familiarity and recognition of or by others in the community) interact with masculinity ideology in many ways. In work with rural men, some of the following considerations should be reviewed.

General Considerations About Rural Men

MASCULINITY TENDS TO BE MORE TRADITIONAL. With more homogeneous populations, fewer people, less rapid change, and more intracommunity contact, masculinity ideology tends to maintain a status quo, unfamiliar with the often radical changes of a more densely populated area. Therefore, adherence to a more traditional code of masculinity with rules, such as "Real men don't cry," should not be seen as abnormal. Emotional expression may in fact be prohibited for rural men.

THERE MAY BE MORE DIVERSITY WITHIN A RURAL MALE CULTURE THAN AMONG SUCH CULTURES. Although rural men tend to be more traditional, there is great variability. As various forms of media expose even the most remote communities and rural areas to other cultures and viewpoints, there is greater opportunity for rural men to challenge traditional views.

PUBLIC IMAGE AND REPUTATION ARE STRONGLY EMPHASIZED. Rural men often live in communities small enough that "everybody knows everybody." It is not uncommon for community members to know personal information about other community members: "A man is as only as good as his word" and "Word travels fast." Knowledge of socially frowned-upon behaviors such as alcoholism, infidelity, or physical abuse can circulate faster through a rural community than through an urban one. As a result, rural men are more likely to try to adhere to a *higher moral code* or else to keep their problems very private.

RURAL MEN ARE OFTEN RELATIONSHIP ORIENTED. As a result of higher visibility and more interaction with a larger percentage of the entire community, rural men interact more *intimately* with people in their communities. This lends itself to a code of being a "good neighbor." Whereas men in urban areas can often live without even knowing who their next door neighbors are, rural men are much more likely to see community members on a more frequent basis: at church, in restaurants, while shopping, at school events. As a result, "the good neighbor doctrine" interacts with masculinity ideology in a way that men are more likely to "pitch in and help" a relative stranger.

RURAL MEN TEND TO BE LESS LIKELY TO SEEK PSYCHOTHERAPY. Some of the basic elements of psychotherapy (i.e., expressing vulnerability, "talking through" problems, gaining access to emotions) conflict with traditional masculinity ideology. Access to professionals is much more limited. A highly visible reputation may be at stake if others in the community discover that a man is seeking psychological help. As a result, the rural man is more likely to discuss problems with his physician or clergyman than with a health care provider from *outside* the community.

RURAL MEN IN GENERAL TEND TO HAVE A MORE TRUSTING ATTITUDE. Perhaps because of the "good neighbor doctrine" and other factors such as lower crime rates, rural men are often less cynical about the intentions of others. A rural man may be more likely to begin a new relationship by trusting a new person until he finds reason to do otherwise (as opposed to slowly building trust). This may prove to be beneficial in establishing a therapeutic relationship, particularly if the provider can reinforce that trust rather than give the client reasons to do otherwise.

Recommendations and Conclusions

Integrating these considerations into clinical work with rural men leads to several recommendations.

Consider Rural Men As a Culture

Although other significant factors are often involved in the man's culture, the rural male ideology (resulting from interaction between the rural setting and masculinity) should be considered as well. Just as with any culture, it is important that the clinician not form assumptions about a rural man and instead learns about his culture to better understand him as an individual.

Gain an Awareness of How the Rural Culture Affects Masculinity

The provider should consider the context of a rural man's environment and how it affects his view of masculinity. The dynamics of a small town or rural area, the "good neighbor doctrine," and a slower process of change from traditional masculinity are some examples.

Adapt Your Style to Accommodate the Rural Man in Therapy

A better therapeutic alliance will be built if the provider can see the rural man's point of view, rather than expecting him to see the provider's. For example, a common mistake many psychologists and other professionals make is criticizing or correcting a more traditional man for not expressing his emotions in therapy. If this does not align with his ideological values of masculinity, focusing sessions on emotions or feelings may only create a distance in the therapeutic alliance and lead to early termination of therapy.

Take a Problem-Solving, Skills-Building Approach

Although this is not a hard rule, rural men tend to respond better to an approach that identifies problems and teaches new skills. As opposed to admitting vulnerability and weakness, a rural man will likely feel more validated and motivated by an approach that will "make him a better man." (For an example of such an approach developed for men, see Levant, 1997b, 1998.)

Build a Therapeutic Alliance on the Foundations of Trust and Respect

Because these are often the foundations of many male relationships, the elements of trust and respect are integral to building a true rapport with rural men.

Be Aware of the Rural Male Value of Self-Reliance

Rural men may be less likely to seek psychotherapy on their own and prefer to "pick themselves up by their own bootstraps." Relying on a professional for help requires a deviation from the rules of rural masculinity ideology; therefore, it will be much more beneficial to help the rural man *build on* his self-reliance than to attempt to *strip it down*.

In this chapter, we introduced the new psychology of men, reviewing the gender role strain paradigm, masculinity ideology, and the three varieties of male gender role strain, and we sketched out their potential application to rural men. It is our hope that this new work will open up areas for assessment, intervention, and applied research in the issues of rural men.

References

Blankenhorn, D. (1995). *Fatherless America: Confronting our most urgent social problem.* New York: Basic Books.

Brod, H. (1987). *The making of the masculinities: The new men's studies.* Boston: Unwin Hyman.

Brooks, G. R. (1990). Post-Vietnam gender role strain: A needed concept? *Professional Psychology: Research and Practice, 21,* 18–25.

Brooks, G. R., & Silverstein, L. S. (1995). Understanding the dark side of masculinity: An interactive systems model. In R. F. Levant & W. S. Pollack (Eds.), *A new psychology of men* (pp. 252–279). New York: Basic Books.

Cohen, T. F. (2001). *Men and masculinity: A text reader.* Belmont, CA: Wadsworth.

David, D., & Brannon, R. (Eds.). (1976). *The forty-nine percent majority: The male sex role.* Reading, MA: Addison-Wesley.

Deutsch, C., & Gilbert, L. (1976). Sex role stereotypes: Effects on perceptions of self and others and on personal adjustment. *Journal of Counseling Psychology, 23,* 373–370.

Eisler, R., & Skidmore, J. (1987). Masculine gender role stress: Scale development and components factors in the appraisal of stressful situations. *Behavior Modification, 11,* 123–136.

Eisler, R. M. (1995). The relationship between masculine gender role stress and men's health risk: The validation of a construct. In R. F. Levant & W. S. Pollack (Eds.), *A new psychology of men* (pp. 207–225). New York: Basic Books.

Gilmore, D. (1990). *Manhood in the making: Cultural concepts of masculinity.* New Haven, CT: Yale University Press.

Harrison, J. (1995). Roles, identities, and sexual orientation: Homosexuality, heterosexuality, and bisexuality. In R. F. Levant & W. S. Pollack (Eds.), *A new psychology of men* (pp. 359–382). New York: Basic Books.

Kimmel, M. S. (2000). *The gendered society.* New York: Oxford University Press.

Kimmel, M. S., & Messner, A. (2001). *Men's lives* (5th ed.). Needham, MA: Allyn & Bacon.

Lazur, R. F., & Majors, R. (1995). Men of color: Ethnocultural variations of male gender role strain. In R. F. Levant & W. S. Pollack (Eds.), *A new psychology of men* (pp. 337–358). New York: Basic Books.

Levant, R. (1996). The new psychology of men. *Professional Psychology: Research and Practice, 27,* 259–265.

Levant, R. F. (1996). The crisis of connection between men and women. *Journal of Men's Studies, 5,* 1–12.

Levant, R. F. (1997a). The masculinity crisis. *Journal of Men's Studies, 5,* 221–231.

Levant, R. F. (1997b). *Men and emotions: A psychoeducational approach* [Videorecording]. Hicksville, NY: Newbridge Communications. (Available from R. F. Levant, Center for Psychological Studies, Nova Southeastern University, 3301 College Ave., Ft. Lauderdale, FL 33314.)

Levant, R. F. (1998). Desperately seeking language: Understanding, assessing and treating normative male alexithymia. In W. S. Pollack & R. F. Levant (Eds.), *New psychotherapy for men* (pp. 35–56). New York: Basic Books.

Levant, R. F., Hirsch, L., Celentano, E., Cozza, T., Hill, S., MacEachern, M., et al. (1992). The male role: An investigation of norms and stereotypes. *Journal of Mental Health Counseling, 14,* 325–337.

Levant, R. F., & Kopecky, G. (1995). *Masculinity reconstructed.* New York: Dutton. (Out of print. Available from R. F. Levant, Center for Psychological Studies, Nova Southeastern University, 3301 College Ave., Ft. Lauderdale, FL 33314.)

Levant, R. F., & Pollack, W. S. (Eds.). (1995). *A new psychology of men.* New York: Basic Books.

Lisak, D. (1995, August). *Integrating gender analysis in psychotherapy with male survivors of abuse.* Paper presented at the Annual Convention of the American Psychological Association, New York.

Messner, M. A. (1992). *Power at play: Sports and the problem of masculinity.* Boston: Beacon Press.

O'Neil, J. M., Good, G. E., & Holmes, S. (1995). Fifteen years of theory and research on men's gender role conflict: New paradigms for empirical research. In R. F. Levant & W. S. Pollack (Eds.), *A new psychology of men* (pp. 207–225). New York: Basic Books.

Pleck, J. H. (1981). *The myth of masculinity.* Cambridge, MA: MIT Press.

Pleck, J. H. (1995). The gender role strain paradigm: An update. In R. F. Levant & W. S. Pollack (Eds.), *A new psychology of men* (pp. 11–32). New York: Basic Books.

Promise Keepers. (1994). *Seven promises of a promise keeper.* Colorado Springs, CO: Focus on the Family Publishing.

Sue, S. (1998). In search of cultural competence in psychotherapy and counseling. *American Psychologist, 32,* 616–624.

Thompson, E. H., & Pleck, J. H. (1995). Masculinity ideology: A review of research instrumentation on men and masculinities. In R. F. Levant & W. S. Pollack (Eds.), *A new psychology of men* (pp. 129–163). New York: Basic Books.

14

Rural Women: Strategies and Resources for Meeting Their Behavioral Health Needs

Mary Beth Kenkel

The purpose of this chapter is to substitute a more realistic portrayal of rural women for the stereotype. To do so is not easy; there is little research on rural women. The few exceptions include the report *The Behavioral Health Care Needs of Rural Women* from the American Psychological Association Committee on Rural Health (Mulder et al., 2000). Asking questions about rural women's behavioral health is an important first step in bringing attention to their needs. The portrait of rural women begins to take shape through the research findings presented in this chapter, but large sections still need to be filled in through future research.

"The worst kind of oppression and inequality occurs to groups that are 'invisible'. If no one has identified rural women as an oppressed class, whence will come the solutions to the problems?" (Cheitman, 1981, p. 19). For years, women living in rural and frontier areas were made "invisible" by the several aspects of their marginal status: being rural residents, being women, and, in some cases, being members of an ethnic minority. Few questions were asked about the needs, problems, strengths, or resources of the women, and even fewer answers were obtained. The picture of rural women, if any picture at all existed, was of a stoic, steady, persevering woman who served as a dependable, comforting helpmate to her spouse and a caretaker of the family and home.

Much about this stereotype of the rural woman is true; it does portray the strengths and roles of many women living in rural communities. However, it also masks differences among rural women and frontier women—differences attributable to income, race, ethnicity, geographical region, education, employment, age, marital status, and sexual orientation. This stereotype also distorts the role of women in the rural workforce because their significant impact on the economy is neglected. Finally, the pressing needs and problems faced by rural women on a daily basis are overlooked.

Dr. Kenkel can be reached at School of Psychology, Florida Institute of Technology, 150 W. University Boulevard, Melbourne, FL 32901, 321-674-8142. E-mail: mkenkel@fit.edu.

Behavioral Health Needs of Rural Women

Rural women are members of a diverse group. They live on farms and reservations, in frontier areas, and in small isolated towns near metropolitan areas. Rural women of differing ethnic backgrounds are located disproportionately throughout regions in the United States; for example, large populations of African Americans are in the rural South; Mexican Americans, in the Southwest; American Indians, in the Western states; Asians and Pacific Islanders, in Hawaii; and Alaska Natives and Aleuts, in Alaska. The profile of rural women changes constantly because of the immigration of urban retirees, relocated urbanites, and migrant and seasonal workers and because of the emigration of young rural residents (Kivett, 1998).

Although rural women are generally poorer and less educated than urban women (Lingg, Braden, Goldstein, & Cooley, 1993), differences in education and income exist within the rural population. About 27% of rural workers, mainly women and minorities, held low-wage jobs in 1999. Low-wage employment was clustered in counties in the South and Great Plains, which tended to have small populations, less diversified economies, and locations remote from urban centers. In 1998, poverty rates continued to vary substantially by race and ethnicity; families headed by a single woman had the lowest median family income of all groups, with 35% of these households classified as poor (more than four times that of families headed by a married couple; U.S. Department of Agriculture, Economic Research Service, 2000). These within-group differences seen across race and region appear to be increasing over time (Hoyt, Conger, Valde, & Weihs, 1997).

Certain themes and values, however, still do dominate the lives of rural women. They value independence and privacy, and they value the space and freedom derived from living in the country. At the same time, rural women have a clear sense of the value of relationships with family and friends. In the family, women's roles are related largely to the maintenance of social relationships; men define the appropriate instrumental tasks. Rural women are involved in ongoing networks of exchange and informal support in their communities and derive much of their identity and satisfaction from these connections with family, friends, and the community. In this context, they often experience challenges trying to meet their own needs while remaining attentive to all the needs of others. Closeness to the land is a prevalent theme, as is a connection with nature and animal life. Work ethic, religion and spirituality, and optimism are key values guiding the lives of rural women (Johnson, 1995; Shenk, 1998).

Because of rural residents' greater involvement in off-farm work, and because of increased ethnic diversity in low-wage industries (Bokemeier & Tickamyer, 1985; Lamphere, 1992), the traditional agrarian values of rural communities are changing (Naples, 1994). Similarly, as rural women pursue more employment opportunities outside the home and off the farm, their values are being tested and undergoing change. Delworth, Veach, and Grohe (1988) identified four value orientations (traditional, conflicted, emerging, and synthesis) related to the stance of women as they dealt with the conflicts between the traditional role of nurturer and emotional leader and the greater independence and instrumentality in the workplace. The pull toward traditional values is strong, usually reinforced by family and the community. However, the *emerging* women were resentful that they were not being recognized as individuals in their own right, experiencing "many of the same conflicts and symptoms often seen in urban middle-class White women in the 1960s: depression, physical symptomatology, and anxiety" (Delworth et al., 1988, p. 426).

Mental Health Issues

Although researchers have sought to demonstrate overall differences between urban and rural populations in the prevalence of psychiatric disorders, the variability within urban and rural populations has made for complex results. In the Epidemiologic Catchment Area Study, rural and urban prevalence rates were compared across psychiatric disorders. The rural prevalence rate was 32%, and the urban rate was only slightly higher, at 34% (Robins & Regier, 1991).

Similarly, studies of women have not revealed rural and urban differences when other relevant sociodemographic variables are controlled. For women in Iowa, depressive symptoms were unrelated to the size of their community (Hoyt et al., 1997). In a study of women older than 55, Craft, Johnson, and Ortega (1998) found that depression was related to feelings of financial hardship but not to urban vs. rural locale. Among the Mexican migrant farmworkers in central California, the prevalence of depression as measured by the Center for Epidemiologic Studies Depression measure (CES-D), was 20%, the same as the normative case rate (Alderete, Vega, Kolody, & Aguilar-Gaxiola, 1999). However, although the overall prevalence rates of rural women's mental health disorders are similar to those for urban women, *how* those needs are (and are not) expressed and *how* to effectively address the needs may vary widely.

Affective disorders are a leading mental health problem for women, rural and urban alike. Major depression and dysthymia affect twice as many women as men. This higher vulnerability may be a result of the particular stresses that many women face, such as major responsibilities at home and work, single parenthood, and caring for children and aging parents (National Institute of Mental Health, 2000). Depression in rural areas follows these same trends. For example, Hoyt et al. (1997) found that increases in depressive symptoms among women in Iowa over a 1-year period were associated with lower levels of income, experiences with financial stress, younger age, greater health limitations, being unmarried, and less sense of personal control. In a study with Mexican American women, Vega, Kolody, Valle, and Hough (1986) found that depression was related to low income, less education, more time in the United States, marital status, and the number of adults in the household. Within a population of farmworkers with very low income and education, depression was higher among those who were divorced, widowed, or separated; among those with higher levels of acculturation; among those who experienced high stress as a result of discrimination; and among those with low levels of social and tangible support (Alderete et al., 1999). Like many other studies, this study shows the importance of social support as a buffer against depression. In addition, the downside of acculturation is revealed. As a person becomes more acculturated and loses a coherent cultural framework, depressive symptoms increase. Other factors associated with depression in rural women include the stressors of poverty, single parenting, isolation, unpredictable and irregular farming income, and the lack of mental health, social, educational, and child care resources (Bushy, 1993; Hauenstein & Boyd, 1994; Haussman & Halseth, 1983; McGrath, Keita, Strickland, & Russo, 1990; Weissman & Klerman, 1987).

In rural areas, women assume the major caregiver roles. Cultural values and norms emphasize this role, and such caregiving is expected by family members (Glasgow, 2000). In a study of chronically mentally ill persons in Mississippi, rural patients were more likely to live with their families and less likely to receive case management or day treatment services than urban patients were (Sullivan, Jackson, & Spritzer, 1996). The home care of a chronically ill relative puts great physical and emotional demands on family members, particularly wives and mothers. They must manage the patient's problematic behavior; handle competition between the caregiver role and other family, marital, and work roles; and deal with the stigma surrounding mental illness, including the community's harsh reactions to poorly understood behavior. There are additional burdens on the family: Little time is available to engage in stress-reducing behaviors, such as relaxing, socializing, or attending to personal interests (Bushy, 1998 Chaftez & Barnes, 1989; Gubman & Tessler, 1987). Rural women with high caregiver stress report higher frustration with an unresponsive treatment system and lower levels of available support for caregiving tasks (Saldana, Dassori, & Miller, 1999).

Because of economic strain on family farms, rural women have sought employment off the farm (Ilg, 1995; Kaiser, 1986). The addition of the off-farm employment does not decrease the woman's home duties and only minimally reduces her farming work. Instead, such women work *three shifts:* the off-farm job (first shift), household responsibilities (second shift), and farm work (third shift). For these women, two major clusters of stressors are apparent: role overload (i.e., having too much to do) and "invisibility" (i.e., a lack of recognition of the woman's efforts and own personal needs). Some women experience role strain because their involvement in off-farm work leads to conflicts with their traditional images of wife and mother. This role strain causes more dissatisfaction and distress (Delworth et al., 1988; Gallagher & Delworth, 1993; Hertsgaard & Light, 1984; Striegel, 1994).

Family life is a source of both stress and support for rural women. After the effects of age, gender, race, and social support were controlled, reported family stress was the strongest predictor of negative health outcomes in a rural clinic (Parkerson, Broadhead, & Tse, 1995). Women report more distress in relation to negative events within the family, whereas financial and work events caused distress for men (Conger, Lorenz, Elder, Simons, & Ge, 1993). Lack of emotional support by their husbands was more important than financial or role-related stressors in determining women's well-being (Giesen, Maas, & Vriens, 1989). Both health care providers and patients increasingly recognize the potent influence of stress on mental and physical health. New instruments are being devised to assess psychosocial stress at major transitions in women's lives. Fetal, infant, and maternal mortality are disproportionately high in rural communities (U.S. Congress, Office of Technology Assessment, 1990). To provide more effective prenatal treatment, the Prenatal Psychosocial Profile, administered to women seeking prenatal care, is used to detect their levels of stress and support (Curry, Burton, & Fields, 1998). The results can be used to help the devise ways to reduce stress and build the support she needs for prenatal and postnatal demands.

Mental Health Treatment

Rural people's willingness to seek mental health treatment is related to several factors. There continues to be more stigma attached to mental health treatment in rural areas than in large population centers, but this appears to be caused more by a fear of discovery by the community than to personal embarrassment or reluctance about using the services (Hoyt et al., 1997). The more negative the labeling, the less likely depressed rural residents are to seek care (Rost, Smith, & Taylor, 1993). Rural women are more willing to seek mental health care than are men; for both, however, prior use of mental health services results in a greater willingness to seek care in the future. For women, prior use of mental health services also results in attachment of fewer stigmas to mental health treatment. These findings suggest that guarantees of privacy and confidentiality are essential in promoting rural individuals' use of mental health services. Encouraging help seeking for mental health problems through such means as public education campaigns and social and professional network referrals is likely to decrease the attitudinal barriers to receiving mental health care.

Challenging the norms of silence and invisibility experienced by many rural women is the aim of a peer group intervention, called the *Listening Partners Program* (Bond, Belenky, & Weinstock, 2000). Directed at poor, rural, isolated, young mothers, the program entails an empowerment perspective to help the women gain a greater voice and promote their own development and that of their families. Individual and group narratives, along with problem solving, are some of the methods used. Participants report positive changes in self-image and agency, increases in social support networks, greater feelings of self-confidence, and more control of their lives.

The use of nurse-facilitated treatment programs for depressed rural women is another method of combating stigma. The Women's Affective Illness Treatment (WAIT) program (Hauenstein, 1996a, 1996b, 1997), designed and delivered by rural psychiatric nurses, addresses the biological, psychological, and social factors involved in depression. Impoverished rural women with major depression disorder are taught skills of self-assessment, stress response reduction, health behavior modification, and relapse prevention. A cognitive–behavioral treatment for rural battered women (Zust, 2000) also entails the use of a holistic approach. Studies of its effectiveness showed posttreatment reductions in clients' depression.

Human Immunodeficiency Virus (HIV) and Acquired Immunodeficiency Syndrome (AIDS)

Although most women with HIV or AIDS reside in urban areas, 6% of the AIDS cases in women reported to the Centers for Disease Control and Prevention in 1994 involved women residing in areas with populations of less than 50,000 (Gwinn & Wortley, 1996). From 1992 to 1995, the number of AIDS cases increased more rapidly in rural areas than in urban areas (30% vs. 25.8%); the largest increases occurred among women, African Americans, and adolescents.

In a study of rural women with HIV or AIDS in five geographical regions, McKinney (1998) found that in most cases (42%–96%, depending on the site), the HIV infection was acquired through heterosexual contact with an infected partner. However, injection and noninjection drug use, especially the use of crack cocaine, puts many rural residents at risk for HIV infection. Intravenous drug use led to HIV infection in 47% of the women patients at a farmworkers' clinic in Washington state. The Centers for Disease Control and Prevention (1995) reported that women with HIV infection are disproportionately Hispanic or African American, and many live in the rural South.

Because members of the staff at rural clinics are usually community members, HIV-infected patients often have concerns about privacy and confidentiality, which results in reluctance to seek testing or information (Frazier & Gabel, 1996; Rounds, 1988). Providers also may underestimate the problem of HIV infection in their communities or may not know how to conduct a thorough risk assessment. Because of the silence and taboos, rural people with HIV or AIDS experience less support; more social isolation; loneliness; fear that others will learn of their condition; less access to medical, mental health, and specialty HIV care; and more maladaptive coping strategies (Berry, McKinney, & Marconi, 1997; Heckman, Somlai, Kalichman, Franzoi, & Kelly, 1998).

In one of the few studies on the experiences and concerns of rural women infected with HIV, Hendrixson (1997) found themes common in all of the basic life domains: spiritual, physical, emotional, social, sexual, and maternal. Because the impact of HIV and AIDS is so pervasive, holistic treatment approaches are indicated. Culturally sensitive prevention and treatment programs for rural women who are members of ethnic minority groups have been developed (Bouey & Duran, 2000; Ortiz-Torres, Serrano-Garcia, & Torres-Burgos, 2000; Torres-Burgos & Serrano-Garcia, 1997).

Occupational Health

Rural women are at risk both for accidental injury because of their work around farm equipment and for cancers resulting from exposure to agricultural chemicals and pesticides (Agency for Health Care Policy and Research, 1996; Grieshop, Villanueva, & Stiles, 1994; McDuffie, 1994). The Rural Information Center (1995) of the U.S. Department of Agriculture has compiled a resource guide on agricultural safety and health. The guide provides information on various aspects of agricultural safety and health that can be of use to health personnel who treat agricultural workers and their families. The guide provides references on chemical, dermatological, electrical, respiratory, machinery, and stress-related dangers; outlines educational, preventive, and rehabilitative programs; and lists audiovisual materials and national and regional agricultural safety organizations.

Violence

Social problems, long associated with big city life, have made significant inroads into rural communities. Overall rates of violent crime—as well as the rates of assault, robbery, and rape—tripled in rural communities from 1965 to 1992 (U.S. Department of Justice, 1965, 1992). In rural communities, perpetrators of rape are much more likely to have been using alcohol at the time of the crime (82%) than are perpetrators in suburban areas (62%) or in central cities (51%; U.S. Department of Justice, 1992). Among all women, the rates of violence by an intimate partner are similar (Bachman, 1994; Bachman & Saltzman, 1995; Websdale & Johnson, 1997). Research in Kentucky also showed few differences in rates of woman-battering, except that rural women reported higher rates of being "shot at," "tortured," and having their hair pulled (Websdale & Johnson, 1995). Gorton and Hightower (1999), studying Latina farmworkers, found that 17% of them reported that a husband, boyfriend, family member, or companion had physically or sexually abused them in the previous year. Pregnant respondents experienced less victimization, and respondents with boyfriends or husbands who used alcohol or drugs experienced higher victimization. A study of abuse in rural Minnesota (Kershner, Long, & Anderson, 1998) among women surveyed at clinics and the supplemental food program offices of Women, Infants and Children (WIC) revealed that in the previous 12 months, 7% had experienced physical abuse; 2%, sexual abuse; and 21%, emotional abuse. Prior abuse was the best predictor of subsequent abuse in the 12-month time period.

In his ethnographic study of woman battering in rural Kentucky, Websdale (1998) stated that the battering of rural women is best understood as part of the "terror of rural patriarchy. Men are more likely to injure or kill women when their supremacy as patriarchs is somehow threatened" (p. 32). Rural women usually are geographically isolated, which makes it difficult for them to escape abusive situations. In addition, they experience nonresponsive policing because local police and sheriffs do not take the battering seriously, feeling they must uphold the patriarchal norms, and so do not interfere in domestic matters or are a part of the "good ol' boys" network with the abusers. Turning to clergy for support sometimes results in the same response, one that supports the marital role and traditional family values over the women's need for safety. Both strong rural, sociocultural norms stressing the value of marriage and traditional gender roles and the difficulty in finding and gaining access to beneficial services, such as transportation, child care services, independent housing, well-paying employment, and social and health services, keep rural victims hostage. As a result, they are even more subordinate and vulnerable to the batterers.

Because rural domestic violence results from a combination of individual, family, and sociocultural factors, a systemic approach for addressing the problem is most effective. A useful resource for designing these programs is provided by the Wilder Research Center (Monsey, Owen, Zierman, Lambert, & Hyman, 1995). Monsey et al. reviewed the literature on violence prevention programs for rape, sexual assault, and domestic violence, as well as assaultive violence, child abuse, child sexual abuse, elder abuse, suicide, and hate crimes.

The report, easily understood by both lay and professional audiences, describes prevention and intervention programs for each form of violence, the programs' effectiveness, and whether they have been shown to be effective in rural communities. The guide then provides a tool—the Community Report Card—that assists rural communities in assessing their risk factors for violence, their current level of violence, and the availability and accessibility of community services. Communities are guided in selecting appropriate intervention strategies and provided ways for monitoring progress over time.

The U.S. Public Health Service's Office of Women's Health (U.S. Department of Health and Human Services) established the National Centers of Excellence (CoEs) in Women's Health in 1996. A brochure (National Centers of Excellence in Women's Health, 2000) highlights CoEs activities related to domestic violence reduction. Program descriptions and contact information are provided. Wallace, Calhoun, Powell, O'Neil, and James (1996) noted that approximately 75% of female American Indian and Alaskan Native homicide victims are killed by someone they know, one third by family members. The Centers for Disease Control and Prevention (2000) has a fact sheet on intimate violence in these populations and provide descriptions of programs specifically designed for American Indian women.

Minority Women

More than 39.6 million women in the United States are members of racial and ethnic minority groups (U.S. Census Bureau, Population Division, 1999). It is unclear how many minorities live in rural areas, but the numbers are believed to be disproportionate to the numbers living in urban areas. Although the number of minority women living in rural communities is large, little is known of their behavioral health care needs. However, information about the health risks and concerns of women of color is being collected and disseminated by the National Women's Health Information Center of the Office on Women's Health of the U.S. Department of Health and Human Services. Through an extensive website (www.4woman.gov), the Center details information on the minority women's use of health services and health status. Extensive references are provided. In addition, all the federal agencies, which are involved in some capacity with women's health research, service delivery, and education, are described, with links to their respective sites.

Conclusions and Recommendations

Both Quantitative Research and Qualitative Research Are Needed

Quantitative studies, especially those that sample a number of geographical regions, can determine the prevalence of rural women's behavioral health needs and can confirm protective and risk factors for those needs. Quantitative studies of the effectiveness and efficiency of treatment methods and models designed for rural behavioral health needs are also necessary. On the other hand, qualitative studies, focus groups, and intensive case studies better capture the realities and particular character and complexities of the needs expressed by rural women. By identifying concepts important to different cultural groups and to the *silenced* rural women, culturally sensitive prevention and treatment services can be designed.

Acknowledge the Critical Role of Relationships in Rural Women's Well-Being and Attitudes

Family life can be a source of stress or support for rural women. Similarly, social networks and social institutions (church, police, schools) can either support or discourage a woman's motivation to make changes. Family and social networks must be mobilized to support women's health-promoting changes. For rural women attempting to adopt new behaviors and/or ones that conflict with the local sociocultural norms, alternative networks may have to be developed. The help and support of community organizations and social institutions are necessary to address widespread problems in the locale, such as domestic violence and HIV and AIDS.

Better Bridges Between Rural Mental Health and Physical Health Services Are Needed

Because of women's reliance on primary care physicians for mental health needs and their own holistic views of health, better links between health and mental health services serve rural women's needs and orientation. These links can be established by colocating services in the same building, forging better referral systems between providers, using the services of mental health specialists within primary care facilities, or having mental health specialists train and consult with primary care physicians on diagnostic and treatment issues. A 1994 national survey by the Maine Rural Health Research Center identified 53 programs linking rural primary and mental health care (Bird, Lambert, Hartley, Beeson, & Coburn, 1998).

References

Agency for Health Care Policy and Research (AHCPR). (1996). *Improving health care for rural populations: Research in action fact sheet* (AHCPR Publication No. 96-P040). Rockville, MD: Author.

Alderete, E., Vega, W. A., Kolody, B., & Aguilar-Gaxiola, S. (1999). Depressive symptomatology: Prevalence and psychosocial risk factors among Mexican migrant farmworkers in California. *Journal of Community Psychology, 27*, 457–471.

Bachman, R. (1994). *Violence against women: A national crime victimization survey report.* (NCJ Report No. 145325). Washington, DC: U.S. Department of Justice Programs.

Bachman, R., & Saltzman, L. E. (1995). *Violence against women: Estimates from the redesigned survey.* Washington, DC: U.S. Department of Justice, Bureau of Justice Statistics.

Berry, D., McKinney, M., & Marconi, K. (1997). A typological approach to the study of rural HIV service delivery networks. *Journal of Rural Health, 13,* 216–225.

Bird, D., Lambert, D., Hartley, D., Beeson, P., & Coburn, A. (1998). Integrating primary care and mental health in rural America. *Administration and Policy in Mental Health, 25,* 287–306.

Bokemeier, J., & Tickamyer, A. (1985). Labor force experiences of non-metropolitan women. *Rural Sociology, 30,* 51–73.

Bond, L. A., Belenky, M. F., & Weinstock, J. S. (2000). The Listening Partners Program: An initiative toward feminist community psychology in action. *American Journal of Community Psychology, 28,* 697–730.

Bouey, P. D., & Duran, B. E. S. (2000). The Ahalaya case-management program for HIV-infected American Indians, Alaska natives, and native Hawaiians: Quantitative and qualitative evaluation of impacts. *American Indian and Alaska Native Mental Health Research, 9,* 36–52.

Bushy, A. (1993). Rural women: Lifestyles and health status. *Nursing Clinics of North America, 28,* 187–197.

Bushy, A. (1998). Health issues of women in rural environments: An overview. *Journal of the American Medical Women's Association, 53*(2), 53–56.

Centers for Disease Control and Prevention. (1995). First 500,000 AIDS cases—United States. *Morbidity and Mortality Weekly Reports, 44,* 849–853.

Centers for Disease Control and Prevention. (2000). *American Indian/Alaskan Natives and intimate partner violence.* Atlanta, GA: National Center for Injury Prevention and Control. Retrieved March 10, 2001, from www.cdc.gov/ncipc/dvp/fivpt/fivpt.htm

Chaftez, L., & Barnes, L. (1989). Issues in psychiatric caregiving. *Archives of Psychiatric Nursing, 3,* 61–68.

Cheitman, E. A. (1981). Heritage and politics of poverty and inequality for rural women. *Journal of Sociology and Social Welfare, 8* 19–28.

Conger, R. D., Lorenz, F. O., Elder, Jr., G. H., Simons, R. L., & Ge, X. (1993). Husband and wife differences in response to undesirable life events. *Journal of Health and Social Behavior, 34,* 71–88.

Craft, B., Johnson, D., & Ortega, S. (1998). Rural urban women's experience of symptoms of depression related to economic hardship. *Journal of Women and Aging, 10*(3), 3–18.

Curry, M. A., Burton, D., & Fields, J. (1998). The prenatal psychosocial profile: A research and clinical tool. *Research in Nursing and Health, 21,* 211–219.

Delworth, U., Veach, S. D., & Grohe, L. (1988). Clinical issues with farm women. *Innovations in clinical practice: A sourcebook, 7,* 423–432.

Frazier, E. M., & Gabel, L. L. (1996). HIV/AIDS in family practice: An approach to care in rural areas. *Family Practice Recertification, 18,* 59–77.

Gallagher E., & Delworth, U. (1993). The third shift: Juggling employment, family, and the farm. *Journal of Rural Community Psychology, 12*(2), 21–36.

Giesen, C., Maas, A., & Vriens, M. (1989). Stress among farmwomen: A structural model approach. *Behavioral Medicine, 15*(2), 53–62.

Glasgow, N. (2000). Rural/urban patterns of aging and caregiving in the United States. *Journal of Family Issues, 21,* 611–631.

Gorton, J., & Hightower, N. R. (1999). Intimate victimization of Latina farm workers: A research summary. *Hispanic Journal of Behavioral Sciences, 21,* 502–507.

Grieshop, J. I., Villanueva, N. E., & Stiles, M. C. (1994). Wash day blues: Secondhand exposure to agricultural chemicals. *The Journal of Rural Health, 10,* 247–257.

Gubman, G. D., & Tessler, R. C. (1987). The impact of mental illness on families. *Journal of Family Issues, 8,* 226–245.

Gwinn, M., & Wortley, P. M. (1996). Epidemiology of HIV infection in women and newborns. *Clinical Obstetrics and Gynecology, 39,* 292–304.

Hauenstein, E. J. (1996a). A nursing practice paradigm for depressed rural women: Theoretical basis. *Archives of Psychiatric Nursing, 10,* 283–292.

Hauenstein, E. J. (1996b). Testing innovative nursing care: Home intervention with depressed rural women. *Issues in Mental Health Nursing, 17,* 33–50.

Hauenstein, E. J. (1997). A nursing practice paradigm for depressed rural women: The Women's Affective Illness Treatment program. *Archives of Psychiatric Nursing, 11,* 37–45.

Hauenstein, E. J., & Boyd, M. R. (1994). Depressive symptoms in young women of the Piedmont: Prevalence in rural women. *Women and Health, 21,* 105–123.

Haussman, M. J., & Halseth, J. H., (1983). Re-examining women's roles: A feminist group approach to decreasing depression in women. *Social Work With Groups, 6,* 105–115.

Heckman, T. G., Somlai, A. M., Kalichman, S. C., Franzoi, S. L., & Kelly, J. A. (1998). Psychosocial differences between urban and rural people living with HIV/AIDS. *Journal of Rural Health 14,* 138–145.

Hendrixson, L. (1997). The psychosocial and psychosexual impact of HIV/AIDS disease on rural women: A qualitative study. *Dissertation Abstracts International: A. Humanities and Social Sciences, 55*(12-A), 5312.

Hertsgaard, D., & Light, H. (1984). Anxiety, depression, and hostility in rural women. *Psychological Reports, 55,* 673–674.

Hoyt, D. R., Conger, R. D., Valde, J. G., & Weihs, K. (1997). Psychological distress and help seeking in rural America. *American Journal of Community Psychology, 25,* 449–470.

Ilg, R.E. (1995). The changing face of farm employment. *Monthly Labor Review,* April, 3–12.

Johnson, S. L. (1995). Life satisfaction of rural farmwomen: An ethnography in Minnesota. *Dissertation Abstracts International: A. Humanities and Social Sciences, 56*(1-A), 379.

Kaiser, A. (1986). Juggling the pieces: Working off the farm. *Farm Woman, 16,* 15.

Kershner, M., Long, D., & Anderson, J. E. (1998). Abuse against women in rural Minnesota. *Public Health Nursing, 15,* 422–431.

Kivett, V. R. (1998). Critical review: Synthesis and recommendations for research, education, and policy. In B. J. McCulloch (Ed.), *Old, female, and rural* (pp. 91–93). New York: Haworth Press.

Lamphere, L. (1992). *Structuring diversity: Ethnographic perspectives on the new immigration.* Chicago: University of Chicago Press.

Lingg, B., Braden, J., Goldstein, A. A., & Cooley, S. G. (1993). Income, poverty, and education. In J. F. Van Nostrand (Ed.), *Vital and health statistics. Common beliefs about the rural elderly* (Series 3: Analytic and Epidemiological Studies, No. 28, Department of Health and Human Services Publication No. [PHS] 93-1412, pp. 25–31). Washington, DC: U.S. Government Printing Office.

McDuffie, H. H. (1994). Women at work: Agriculture and pesticides. *Journal of Occupational Medicine, 36,* 1240–1246.

McGrath, E., Keita, G. P., Strickland, B. R., & Russo N. (1990). *Women and depression: Risk factors and treatment issues.* Washington, DC: American Psychological Association.

McKinney, M. (1998). Service needs and networks of rural women with HIV/AIDS. *Community Health Solutions, Inc., 12,* 471–480.

Monsey, B., Owen, G., Zierman, C., Lambert, L., & Hyman, V. (1995). *What works in preventing rural violence: Strategies, risk factors, and assessment tools.* St. Paul, MN: Amherst H. Wilder Foundation.

Mulder, P. L., Kenkel, M. B., Shellenberger, S., Constantine, M., Streiegel, R., Sears, S. F., et al. (2000). *Behavioral health care needs of rural women.* Washington, DC: American Psychological Association, Committee on Rural Health. Retrieved March 19, 2001, from http://www.apa.org/rural/ruralwomen.pdf

Naples, N. (1994). Contradictions in agrarian ideology: Restructuring gender, race-ethnicity and class. *Rural Sociology, 59,* 110–135.

National Centers of Excellence in Women's Health. (2000, May). *Domestic violence initiatives.* Washington, DC: U.S. Department of Health and Human Services.

National Institute of Mental Health. (2000, August). *Depression: What every woman should know* (NIH Publication No. 00-4479). Washington, DC: National Institute of Health.

Ortiz-Torres, B., Serrano-Garcia, I., & Torres-Burgos, N. (2000). Subverting culture: Promoting HIV/AIDS prevention among Puerto Rican and Dominican women. *American Journal of Community Psychology, 28,* 859–881.

Parkerson, G. R., Jr., Broadhead, W. E., & Tse, C. K. (1995). Perceived family stress as a predictor of health related outcomes. *Archives of Family Medicine 4,* 253–260.

Robins, L. N., & Regier, D. A. (1991). *Psychiatric disorders in America: The Epidemiologic Catchment Area Study.* New York: Free Press.

Rost, K., Smith, R., & Taylor, J. (1993). Rural-urban differences in stigma and the use of care for depressive disorders. *Journal of Rural Health, 9,* 57–62.

Rounds, K. A. (1988). Responding to AIDS: Rural community strategies. *Social Casework, 69,* 360–365.

Rural Information Center. (1995, January). *Agricultural safety and health: A resource guide* (Rural Information Center Publication Series, No. 40.) Beltsville, MD: U.S. Department of Agriculture.

Saldana, D. H., Dassori, A. M., & Miller, A. L. (1999). When is caregiving a burden? Listening to Mexican American women. *Hispanic Journal of Behavioral Sciences, 21,* 283–301.

Shenk, D. (1998). Subjective realities of rural older women's lives: A case study. In B. J. McCulloch (Ed.), *Old, female, and rural* (pp. 7–24). New York: Haworth.

Striegel, M. R. (1994). *Sustainable agriculture and its influence on life satisfaction of farm women.* Unpublished master's thesis, University of Iowa, Iowa City.

Sullivan, G., Jackson, C. A., & Spritzer, K. L.(1996). Characteristics and service use of seriously mentally ill persons living in rural areas. *Psychiatric Services, 47,* 57–61.

Torres-Burgos, N., & Serrano-Garcia, I. (1997). Empowerment and HIV/AIDS: A prevention project for young heterosexual Puerto Rican women. In M. Montero (Ed.), *Memorias de psicologia comunitaria del XXV Congreso Interamericano de Psicologia* [Psychology and Community: Proceedings of the XXV Interamerican Congress of Psychology] (pp. 366–371). Caracas, Venezuela: Litopar

U.S. Census Bureau, Population Division. (2001). *Resident population estimates of the United States by age and sex: April 1, 1990 to October 1, 1999.* Retrieved November 26, 1999, from www.census.gov/population/estimates/nation/intfile2-1.txt

U.S. Congress, Office of Technology Assessment. (1990). *Health care in rural America* (OTA Publication No. OTA-H-434). Washington, DC: U.S. Government Printing Office.

U.S. Department of Agriculture, Economic Research Service. (2000, December). Socioeconomic conditions. *Rural Conditions and Trends, 11*(2). Retrieved March 17, 2001, from http://www.ers.usda.gov/publications/rcat/rcat112/

U.S. Department of Justice (1965). *Sourcebook of criminal justice statistics.* Washington, DC: Bureau of Justice Statistics.

U.S. Department of Justice (1992). *Sourcebook of criminal justice statistics.* Washington, DC: Bureau of Justice Statistics.

Vega, W. A., Kolody, B., Valle, J. R., & Hough, R. (1986). Depressive symptoms and their correlates among immigrant Mexican women in the United States. *Social Science and Medicine, 22,* 642–645.

Wallace, J., Calhoun, A., Powell, K., O'Neil, J., & James, S. (1996). *Homicide and suicide among Native Americans, 1979–1992.* Atlanta, GA: Centers for Disease Control and Prevention, National Center for Injury Prevention & Control. Retrieved March 19, 2001, from www.cdc.gov/ncipc/pub-res/hombook.pdf

Websdale, N. (1998). *Rural woman battering and the justice system: An ethnography.* Thousand Oaks, CA: Sage.

Websdale, N., & Johnson, B. (1995, August). *A comparison of the forms and levels of domestic violence in urban and rural areas of Kentucky.* Paper presented at the annual conference of the Society for the Study of Social Problems, Washington, DC.

Websdale, N., & Johnson, B. (1997). The policing of domestic violence in rural and urban areas: The voices of battered women in Kentucky. *Policing and Society, 6,* 297–317.

Weissman, M. M., & Klerman, G. L. (1987). Gender and depression. In R. Formanek & A. Gurian (Eds.), *Women and depression: A lifespan perspective.* New York: Springer.

Zust, B. L. (2000). Effect of cognitive therapy on depression in rural battered women. *Archives of Psychiatric Nursing, 14,* 51–63.

15

Rural Geriatrics and Gerontology

Susan Guralnick, Kathy Kemele,
B. Hudnall Stamm, and Sister Anthony Marie Greving

Older people represent a disproportionately large percentage of the population in rural and frontier areas, owing to decades of emigration to urban centers by job-seeking younger adults. Many older rural adults are characterized by self-reliance, hardiness, and a preference for informal networks of support. Older adults who live in rural and nonmetropolitan areas typically have fewer financial resources and significantly poorer health status than do their urban counterparts. In this chapter, we review health and functional status, health services utilization, and health promotion. We conclude with recommendations for the use of telehealth, health promotion, and the appropriate use of the services of health providers, including nonphysician providers.

Researchers and policy writers have used ages ranging from 50 to 85 years and older to denote old age. Age 65, the most commonly used number in the United States, became the de facto marker in 1935 with the establishment of the Social Security Act, in which 65 years was designated as the age of retirement. In 1983, members of the National Commission on Social Security Reform recognized increases in average life expectancy and gradually increased retirement age eligibility from 65 to 67 years of age (starting in 2000; www.ssa.gov/history/pdf/histdev.pdf). Despite this, researchers studying older adults typically use the chronological age of 65 to designate *old.*

According to the numbers of people aged 65 and older and the metropolitan versus nonmetropolitan definitions of *rural* and *old,* 27% of older adults in the United States live in rural, nonmetropolitan areas (U.S. Bureau of the Census, 1994), which is a far higher proportion than their 12% share of the total U.S. population suggests; in contrast, 43% of older adults live in suburbs, and 30% live in cities. Because the greatest share of rural territory is in the Midwest and West, it is not surprising that state-by-state figures indicate that the numbers of rural older adults in many states far exceed the national average (e.g., in Alaska, the proportion is 32.5%; in Idaho, 42.2%; and in Montana, 44.3%).

Because of individual variables such as physiological changes, health status, psychological well-being, ethnicity, lifestyle behaviors, and life events,

Dr. Guralnick can be reached at Medicine/Gerontology and Geriatric Medicine, 1910 Fairview Ave E., Suite 203, Seattle, WA 98102-3699. E-mail: sgural@u.washington.edu

older adults are the most heterogeneous group in U.S. society. As a group, rural elderly persons are perhaps even more diverse than their urban counterparts, defying researchers' ability to categorize them. Gerontologists have long recognized that each generation experiences the aging process differently, as the culmination of many decades of life events shapes physical, mental, and social health. Self-reliance, hardiness, and a preference for informal networks of support appear to characterize a majority of rural older adults. In addition to these common characteristics, decades of emigration to urban centers by job-seeking, younger adults, coupled with immigration by retirees seeking the beauty and tranquility of rural life, have led to a "silvering" of and a change in the present-day population. The needs and attitudes of those who have aged in place may be different from those of younger and often more affluent retirees.

Being Elderly in Rural America

Demographics of the Aging Rural Population

Older adults who live in rural and nonmetropolitan areas typically have lower incomes (Hooyman & Kiyak, 1999) and significantly poorer health status (Cordes, 1989; Lubben, Weiler, Chi, & DeLong, 1988; Norton & McManus, 1989; Schoenberg & Coward, 1998) than do their urban counterparts. In the United States, Social Security provides a basic level of economic support to older adults, and Medicare, governmental health insurance for the elderly and disabled, provides coverage for acute health care and some preventive services. However, Medicare does not provide coverage for prescription drugs, hearing aids, home care, support services, or long-term care except for a limited rehabilitation benefit after a 3-day hospital stay. For many rural elderly residents, purchasing these uncovered health care costs can erode the financial support provided by Social Security.

These gaps in coverage result in difficulties for rural elderly residents in that most rural communities have a fragile infrastructure unable to provide the safety net that people would like or assume is present. Rural communities have fewer community-based resources—such as transportation, community centers, home care services, and meal programs—that can support individuals in their homes or foster social contact. As a result, many rural older adults experience low levels of social support and high levels of isolation, which are significant health risks. Extreme loneliness can be a significant predictor of admission to nursing homes for older rural men and women (Russell, Cutrona, de la Mora, & Wallace, 1997), and social isolation and fewer social ties result in higher mortality, especially if sustained over 3 years (Cerhan & Wallace, 1997). Because of limited support networks and fewer options for care, rural older persons tend to enter nursing homes at earlier ages, and in greater numbers, than do their urban counterparts. This problem is particularly severe for rural women, almost half of whom live alone (McCullock, 1998).

Adults in rural areas are 36% more likely to report their health status as fair or poor than are adults in urban areas (U.S. Department of Health and Human Services, 2000). Eighty-seven percent of rural elderly residents have at least one chronic condition (Johnson & Taylor, 1991). In comparison with elderly persons living in metropolitan areas, rural older adults report poorer emotional well-being, more chronic illness, greater physical impairment and functional limitations. Also, they have more difficulty performing activities of daily living (ADLs)—bathing, dressing, toileting, eating, and transferring (getting out of a bed or chair)—as well as instrumental activities of daily living (IADLs), such as shopping, cooking, and paying bills (Coward & Dwyer, 1991; Mainous & Kohrs, 1995; Ortega, Mueller, & Metroka, 1995). Data suggest that rates of mortality from major health problems (cardiovascular and cerebrovascular disease, diabetes, and accidents) are higher in rural areas (Cooper, 1988; Schorr, Crabtrees, & Wetterau, 1989; U.S. Department of Health and Human Services, 2000). People are less likely to use preventive screening services, to exercise regularly, or to wear seat belts (U.S. Department of Health and Human Services, 2000). As reported in *Health Care in Rural America* (U.S. Congress, Office of Technology Assessment, 1990), some chronic, age-related diseases, such as heart disease, hypertension, diabetes, arthritis, and certain vision and hearing impairments, are especially prevalent in rural populations.

Several possible explanations for findings of poor health include a reluctance of rural older adults to seek early medical care, lack of health screening programs, inadequate health promotion programs, ineffective treatment programs, a lack of money to pay for preventive or restorative health care, and more limited access to transportation (Mockenhaupt & Muchow, 1994). Despite attempts to offset urban–rural differences in health and social services, significant gaps remain (Hooyman & Kiyak, 1999). In the following sections, we more closely examine health and functional status, cardiovascular disease, nutrition, cognitive impairment, mental health, depression, health services utilization, and health promotion as they relate to rural elderly persons.

Health and Functional Status

More rural than urban elderly persons negatively assess their personal health status. This negative assessment, which is strongly associated with physical illness, functional disability, life satisfaction, and objective health status measures (e.g., physical examinations), means that rural elderly persons have a higher risk of mortality at all ages than do urban elderly persons (Van Nostrand, Furner, Brunelle, & Cohen, 1993). Lower self-rating of health in older adults is also correlated with depressive symptoms and is a robust predictor of overall mortality. At least one group of investigators has found this to be true in rural subjects across multiple levels of disability (Mulsant, Ganguli, & Seaberg, 1997). Functional status, divided in the geriatric literature into ADLs and IADLs, is the best overall indicator of health and is frequently assessed through self-report. It is important to note that rural older adults equate health with the ability to work on an instrumental activity (Hornberger & Cobb, 1998), whereas urban residents focus on cosmetic items, life prolongation, or the provision of comfort. This may be a reflection of rural occupations, which requires a person to be active and productive, or a reflection of the emphasis that rural elderly persons place on self-reliance.

CARDIOVASCULAR DISEASE. In the 1960s and 1970s, urban older adults had higher rates of cardiovascular disease than did their rural counterparts. By the early 1980s, this trend reversed, with living in a rural area directly correlating with cardiovascular mortality. This reversal may be related to poorer socioeconomic status, higher rates of obesity, or a high prevalence of diabetes, all of which are risk factors for heart disease and stroke. Pearson and Lewis (1998) decided that rural residents are characterized by a "slow adoption" of lifestyle changes; thus, trends toward tobacco use and high fat consumption were adopted later among rural residents than among than among city dwellers. Similarly, behaviors reversing these negative health trends have been adopted more slowly in rural communities. Increased prevalence of cardiovascular disease in rural areas may also reflect the aging of the population, inasmuch as younger rural inhabitants migrate to cities. Despite these changes and restricted access to health care services, or perhaps as an artifact of the "slow adoption," a 24-year review by Hayward, Pienta, and McLaughlin (1997) revealed that overall mortality rates for older rural American men were lower than those of their urban counterparts. Other powerful predictors in the study included tobacco avoidance, higher socioeconomic status at midlife, and a robust support system. Data on the mortality rates for women have not yet appeared in the literature.

For rural African Americans, data suggest that the prevalence of smoking, elevated blood cholesterol levels, and sedentary lifestyle are the same as for urban dwellers. However, diabetes, hypertension, and obesity rates are higher, which suggests that rural African Americans are at greater risk for mortality from cardiovascular disease (Gillum, 1997; Jenson, Kita, Fish, Heydt, & Frey, 1997). Gillum (1997) found higher rates of mortality from stroke in rural African Americans.

NUTRITION. Americans in general have poor nutrition profiles; many are overweight, and many others suffer from undernutrition. Rural inhabitants are not exempt from this problem. Jenson et al., in 1997, reported that in general rural women had high body mass indices and elevated blood cholesterol levels; more than 50% met criteria for being overweight and 10% for obesity. Numerous nutrition problems were seen, including poor appetite, low income, and eating alone, which are correlated with poor nutrition. More than 50% of study participants did not follow food pyramid guidelines. Another group of investigators (Wolfe, Olson, Kendall, & Frongillo, 1998) found that rural older adults were less likely to report food insufficiency and hunger, but they often supplemented their diets with hunting or fishing or participated in food programs. In addition, a substantial number of rural elder persons routinely skip one or two meals (Lee, Templeton, & Wang, 1996), which significantly reduces their nutrient intake and the quality of their diets, placing them at risk for developing chronic diet-related degenerative problems.

COGNITIVE IMPAIRMENT. The prevalence of cognitive impairment is essentially unknown in the elderly rural population because it has barely been studied in the United States. In addition to the limited time that primary care providers may have to assess cognition in a high-volume rural practice, there is the possibility that demented patients and their families may not recognize the illness or seek care. Specialists are usually not available in rural clinics to assist in diagnosis and management. Depression, the most common mental health problem in later life (Okwumabua, Baker, Wong, & Pilgrim, 1997), is frequently seen in the rural population and may be mistaken for or coexist with dementia. Well-validated, positive scores on rapid-screening dementia assessment instruments, such as the Folstein Mini-Mental State Examination (MMSE), are heavily influenced by education level, which may lower scores for older rural people, most of whom have completed fewer than 8 years of formal education (Keefover Rankin, & Shaw, 1996). In addition, tests that require intact vision and hearing may contain cultural or urban biases. The rapid growth of the *oldest old* (the group with the highest rates of dementia), a higher probability for nursing home placement than among urban older persons, and the advent of medical therapies for dementias such as Alzheimer's disease mandate further study of cognitive impairment in the rural population.

MENTAL HEALTH. Although little is known about mental health in rural older adults, more information is available about mental health than about cognitive impairment. Rural senior citizens wait longer to obtain formal health care services, including those provided for mental health problems. They tend to attach more stigma to mental health disorders than do their urban counterparts and are less likely to have ready access to specialty providers and counselors (Davis et al., 1992). For diagnosis and therapy, they are more likely to rely on their overburdened primary care providers, who may not be comfortable treating mental health concerns. The issue of confidentiality also needs to be considered in rural communities.

As has already been seen, functional ability is the key to remaining in the community and is a strong indicator of mortality. Hayward et al. (1997) found that, in rural areas, functional impairment is more strongly associated with psychological stress than with medical illness, whereas psychiatric distress is also associated with severe medical disorders.

Depression is the most examined mental health problem in the rural older adult group, and its prevalence seems to mirror that in urban elderly persons. In a study on antidepressant use by rural elderly residents (Ganguli, Mulsant, Richards, Stoehr, & Mendelsohn, 1997), women with five or more depressive symptoms and those using more than five prescription drugs were most likely to be treated, usually by their primary care providers. Underdetection of depression by rural physicians does not appear to be an issue, inasmuch as they report that 20% of the patients in their practices suffer from the disorder (Rost, Humphrey, & Kelleher, 1994). However, because the true overall prevalence is unknown, there may be many in the community who do not seek attention. Because the availability of psychotherapy is very limited and medications alone have a positive effective, even if it is less than that derived from a combination of medication and psychotherapy, antidepressants, especially the selective serotonin inhibitors, are the mainstays of rural therapy. As noted earlier, extreme loneliness, a factor in depressive illness, is a predictor of nursing home admission and is very common among older people living in rural areas.

Health Services Utilization

A number of investigators have attempted to compare urban with rural utilization of formal health care services. Their findings have varied, depending on the specific population and locale as well as on the type of service studied. In general, rural areas are marked by a greater reliance on informal support from family and community and with less emphasis on professionals. Rural hospitals are often the system "portal of entry" for rural elderly residents, but since the mid-1980s, many community hospitals have closed because dwindling Medicare reimbursements and escalating costs have forced them out of business. The effects of hospital closure on a rural community go far beyond the loss of an essential health care resource, inasmuch as the entire region suffers economically through loss of employment and business opportunities. This may further exacerbate the out-migration of young individuals to urban centers, with the subsequent loss of informal support for elderly residents. The full long-term effects of the closure of rural hospitals are yet to be seen.

Rural areas are characterized by a lack of other health care services, namely emergency services, adult daycare, counseling and mental health services, housing, and transportation. Because older farm workers are at highest risk for accidental injuries, the paucity of emergency services is of particular concern (Olenchock & Young, 1997). Although lack of health insurance is usually not a problem for older adults, because most participate in Medicare, rural elderly residents are infrequently enrolled in Medicare health maintenance organizations and often do not have secondary insurers (Medigap policies). Rural counties are also marked by a relative lack of physicians and other health care providers. This leads to longer waits for access to care. Indeed, one study revealed that most rural older men had not seen a physician in many years (Mortison, 1996). Even in areas with adequate hospital and physician services, there is a shortage of other service providers, such as audiologists, physical therapists, and mental health counselors (Cheh & Phillips, 1993; Ives, Bonino, Traven, & Kuller, 1995). Despite a high value placed on care in the home, rural elderly persons are also less likely to receive home health services after hospitalization, often because the services are unavailable. When home services are available, rural elderly residents receive fewer visits than do their urban counterparts (Cheh & Phillips, 1993). These lower rates may be characteristics of the home health industry more than of the elderly persons they serve. Rural agencies cannot accommodate as many patients per caregiver or operate as cost effectively as their urban counterparts, because of the long distances that caregivers must drive between appointments.

The effect of this fragmented, understaffed, and underfunded system is seen in the higher utilization rates of nursing homes for rural older adults. Despite a national trend for nursing home residents to be older and sicker rural elderly persons enter homes at younger ages and are somewhat less physically disabled than their urban peers (Duncan, Coward, & Gilbert, 1997). Their care may be custodial in nature, which perhaps reflects the dearth of less costly assisted-living centers and home health services commonly found in cities. Although there is little information regarding caregiving burden specific to rural areas, it is known that socialization opportunities and respite services, which may be less available in rural areas, help to decrease perceived caregiver burden. Perhaps the more prevalent use of nursing homes is also related to caregiver concerns.

Health Promotion

In a system oriented toward acute care needs, health promotion tends to be neglected in all areas. As a group, rural elderly persons may be less likely than their urban peers to place a priority on health promotion activities, inasmuch as health is seen as the ability to work. A few studies have shown that although rural residents respond to health promotion projects recommended by their primary care providers, baseline usage rates continue to remain low. In 1996, a 3-year study (Ives & Lave, 1996) of rural women revealed that only 44.6% of older women had had a mammogram and fewer than 15% had had a Pap smear. At a time when both mammograms and Pap smears were covered by Medicare Part B, 50% of rural women used neither. It is noteworthy that the authors of the study believed that the response rate was falsely elevated by the nature of the study itself and that true rates were much lower. The authors speculated that low education levels in rural communities played a large role, as did a fear of cancer. Another 1995 study indicated that education level was an important factor, showing that better educated rural older adults were more likely to participate in health promotion activities. Promotion activities requiring little effort, such as pneumonia or influenza vaccination programs, appeal to older rural adults (Lave, Ives, Traven, & Kuller, 1995).

Conclusions and Recommendations

Collect Data on the Demographics, Habits, and Health Care Needs and Preferences of Rural Elderly People and Their Families

As record numbers of baby boomers age, a more thorough understanding of rural elderly residents and their health care needs will prove essential to the appropriate allocation of ever scarcer health resources. In the late 1980s, managed care arose as one potential solution to control rising costs, but it has been slow to move into rural areas because it operates on principles of concentrated populations. In most rural areas, fee-for-service arrangements are still the most common methods of reimbursement. There is an overwhelming need for more research into the health care needs and preferences of rural older adults. The prevalence of such common diseases as dementia and osteoarthritis, both of which are known precipitators of disability in older adults, is still unclear.

Establish Systems of Care That Are Effective in Rural and Frontier Areas

Good data will allow researchers and health care and social service providers to understand the concerns and health care needs of the elderly and their families. This will enable them to begin to design and test a system that can provide cost-effective, high-quality care. A successful system will be cost effective and high quality and will reach rural and frontier areas, addressing the unique needs of the elderly in those regions.

Implement and Support Rural Assisted-Living Facilities

The "silvering" of America presents challenges for the entire health care system, and the most vulnerable patients, the rural elderly, will face the greatest hurdles to gaining access to appropriate care. Of particular concern for rural dwellers is the lack of assisted-living facilities. The reliance on the nursing home for custodial care of rural elderly residents is costly, not only for the older adult, many of whom equate nursing home placement with death, but also for society, which frequently assumes the cost of expensive, skilled nursing facility care through the Medicaid program. Health care and social service providers need to understand how best to support the rural caregiver to allow rural older adults to perhaps age-in-place, avoiding nursing home placement and receive needed care at home.

Utilize Telehealth to Provide and Support Care in the Community

Telehealth networks for rural and frontier areas are a crucial adjunct of the assisted-living program and an element that will prove helpful across the health care system. Telehealth may increase elderly persons' ability to age in place. In addition to giving the hometown provider access to specialty care for complex cases, telehealth consultation in the home and as a support for home health providers may reduce some travel costs associated with caring for elderly persons who are widely dispersed geographically. It may also offer opportunities to incorporate distant family members in the care process by regularly linking the rural elderly person, caregivers, and the distant family member through technology rather than by infrequent visits.

Build a Decentralized System That Functions Within a National System

By virtue of the unique character of each rural and frontier region, any successful system must be decentralized, with the national system guiding and supporting the individual programs that will create a system appropriate to the needs of patients and their families and significant others. Because of the rural elderly population's diversity, there cannot be a one-size-fits-all solution to their health care needs. After discussion with a community's older residents and their families, as well as local health care and business leaders, the system of care will need to be designed according to each area's own require-ments. The national system should facilitate research and coordination of local and state programs of care.

References

Cerhan, J. R., & Wallace, R. B. (1997). Change in social ties and subsequent mortality in rural elders. *Epidemiology, 8,* 475–481.

Cheh, C., & Phillips, B. (1993). Adequate access to post-hospital home health services: Differences between urban and rural areas. *Journal of Rural Health, 9,* 262–269.

Cooper, J. K. (1988). A national rural geriatrics program. *Journal of Rural Health, 4*(30), 5–8.

Cordes, S. M. (1989). The changing rural environment and the relationship between health services and rural development. *Health Services Resources, 23,* 757–781.

Coward, R. T., & Dwyer, J. W. (1991). *Health programs for elders in rural America: A review of the life circumstances and formal services that affect the health and well-being of elders.* Kansas City, MO: National Resources Center for Rural Elderly.

Davis, D. C., Henderson, M. C., Boothe, A., Douglass, M., Faria, S., Kennedy, D., et al. (1992). Health beliefs and practices of rural elders. *Caring, 11*(2), 22–28.

Duncan, R. P., Coward, R. T., & Gilbert, G. H. (1997). Rural–urban comparisons of age and health at the time of nursing home admission. *Journal of Rural Health, 13,* 118–125.

Ganguli, M., Mulsant, B. B., Richards, S., Stoehr, G., & Mendelsohn, A. (1997). Antidepressant use over time in a rural older adult population: The MoVIES project. *Journal of the American Geriatrics Society, 45,* 1501–1503.

Gillum, R. F. (1997). Secular trends in stroke mortality in African Americans: The role of urban-ization, diabetes and obesity. *Neuroepidemiology, 16,* 180–184.

Hayward, M. D., Pienta, A. M., & McLaughlin, D. K. (1997). Inequality in men's mortality: The socio-economic gradient and geographic context. *Journal of Health and Social Behavior, 38,* 313–330.

Hooyman, N. R., & Kiyak, H. A. (1999). *Social gerontology: A multidisciplinary perspective* (5th ed.). Boston: Allyn & Bacon.

Hornberger, C. A., & Cobb, A. K. (1998). A rural vision of a healthy community. *Public Health Nursing, 15,* 363–369.

Ives, D. G., Bonino, P., Traven, N. D., & Kuller, L. H. (1995). Characteristics and comorbidities of rural older adults with hearing impairment. *Journal of the American Geriatrics Society, 43,* 803–806.

Ives, D. G., & Lave, J. R. (1996). Mammography and Pap smear use by older rural women. *Public Health Reports, 111,* 244–251.

Jenson, G. L., Kita, K., Fish, J., Heydt, D., & Frey, C. (1997). Nutrition risk screening character-istics of rural older persons: Relation to functional limitations and health care charges. *American Journal of Clinical Nutrition, 66,* 819–828.

Johnson, A., & Taylor, A. (1991). *Prevalence of chronic diseases: A summary of data from the Survey of American Indians and Alaska Natives* (Agency for Health Care Policy and Research Publication No. 91-0031). Rockville, MD: Agency for Health Care Policy and Research.

Keefover, R. W., Rankin, E. D., & Shaw, J. (1996). Dementing illnesses in rural populations: The need for research and challenges confronting investigators. *Journal of Rural Health, 12,* 178–187.

Lave, J. R., Ives, D. G., Traven, N. D., & Kuller, L. H. (1995). Participation in health promotion programs by the rural elderly. *American Journal of Preventive Medicine, 11*(1), 46–53.

Lee, C. J., Templeton, S., & Wang C. (1996). Meal skipping patterns and nutrient intakes of rural southern elderly. *Journal of Nutrition for the Elderly, 15*(2), 1–14.

Lubben, J. E., Weiler, P. G., Chi, I., & DeLong, F. (1988). Health promotion for the rural elderly. *Journal of Rural Health, 4,* 85–96.

Mainous, A. G., III, & Kohrs, F. P. (1995). A comparison of health status between rural and urban adults. *Journal of Community Health, 20,* 423–431.

McCullock, J. B. (1998). Old, female, and rural. *Journal of Women and Aging, 10*(4), 1–5.

Mockenhaupt, R., & Muchow, J. A. (1994). Disease and disability prevention and health promo-tion for rural elders. In J. Krout (Ed.), *Providing community-based services to the rural elderly* (pp. 183–201). Thousand Oaks, CA: Sage.

Mortison, R. (1996). Improving rural health care in South Dakota. *South Dakota Journal of Medicine, 49,* 452–456.

Mulsant, B. H., Ganguli, M., & Seaberg, E. C. (1997). The relationship between self-rated health and depressive symptoms in an epidemiological sample of community-dwelling older adults. *Journal of the American Geriatrics Society, 45,* 954–958.

Norton, C. H., & McManus, M. A. (1989). Background tables on demographic characteristics, health status, and health services utilization. *Health Services Resources, 23,* 725–755.

Okwumabua, J. O., Baker, F. M., Wong, S. P., & Pilgrim, B. O. (1997). Characteristics of depressive symptoms in elderly urban and rural African Americans. *Journals of Gerontology Series A: Biological Sciences and Medical Sciences, 52,* M241–M261.

Olenchock, S. A., & Young, N. B. (1997). Changes in agriculture bring potential for new health and safety risks. *Wisconsin Medical Journal, 96*(8), 10–11.

Ortega, S., Mueller, K., & Metroka, M. (1995). Health insurance status and ill health: Implications for health professionals. *Journal of Nursing Care Quality, 1*(10), 46–54.

Pearson, T. A., & Lewis, C. (1998). Rural epidemiology: Insights from a rural population laboratory. *American Journal of Epidemiology, 148,* 949–957.

Rost, K., Humphrey, J., & Kelleher, K. (1994). Physician management preferences and barriers to care for rural patients with depression. *Archives of Family Medicine, 3,* 409–414.

Russell, D. W., Cutrona, C. E., de la Mora, A., & Wallace R. B. (1997). Loneliness and nursing home admission among rural older adults. *Psychology and Aging, 12,* 574–589.

Schoenberg, N. E., & Coward, R. T. (1998). Residential differences in attitudes about barriers to using community-based services among older adults. *Journal of Rural Health, 14,* 295–304.

Schorr, V., Crabtrees, D., & Wetterau, P. (1989). Differences in rural and urban mortality: Implications for health education and promotion. *Journal of Rural Health, 5,* 67–79.

U.S. Bureau of the Census. (1994). *Population profile of the United States: 1993.* Washington, DC: U.S. Government Printing Office.

U.S. Congress, Office of Technology Assessment. (1990). *Health care in rural America* (Office of Technology Assessment Publication No. OTA-H-34). Washington, DC: U.S. Government Printing Office.

U.S. Department of Health and Human Services. (2000). *Healthy people 2010: Understanding and improving health* (2nd ed.). Washington, DC: U.S. Government Printing Office. Retrieved March 19, 2001, from http://www.health.gov/healthypeople/Document/tableofcontents.htm

Van Nostrand, J. F., Furner, S. E., Brunelle, J. A., & Cohen, R. A. (1993). Common beliefs about the rural elderly: What do national data tell us? *Vital and Health Statistics 3*(28), 51–62.

Wolfe, W. S., Olson, C. M., Kendall, A., & Frongillo, E. A. (1998). Hunger and food insecurity in the elderly. *Journal of Aging and Health, 10,* 327–350.

16

Individuals With Serious Mental Illnesses in Prison: Rural Perspectives and Issues

Robert K. Ax, Thomas J. Fagan, and Shelia M. B. Holton

Rural prisons and jails are the contemporary manifestation of a long tradition of exiling persons with serious mental illness from society. Powerful social and economic forces effectively distance these already disenfranchised individuals from the community. In this chapter, we discuss issues specific to the treatment of persons with serious mental illness in rural prisons and jails. Telehealth technology has particular relevance to treatment in these facilities. Ideally, a range of community services would reduce the initial involvement of individuals with serious mental illness in the criminal justice system. If rehabilitation is once again to be a priority in American prisons, mental health professionals must become reinvolved in policymaking.

Although no one would argue that prisons should not house individuals who pose an obvious threat to society, since the mid 1990s there has been a considerable increase in the number of incarcerated mentally ill and substance-abusing individuals. A study of public beliefs about mental illness revealed that people reported an unrealistic fear of persons with mental illness and a strong desire to maintain social distance from these individuals (Link, Phelan, Bresnahan, Stueve, & Pescosolido, 1999). There were approximately 283,000 mentally ill inmates in American prisons and jails in 1998 (Ditton, 1999).

This shift from housing mentally ill individuals in mental institutions to housing them in correctional facilities coincides roughly with the passage of the Mental Retardation Facilities and Community Mental Health Centers Act of 1963. Before this act was passed, the average daily census of individuals hospitalized in public mental institutions hovered at about 600,000 (Torrey, 1988). After the act's passage, the average daily census began a dramatic drop. Butterfield (1999) noted that the number of patients in state hospitals was only 69,000 by 1995. Shortly after deinstitutionalization began, many patients, when released from hospitals, began to find their way into correc-

---

The views expressed in this chapter are those of the authors only and do not represent the official policy or opinions of the Federal Bureau of Prisons.

Dr. Ax can be reached at 5610 Chatmoss Rd, Midlothian, VA 23112. E-mail: shrinkart@aol.com

tional settings (Abramson, 1972; Bassuk & Gerson, 1978). Persons with serious mental illness (SMI) were more likely than offenders without SMI to be arrested for certain kinds of crimes (L. Teplin, 1984) and were more likely than nondisordered offenders to be arrested for less serious infractions (Valdeserri, Carroll, & Hartl, 1986). Some data indicate that a similar trend characterizes the treatment of children. Martz (1999; personal communication, 2000) reported that, between 1993 and 1999, the proportion of incarcerated boys in Virginia needing mental health treatment increased from 33% to 47%, and the proportion of incarcerated girls needing treatment climbed from 42% to 57%.

Incarcerating persons with mental illness is not a new phenomenon but rather part of a long tradition of disenfranchising the different and powerless. The ancient Greeks and Romans feared that the evil spirits thought to cause mental illness could possess others with whom those people came in contact. To prevent such possession, those with serious mental illness who could not be cared for by family members were allowed to wander, essentially becoming street people (Porter, 1999). During the 15th century, in Germany, the mentally ill or retarded were sometimes driven out of towns. More generally, it was also during this time that confinement in madhouses and the association of mental illness with witchcraft (which, in turn, heightened the fear that mentally ill people aroused among the public) became common in Europe (Porter, 1999). Over the next 200 years, institutions were created to accommodate the needs of different groups of disadvantaged individuals, but these facilities subsequently achieved a common function: that of simple exclusion and containment of the marginalized (Foucault, 1965/1988). People with mental illnesses were often housed with criminals and the poor.

In the attitudes of the American colonists toward persons with serious mental illness, a similar process of disenfranchisement, exclusion, and loss of identity began: "From their perspective, insanity was really no different from any other moral disability; its victim, unable to support himself, took his place as one more among the needy" (Rothman, 1971, p. 4–5).

Insane asylums became common in the United States during the Jacksonian era (circa 1820–1840) and, for a time, were settings in which humane care were provided. By 1860, however, the guiding philosophy of these institutions had shifted from rehabilitative to largely custodial, partly fueled by an increasing population of patients from the poor and immigrant classes, who were thought to be untreatable (Rothman, 1971). Hence, the status of the insane had been transformed, not by a transition from one system (mental health) to another (criminal justice), as is often now the case, but simply by enhancing their identification with the lower socioeconomic classes. They came to be perceived more as members of a larger social underclass than as impaired individuals with special needs; they were seen no longer as sick so much as a threat to economic and social stability.

Institutionalized banishment or exile has also been a common practice for dealing with criminals and other devalued persons for hundreds of years. This alternative to execution and local incarceration included the transportation of criminals from the British Isles to Australia (Robson, 1994) and the American colonies (Shaw, 1966) and from France to Algeria and French Guiana (Forster, 1996). Russia provided internal exile through its network of corrective labor camps (Dallin & Nicolaevsky, 1947). In 1980, Fidel Castro opened the port of

Mariel, Cuba, and allowed any citizen to leave. In this mass exodus, Castro allowed political dissidents to leave Cuba and also used this as an opportunity to reduce his prison and mental hospital populations.

It is evident and unfortunate that prisons are now housing larger numbers of mentally ill individuals at a time when support for rehabilitative services within the correctional environment is at an all-time low. Furthermore, a trend toward building prisons in rural areas, which often means sending inmates greater distances from their homes, as well as toward the use of longer and determinate sentences echo the practice of exiling the disenfranchised.

Jails Versus Prisons

Jails are typically considered short-term facilities. They house individuals awaiting trial and offenders who are serving relatively short sentences (e.g., 1 year or less). Most jails are relatively small and are locally operated by county sheriffs' departments. Prisons, on the other hand, maintain individuals serving longer sentences. They are usually larger than jails and are operated by states, the federal government, or private correctional companies. There are a few additional noteworthy distinctions between jails and prisons. Jails tend to have a more direct interface with the surrounding community. When people are arrested, they usually are confined first in local jails. Upon entering a jail, a person's background, including mental health history, may be largely unknown. They may also be intoxicated at the time of incarceration and dealing with the initial shock of arrest and confinement. This is much less true in prisons. In prisons, newly admitted inmates have already been stabilized, detoxified, assessed for the existence of mental illness and substance abuse, and had a chance to cope with the initial shock of incarceration.

In their review of the literature on suicide in correctional settings, Lester and Danto (1993) found that suicides occurred much more commonly in jails than in prisons or the general population; they cited estimates of up to 187.5 per 100,000. Consequently, to the extent that jails are the sites at which offenders with mental illnesses are incarcerated, it becomes especially important to have adequate suicide screening programs in place at these facilities.

Offenders With Mental Illnesses in Rural Areas

Although prisons have been built in both rural and urban areas, there is a tendency to construct prisons in areas where space is readily available and where the public is supportive. In practice, this means that many prisons are constructed in rural areas, where jobs are scarce (Federal Bureau of Prisons, 1999; Schlosser, 1998; Traylor, personal communication, 1999).

Rural Prisons and Jails

Several problems arise when urban criminal offenders are confined in rural prisons. Confinement in a distant correctional facility often involves the effective separation of inmates from their previous social identities and support systems. They are less likely to be able to receive visits from family members and attorneys. When visits are arranged, they often involve greater expenses to families that are ill equipped to manage the increased fiscal demands. These offenders are also farther from the local media, representatives of which might take an interest in their legal cases.

Culture clash with locally recruited staff may further increase a prisoner's sense of alienation. This is especially true when inmates from one part of a state are moved to another part of the state or when federal offenders from one state are housed in a different state. This may also occur when inmates are "boarded out" to another state correctional system. In 1996, for example, private prisons in Texas housed inmates from 14 different states (Schlosser, 1998) and in 1998, prison inmates from 18 states were sent to systems in other states (Costello, 1999). Perhaps the greatest chance for culture clashes occurs in the federal prison system, in which individuals from many countries are housed together. As just one example, in the institution in which one of us (Robert K. Ax) works, there are over 40 nationalities represented within the inmate population.

Racial issues are also a factor in comparisons of rural and urban prisons and jails. Haney and Zimbardo (1998) noted that African Americans constitute 48% of those confined in state prisons, although such offenders account for less than 6% of the total population of the United States. In rural Mississippi, African Americans with mental illnesses were three times as likely to be held in jail without charges while awaiting transportation to a state hospital as were White people with similar mental disorders (Sullivan & Spritzer, 1997). In two studies of incarcerated women, one study in an urban jail (Teplin, Abram, & McClelland, 1996) and the other in a prison (Jordan, Schlenger, Fairbank, & Caddell, 1996), rates of mental illness were higher among non-Hispanic White women than among non-White inmates.

Prevalence Rates of Mental Disorders Among People Who Are Incarcerated

Questions have not yet been resolved about the incidence of serious mental illness in urban versus rural corrections facilities. There are few studies of rural prison and jail inmates. It is important to note that jails' and prisons' prevalence rates for mental disorder have different meanings. In general, mental disorder prevalence rates in jails more closely reflect those of the local community, whereas prisons have larger catchment areas, which may be regional, national, or even, in the case of some state systems and the federal prison system, international in scope.

In studies of mental illness and substance abuse among incarcerated people, researchers use different populations (e.g., men vs. women), prevalence rate time frames (e.g., serious mental illness present during interview vs. in the past 2 weeks vs. in the past 6 months vs. over the lifetime), and differently defined illness categories, or they do not use certain categories (e.g., Jordan et al. [1996] did not assess for schizophrenia or manic episode in their study of female prison inmates). The weight of evidence indicates that rates of serious mental illness and substance abuse are much higher in incarcerated people than they are in the general population, in both rural and urban settings (Chiles, Von Cleve, Jemelka, & Trupin, 1990; Ditton, 1999; Duclos et al., 1998; James, Gregory, Jones, & Rundell, 1980; Jordan et al., 1996; Kessler et al., 1994; National Center on Addiction and Substance Abuse [CASA], 1998; Regier et al., 1990; Teplin, 1990; Teplin et al., 1996). Incarcerated seriously mentally ill individuals are also at greater risk of having a comorbid substance abuse disorder than is the general population. For example, Regier et al. (1990) found that 92.3% of prisoners diagnosed with schizophrenia also had addictive disorders, in comparison with 47% of nonincarcerated individuals with schizophrenia. However, one study conducted in a rural Northeastern state revealed high rates among individuals incarcerated in prisons, which was consistent with other studies, but it revealed only slight increases in mental illness rates among those in rural jails in relation to the general population (Powell, Holt, & Fondacaro, 1997). Conclusions about SMI incidence rates in rural prison and jail settings are premature at this point, in the absence of additional data.

Access to Care

Inmates in rural prisons and jails face the same difficulties as residents of rural areas in acquiring adequate mental health care. Sullivan and Spritzer (1997) identified a phenomenon they called "rural criminalization." They found that many rural people in their sample had been held in jail—often for more than 5 days—without being charged with a crime; instead, they were awaiting transportation to state hospitals for admission. Accordingly, Sullivan and Spritzer suggested that there was a need for public mental health and law enforcement officials to cooperate in providing appropriate care for persons awaiting inpatient hospitalization, including outpatient crisis intervention. Until psychiatrists and psychologists begin to practice in rural areas in greater numbers, which currently seems unlikely, this task will devolve on paraprofessionals and the cross training of law enforcement personnel in mental health crisis intervention procedures.

Alternatives and Possible Solutions

JAIL AND PRISON-BASED PROGRAMS. Whether inmates arrive in a prison or jail with a mental illness or develop a mental illness during incarceration, it is clear that having a range of mental health programs available to the inmate population provides a first step in addressing the needs of incarcerated mentally ill offenders. Morris, Steadman, and Veysey (1997) found that screening and suicide prevention were the most common mental health services provided (88.3 % and 79.4 % of all jails surveyed, respectively). Other services supplied by at least half of the jails surveyed were follow-up evaluation, crisis intervention, inpatient treatment, and psychotropic medications. Availability of services was typically greater at larger jails. Morris et al. indicated that discharge planning for mentally ill detainees was commonly the weakest component of jail programs, but they singled out one facility as a positive role model: the Fairfax County Jail in Virginia, which provided detainees with referrals to mental health centers and also emphasized maintenance of family ties while they were incarcerated.

As previously noted, jails are typically short-term facilities for pretrial detainees and for individuals sentenced to less than a year's imprisonment. It is thus understandable that psychotherapy and counseling were provided at only a third of the facilities surveyed, whereas inpatient care was made available by nearly two thirds of the jails. The use of outside providers for correctional mental health services appears to be a growing trend in the United States. Morris et al. (1997) reported that several of the jails had contracted for mental health services with local medical schools or private correctional services (e.g., Correctional Medical Services).

Morgan, Winterowd, and Ferrell (1999) conducted a national survey of group therapy services in state prisons. Data indicated that about 20% of male inmates were receiving some type of group therapy service. Common group goals included the development of stress management skills, reducing addictive behaviors and preventing relapse, and preparation for life outside of prison. Offenders with mental illnesses may benefit from assistance with practical postrelease issues such as job-finding skills, because not all qualify for disability benefits but would be capable and anxious to work. Finn (1999) described several programs that assist ex-offenders in obtaining jobs.

Many of those incarcerated need substance abuse treatment. People with serious mental illness may have comorbid substance abuse problems and are frequently arrested because of their drug abuse or related behaviors. In 1998, at CASA at Columbia University, the results of a 3-year study on the American prison and jail population showed an 80% prevalence rate of drug and alcohol abuse among incarcerated men and women. CASA's analysis revealed that at least 81% of state inmates, 80% of federal inmates, and 77% of local jail inmates had used an illegal drug regularly (at least weekly for a period of at least 1 month). In addition, they had been incarcerated for selling drugs or possession or driving under the influence of alcohol or drugs when they committed their crimes, committed their offenses to get money for drugs, had a history of alcohol abuse, or were characterized by some combination of these offenses. Ditton (1999) reported that 6 in 10 inmates with SMI were under the influence of alcohol or drugs when they committed offenses for which they were currently incarcerated. Substance abuse in the general population is relatively low, but individuals with mental disorders are much more likely to abuse alcohol and illicit drugs.

However, in the CASA (1998) report, it was noted that only a minority of state and federal prison inmates with substance abuse problems were receiving treatment:

> In state prisons in 1991, fewer than half (44%) of regular drug users had received any kind of drug treatment in prison as of the time they were interviewed. In federal prison in 1991, regular drug users were slightly less likely to receive drug treatment (40%). (pp. 115–116)

Camp and Camp (1998) noted that only about 14% of the inmate population in 1997 was receiving any type of substance abuse treatment. However, this does not mean that programs were unavailable. Typically, mental health professionals do not mandate treatment. Prison treatment programs may be meeting the current demand for services but would probably not be adequate to meet the actual need for services if such services were uniformly required of prisoners with drug abuse histories. Courts, probation officers, prison policies, or other entities may mandate participation in treatment. In a review of published studies, Farabee, Prendergast, and Anglin (1998) found mixed support for "coerced" participation in treatment by drug offenders. It is not clear that mandated treatment, at least within a prison setting, would accomplish anything other than drive up the numbers of individuals whom prisons can show as participating in substance abuse treatment.

Nonetheless, it is evident that mental health programming can have a positive effect on the overall atmosphere of a prison. Mental health programs offer inmates a release for frustrations that might otherwise be acted out on prison staff or other inmates. These programs offer inmates many opportunities to learn prosocial values and methods of dealing with routine problems.

TELEHEALTH: ENHANCING PRISON-BASED MENTAL HEALTH TREATMENT. Emerging telehealth technology has considerable potential value in helping provide health care, especially mental health services, to prison inmates in rural areas that are underserved by health care professionals. The Federal Bureau of Prisons has committed to a telehealth program that has brought all of its facilities online within a few years (Abt Associates, Inc., 1999). This will enable the agency to leverage the skills of staff health care specialists, allowing them to consult at facilities around the country without leaving their respective institutions. The agency's pilot program revealed high levels of acceptance for consultations with remote providers within a patient sample that included seriously mentally ill patients and those with Axis II disorders (Magaletta, Fagan, & Ax, 1998). Just as important was the fact that the providers were satisfied with the experience, although some were initially ambivalent. Graham (1996) found preliminary evidence that the use of telehealth consultations with psychiatrists in a rural hospital resulted in a reduced incidence of SMI patients' rehospitalization. This use of telepsychiatry could be especially effective in rural jails and prisons, including some of the institutions within the federal prison system, in which rehospitalization can be a lengthy and cumbersome process.

Telehealth has other benefits in these settings, including the preservation of security (e.g., avoiding travel by inmates to see community providers) and having equipment that can serve dual functions: for use in health care and in teleconferencing and distance learning. More important, it offers the opportunity to bridge cultural gaps by obtaining consultative services with providers who are familiar with the practices and belief systems and who speak the languages of seriously mentally ill inmates foreign to the local culture. Telehealth can prevent provider burnout (Ramsbottom-Lucier, Caudill, Johnson, & Rich, 1995; Stamm, 1999; Stamm & Pearce, 1995), a problem to which mental health professionals working in rural prisons may be particularly vulnerable.

Telehealth may also be used as a means of improving the quality of services offered to inmates. Morgan et al. (1999) found that a variety of providers offering group therapy in their study were nonpsychologists, including *nonprofessionals,* and, furthermore, that 20% of therapists responded that there was no supervision of group work available at their correctional facilities. In this context, telehealth can increase the availability of supervisors in facilities where nonprofessionals provide services or where new therapists require supervision for various kinds of direct services.

DIVERSION PROGRAMS. Jail diversion programs provide a mental health disposition of charges outside a jail through dismissal of or reduction in charges. These programs typically involve the mechanisms of screening detainees for mental disorder, evaluation of those identified with mental disorders, and negotiation with the courts and other relevant parties to place these individuals into other community-based treatment programs (Steadman, Barbera, & Dennis, 1994). The actual number of such programs in the United States is unknown but is probably quite small at this time.

On the basis of the results of a mail survey and a telephone survey of randomly selected jail programs, Steadman et al. (1994) identified only 21 that had a program that fit their definition of a diversion program. Extrapolating from this data, they further estimated that there were only about 52 diversion programs in the 1,100 or more U.S. jails with a housing capacity of more than 50 pretrial inmates. This number proved to be an overestimate. In a follow-up study, Steadman, Morris, and Dennis (1995) selected 18 of the sites for in-person visits, at which point they discovered that five of these sites "did not actually have a diversion program" (p. 1633). This suggests that jail administrators may be overgenerous in estimating the qualities of their programs or that Steadman et al. defined diversion so narrowly as to miss the actual nature and extent of programs available to mentally ill jail detainees.

Some model programs exist. Steadman et al. (1995) identified six factors characterizing the most effective diversion efforts: integrated services (i.e., coordinated activities among criminal justice and mental health agencies); regular meetings of interagency administrative staff and separate meetings of direct services providers; boundary spanners, liaisons who coordinate across agencies; strong leadership; early identification of mentally ill detainees who meet criteria for the diversion program; and distinctive case management services, preferably provided by individuals with knowledge and experience in the areas of criminal justice and mental health.

Cost effectiveness was not assessed for these programs. However, in the current climate of concern about the expenses of incarceration, this is an important consideration. Cost savings can be calculated in dollar amounts or in more subjective terms that may or may not be seen to be of value to the community, such as reduction in days that individuals with mental illnesses are incarcerated. Alternative sentencing programs unrelated to mental health issues are increasingly common. For example, Yesterday's Rose in Washington, D.C., provides misdemeanants with an opportunity to perform community service instead of going to prison (Loose, 1999). The public receives value in terms of services performed and avoids the costs of incarcerating successful program participants. However, the feasibility of such programs is uncertain at best for those diverted from prison in rural areas because of mental illness, inasmuch as personnel and resources are likely to be more limited in these settings than in larger cities.

Diversion programs are obviously most effective in larger communities with adequate community-based mental health and substance abuse programs. They make far less sense in communities in which adequate treatment services are either not available or are already overtaxed, as might be the case in many rural areas. In fact, Sullivan and Spritzer (1997) asserted that diversion programs are inappropriate for rural areas and suggested instead "an intervention that makes available appropriate medical and mental health attention for those persons with SMI awaiting inpatient treatment" (p. 11). Assuming diversion programs are not feasible in rural areas, other interventions are necessary to reduce the involvement of persons with serious mental illness with the criminal justice system. However, because a central thesis of this chapter is that many seriously mentally ill individuals in rural prisons are displaced from their communities of origin, it is thought that properly designed and adequately funded diversion programs can help avoid the effective exiling of many mentally ill individuals from more urban areas to these facilities.

What diversion programs do suggest is that, with better risk assessment early in the criminal justice process, it may be possible to determine which individuals need incarceration and which may benefit from alternatives. Community education could reinforce the idea that not every offender must be incarcerated. Treatment can work for some individuals and is cheaper and more productive. Effective risk assessment is critical for the success of diversion programs.

Any detailed discussion is beyond the scope of this chapter. Suffice it to say that ideal programs will prevent the development of mental illness or substance abuse or provide early intervention before individuals become seriously debilitated or are arrested. In rural areas, where traditional mental health and substance abuse treatment services are less available and less accessible, the focus will probably be on self-help; the use of nonpsychologists and nonpsychiatrists as mental health professionals; and imaginative uses of technology, such as telehealth and Internet support groups.

Conclusions and Recommendations

Exiling individuals, especially those with mental disorders or substance abuse problems, to prisons far from their communities does not appear to accomplish anything more, in terms of its direct effect on them, than the further disenfranchisement of an already alienated population. Perhaps more tragic is the fact that they find themselves in an environment that is not designed primarily to meet their mental health needs. At the same time, the underlying socioeconomic factors that dictate this reality must be acknowledged.

Reintroduce Psychological Intervention With Adjunct Rehabilitation Programs

According to Haney and Zimbardo (1998), there is a need for psychologists to become reinvolved in prison policy issues. The future of U.S. prisons will be shaped by public opinion, economics, and legislative mandates. Prisons are not to blame for the reduced emphasis on reform and rehabilitation. Prison systems are entirely reactive to the courts, the legislature, and the public. They and their policies reflect societal attitudes. Hence, prison reform and the treatment of the mentally ill in prisons are as much questions of social policy as of social science.

Advocate for Patients and Providers

Mental health professionals working within this system must view themselves both as advocates for the patients and as therapists. Psychologists and other mental health professionals seeking to improve the quality of care in prisons or to create viable alternatives to incarceration, or both, must be effective advocates for those issues rather than merely collect data and present it to their colleagues.

Differentiate Between Mental Illness and Criminal Offenses

A public awareness program aimed at informing the public and explicating the differences between people who are mentally ill and criminal offenders can facilitate the creation of a less expensive and more effective alternative form of care for the incarcerated mentally ill patient. The economics of incarceration certainly compel a consideration of less costly and potentially more beneficial alternatives to confinement, especially for nonviolent mentally ill offenders and substance-abusing offenders. However, mental health professionals looking for alternatives to incarceration must realize that the public perceives a subjective value in incarcerating mentally ill and substance-abusing offenders, (e.g., they feel safer and believe that prisons protect society from the mentally ill or substance-abusing offender). In lobbying for implementation of diversion programs in a community, under the assumption that these programs are appropriate for a given municipality, advocates would first need to address people's perceptions that the mentally ill are dangerous or that they threaten society and, as a result, need to be separated from the public. Finally, decisions must be made as to placement for mentally ill offenders and whether they should be sentenced and treated in the same system as offenders who are not mentally ill.

Identify Goals of Mental Health Professionals Working With Mentally Ill Offenders

What should be the goals of mental health professionals who work with mentally ill offenders? Mental health professionals must also address several other difficult questions posed by diversion programs. Should mentally ill offenders be diverted from prison? (This, too, is a question to which the general public and the mental health professions may have different answers.) If so, where should they go and for how long? Steadman et al. (1994) pointed to a problem of high recidivism rates of individuals diverted to mental health dispositions in some of the programs surveyed. If they are sent to hospitals, should the goal of treatment be to help them recover sufficiently to return to the community or to proceed to incarceration? If individuals with serious mental illness are diverted to community-based treatment programs, how do health care providers avoid creating the "false positive" problem of malingerers—people feigning mental illness (some of whom do so quite well) in order to avoid legitimate incarceration?

Identify Programs That Support and Reintegrate Mentally Ill Offenders Into the Community

What, if any, other programs should be implemented to support and reintegrate mentally ill offenders into society? Another question that mental health professionals can help answer is whether they could implement other programs that would reduce the likelihood that these individuals would become involved in the criminal justice system. For example, enhanced support services, including Fairweather Lodges (Fairweather, Sanders, Maynard, & Cressler, 1969), might bridge the gap between total institutional care, as in hospitals, and the relative paucity of services on which most mentally ill now rely. These long-term, largely autonomous, and supportive living arrangements might allow many individuals, who neither meet the criteria for psychiatric hospitalization nor have the capacity for independent living, to remain in the community and avoid becoming involved in drug abuse or other criminal activities that lead to incarceration.

A final question for psychologists and other mental health professionals to ponder is whether the role of rehabilitation should once again be ascendant in the mission of the American prison. If the answer to this question is to be yes, then the debate must go beyond the profession to the public and the legislature. Again, Haney and Zimbardo's (1998) comments are relevant to the role of mental health care professionals in these debates:

> Historically, psychologists once contributed significantly to the intellectual framework on which modern corrections was built. . . . In the course of the past 25 years, they have relinquished voice and authority in the debates that surround prison policy. Their absence has created an ethical and intellectual void that has undermined both the quality and the legitimacy of correctional practices. It has helped compromise the amount of social justice our society now dispenses. (p. 721)

References

Abramson, M. F. (1972). The criminalization of mentally disordered behavior: Possible side-effect of a new mental health law. *Hospital and Community Psychiatry, 23,* 101–105.

Abt Associates, Inc. (1999). *Telemedicine can reduce correctional health care costs: An evaluation of a prison telemedicine network.* Washington, DC: Department of Justice.

Bassuk, E. L., & Gerson, S. (1978). Deinstitutionalization and mental health services. *Scientific American, 238,* 46–53.

Butterfield, F. (1999, July 12). Experts say study confirms prison's new role as mental hospital. *The New York Times,* p. A10.

Camp, C. G., & Camp, G. M. (1998). *The corrections yearbook 1998.* Middletown, CT: Criminal Justice Institute.

Chiles, J. A., Von Cleve, E., Jemelka, R. P., & Trupin, E. W. (1990). Substance abuse and psychiatric disorders in prison inmates. *Hospital and Community Psychiatry, 41,* 1132–1135.

Costello, A. (1999, September 22). Long distance service providers. *Morning Edition* [Radio broadcast]. New York: National Public Radio.

Dallin, D., & Nicolaevsky, B. I. (1947). *Forced labor in Soviet Russia.* New Haven, CT: Yale University Press.

Ditton, P. M. (1999, July). *Mental health and treatment of inmates and probationers. Bureau of Justice Statistics special report.* Retrieved March 13, 2001, from http://www.ojp.usdoj.gov /bjs/abstract/mhtip.htm

Duclos, C. W., Beals, J., Novins, D. K., Martin, C., Jewett, C. S., & Manson, S.M. (1998). Prevalence of common psychiatric disorders among American Indian adolescent detainees. *Journal of the Academy of Child and Adolescent Psychiatry, 37,* 866–873.

Fairweather, G. W., Sanders, D. H., Maynard, H., & Cressler, D. L. (1969). *Community life for the mentally ill.* Chicago: Aldine.

Farabee, D., Prendergast, M., & Anglin, M. D. (1998). The effectiveness of coerced treatment for drug-abusing offenders. *Federal Probation, 62,* 3–10.

Federal Bureau of Prisons. (1999). [Facilities executive summary report.] Unpublished raw data.

Finn, P. (1999, July). Job placement for ex-offenders: A promising approach to reducing recidivism and correctional costs. *National Institute of Justice Journal, 240,* 3–11.

Forster, C. (1996). *France and Botany Bay: The lure of a penal colony.* Carlton, Victoria, Australia: Melbourne University Press.

Foucault, M. (1988). *Madness and civilization: A history of insanity in the age of reason.* New York: Vintage Books. (Original work published 1965)

Graham, M. A. (1996). Telepsychiatry in Appalachia. *American Behavioral Scientist, 39,* 602–615.

Haney, C., & Zimbardo, P. (1998). The past and future of U.S. prison policy: Twenty-five years after the Stanford prison experiment. *American Psychologist, 53,* 709–727.

James, F. P., Gregory, D., Jones, R. K., & Rundell, O. H. (1980). Psychiatric morbidity in prisons. *Hospital and Community Psychiatry, 31,* 674–677.

Jordan, B. K., Schlenger, W. E., Fairbank, J. A., & Caddell, J. M. (1996). Prevalence of psychiatric disorders among incarcerated women: II. Convicted felons entering prison. *Archives of General Psychiatry, 53,* 513–519.

Kessler, R. C., McGonagle, K. A., Zhao, S., Nelson, C. B., Hughes, M., Eshleman, S., et al. (1994). Lifetime and 12-month prevalence of *DSM–III–R* psychiatric disorders in the United States: Results from the National Comorbidity Survey. *Archives of General Psychiatry, 51,* 8–19.

Lester, D., & Danto, B. L. (1993). *Suicide behind bars: Prediction and prevention.* Philadelphia: Charles Press.

Link, B. G., Phelan, J. C., Bresnahan, M., Stueve, A., & Pescosolido, B. A. (1999). Public conceptions of mental illness: Labels, causes, dangerousness, and social distance. *American Journal of Public Health, 89,* 1328–1333.

Loose, C. (1999, July 18). Acting on their convictions. *Washington Post,* pp. A1, A14.

Magaletta, P., Fagan, T., & Ax, R. K. (1998). Advancing psychology services through telehealth in the Federal Bureau of Prisons. *Professional Psychology: Research and Practice, 29,* 543–548.

Martz, M. (1999, November 28). Mentally ill imprisoned for treatment. *Richmond Times-Dispatch,* pp. A1, A9.

Morgan, R. D., Winterowd, C. L., & Ferrell, S. W. (1999). A national survey of group psychotherapy services in correctional facilities. *Professional Psychology: Research and Practice, 30,* 600–606.

Morris, S. M., Steadman, H. J., & Veysey, B. M. (1997). Mental health services in United States jails. *Criminal Justice and Behavior, 24,* 3–19.

National Center on Addiction and Substance Abuse. (1998, January). *Behind bars: Substance abuse and America's prison population.* New York: Columbia University and National Center on Addiction and Substance Abuse.

Porter, R. (1999). *The greatest benefit to mankind: A medical history of humanity from antiquity to the present.* New York: W. W. Norton.

Powell, T. A., Holt, J. C., & Fondacaro, K. M. (1997). The prevalence of mental illness among inmates in a rural state. *Law and Human Behavior, 21,* 427–438.

Ramsbottom-Lucier, M. T., Caudill, T. S., Johnson, M. M. S., & Rich, E. C. (1995). Interactions with colleagues and their effects on the satisfaction of rural primary care physicians. *Journal of Rural Health, 11,* 185–191.

Regier, D. A., Farmer, M. E., Rae, D. S., Locke, B. Z., Keith, S. J., Judd, L. L., et al. (1990). Comorbidity of mental disorders with alcohol and other drug abuse: Results from the Epidemiologic Catchment Area (ECA) Study. *Journal of the American Medical Association, 264,* 2511–2518.

Robson, L. L. (1994). *The convict settlers of Australia.* Carlton, Victoria, Australia: Melbourne University Press.

Rothman, D. (1971). *The discovery of the asylum: Social order and disorder in the New Republic.* Boston: Little, Brown.

Schlosser, E. (1998, December). The prison-industrial complex. *Atlantic Monthly, 282*(6), 51–77.

Shaw, A. (1966). *Convicts and the colonies: A study of penal transportation from Great Britain and Ireland to Australia and other parts of the British Empire.* London: Faber & Faber.

Stamm, B. H. (1999). Creating virtual community: Telehealth and self-care updated. In B. H. Stamm (Ed.), *Secondary traumatic stress: Self-care issues for clinicians, researchers and educators* (2nd ed., pp 179–208). Lutherville, MD: Sidran Press.

Stamm, B. H., & Pearce, F. W. (1995). Creating virtual community: Telemedicine applications for self-care. In B. H. Stamm (Ed.), *Secondary traumatic stress: Self-care issues for clinicians, researchers and educators* (pp. 179–210). Lutherville, MD: Sidran Press.

Steadman, H. J., Barbera, S. S., & Dennis, D. L. (1994). A national survey of jail diversion programs for mentally ill detainees. *Hospital and Community Psychiatry, 45,* 1109–1113.

Steadman, H. J., Morris, S. M., & Dennis, D. L. (1995). The diversion of mentally ill persons from jails to community-based services: A profile of programs. *American Journal of Public Health, 85,* 1630–1635.

Sullivan, G., & Spritzer, K. (1997). The criminalization of persons with serious mental illness living in rural areas. *Journal of Rural Health, 13,* 6–13.

Teplin, L. (1984). Criminalizing mental disorder: The comparative arrest rate of the mentally ill. *American Psychologist, 39,* 794–803.

Teplin, L., Abram, K., & McClelland, G. (1996). Prevalence of psychiatric disorders among incarcerated women: Pretrial jail detainees. *Archives of General Psychiatry, 53,* 505–512.

Teplin, L. A. (1990). The prevalence of severe mental disorder among male urban jail detainees: Comparison with the Epidemiologic Catchment Area Program. *American Journal of Public Health, 80,* 663–669.

Torrey, E. F. (1988). *Nowhere to go: The tragic odyssey of the homeless mentally ill.* New York: Harper & Row.

Valdiserri, E. V., Carroll, K. R., & Hartl, A. J. (1986). A study of offenses committed by psychotic inmates in a county jail. *Hospital and Community Psychiatry, 37,* 163–165.

17

Veterans Health Administration: Reducing Barriers to Access

Judith A. Lyons

There are numerous formal memorials to the sacrifices made by fallen warriors and surviving veterans. Sometimes overlooked is the degree to which our nation's prosperity stands as a living memorial to those who served their country. At the time many of these veterans served, they did so with the understanding that they would share in this prosperity through the promised benefit of future medical care. Many who served a full career expected to retire with full medical care for their families also (Shows, 2000). That expectation has been fulfilled in some cases but not in all.

In this chapter, I discuss the complexities of providing health care to rural veterans. In the initial sections, I describe the veteran population and veterans' health care system. I then review reforms designed to manage costs and increase access for a broader range of veterans, particularly in those rural areas. In the next section, I focus on provision of care for posttraumatic stress disorder (PTSD), a disorder for which many veterans require specialized treatment. I close the chapter with conclusions and recommendations. Throughout the chapter, consideration is given to the importance of family services.

Rural Veterans

The United States Veteran Population

The sheer volume and the changing demographics of the U.S. veteran population present a challenge to health care planners. According to the U.S. Department of Veterans Affairs (VA; formerly known as the Veterans Administration), there are 24.8 million living American veterans (DVA, 2000b). Approximately 25% of the American adult male population is veterans. Although women currently constitute only 4.8% of the veteran population, their number has been increasing. As a result, the median age of female veterans is younger (46.0 years) than that of male veterans (58.8 years).

Dr. Lyons can be reached at the G. V. (Sonny) Montgomery Veterans Affairs Medical Center, 1500 Woodrow Wilson Drive, Jackson, MS 39216. E-mail: judith.lyons@med.va.gov. This work is supported by South Central Mental Illness Research, Education and Clinical Center (VISN 16). Dr. Lyons is also on faculty at University of Mississippi Medical Center.

Although the veteran population is projected to decrease by nearly 7% per year, the female veteran population is projected to increase by nearly 20% between 1990 and 2020. The number of veterans aged 65 and older is also projected to increase, from 26% in 1990 to 53% by 2020. It is estimated that 23% of veterans reside in rural areas (DVA, 2000c), with an ongoing shift away from large population centers (DVA, 2000b).

Researchers consistently find that veterans have poorer physical and mental health than do nonveterans (Kazis et al., 1998, 1999; Skinner et al., 1999). Rates of depression among patients in the VA medical system have been found to be up to five times higher than rates in the private sector (Kazis et al., 1998). Reductions in military forces mean that the average age of veterans will continue to increase, with a concomitant increase in medical burden (Ashton et al., 1994). The largest cohort, 8.1 million Vietnam War era veterans, is now in their 50s (DVA, 2000b). In comparison with veterans already older than 65 (which would include Korean War and World War II era veterans), younger veterans (predominantly Vietnam War veterans; Kazis et al., 1998, 1999) and female veterans (Skinner et al., 1999) have been found to have the most serious mental health needs. Thus, in spite of decreasing numbers, the veteran medical and mental health burden is steadily increasing and will continue to require the careful consideration of health care policymakers.

The Veterans Health Administration

Many continue to know the VA as the Veterans Administration, but it is now formally the Department of Veterans Affairs. The Veterans Health Administration (VHA) is the health care arm of VA. It has grown from 54 hospitals in 1930 to its current mix of 173 medical centers, more than 400 community-based outpatient clinics, 131 nursing home care units, 39 domiciliary arrangements, and 205 Vet Centers (DVA, 2000a; Miller, 2001). It is the largest health care system in the world and the largest health care provider for the homeless (West, 1999). More health care personnel are trained within VA than in any other organization (DVA, 2000a; West, 1999).

As other industrialized nations have developed universal health care systems, they have merged veterans' care into the general system. However, veterans groups have lobbied adamantly for maintaining a separate system in the United States (American Legion, 2000; Iglehart, 1996). As chair of the Health Subcommittee on Veterans, Congressman Cliff Stearns (R-Florida; 1999) described the unique obligation our government has in regard to veterans' health care: ". . . this is one group of individuals the government has entered into a contract with to provide services. So it isn't a case of an entitlement; it's a contract that we have with them" (p. 58). During his tenure as Secretary of Veterans Affairs, Togo West, Jr. (1999), offered additional reasons for maintaining a special system for veterans, rather than distributing vouchers for medical care: First, veterans have their own unique culture with experiences that are foreign to most civilians. Second, transfer of care to the state health systems would overburden the states. Third, it is feared that veterans, being older and sicker than the general population, would not find their needs met by other systems. Finally, alternative sources of care do not offer comparable specialization in conditions such as spinal cord injury and PTSD.

PATTERNS OF VETERANS HEALTH ADMINISTRATION UTILIZATION. To understand the factors that affect access for rural veterans and their families, it is important to understand that federal legislation regulates access for all users of VHA services. Therefore, before addressing issues of travel distance and access to specialized services for PTSD, I present an overview of general utilization issues and regulatory reforms.

"Service-connected disability" status is a key concept inherent in legislation regarding VHA eligibility. If VA rules that an individual is "disabled by injury or disease incurred or aggravated during active military service" (DVA, 2000d, p. 13), a rating is given to indicate the percentage to which the individual is currently disabled. Monthly monetary compensation is based on this percentage. Degree of disability has historically been the key to various other benefits, such as vocational rehabilitation and health care. Although access to care is no longer limited to veterans with service-connected disabilities to the extent that it was in the past, service-connected status is still used to determine prioritization for care and whether a veteran's spouse and children are also eligible. Care for service-connected conditions has always been provided at no charge to the veteran, and veterans receive a modest 11-cents-per-mile travel reimbursement for service-connected care.

Not surprisingly, service-connected status is predictive of VHA utilization. The veterans most likely to use VHA are men who served during wartime, are sick, have service-connected disability status, lack other health insurance, are of a minority race, or are seeking care for substance abuse and other psychiatric problems (Mooney, Zangziger, Phibbs, & Schmitt, 2000; Rosenheck & Massari, 1993; Strauss, Sack, & Lesser, 1985; Virgo, Price, Spitsnagel, & Ji, 1999).

VHA has traditionally been a major provider of mental health care, which is the fastest growing segment of VHA care (Hoff & Rosenheck, 1997). In 1986, VHA provided 11% of all inpatient mental health care and 8% of all formal outpatient care provided nationwide. The highest per capita VHA utilization rates for these mental health services were in states with small or rural populations, including Maine, South Dakota, Wyoming, and West Virginia (Sunshine, Witkin, Atay, & Manderscheid, 1991). From 1980 to 1990, there was a 10% increase in the number of veterans admitted to VHA for inpatient psychiatric care, with a 59% increase among veterans younger than 45 (those who served during the Vietnam War and subsequent eras). It was speculated that the incidence of PTSD and changes in eligibility regulations that increased access to substance abuse care were among the factors contributing to the growing demand for psychiatric admissions (Ashton et al., 1994). Ashton, Petersen, Wray, and Yu (1998) found that 23% of VHA admissions, 43% of inpatient days of care, and 16% of outpatient visits during 1994 were for psychiatric care; the percentage of psychiatric hospitalizations was four times that reported in other hospital systems. During 1998, 8.7% of the veterans who were eligible for VHA care used VHA mental health services (Fontana, Rosenheck, Spencer, Gray, & DiLella, 1999).

VHA utilization rates have increased more for women than for men since 1980; however, it remains true that disproportionately fewer women use VHA (Weiss & Ashton, 1994). Further analyses revealed that the gender difference is attributable largely to less use of psychiatric care, particularly substance abuse care, by women veterans (Hoff & Rosenheck, 1997, 1998). Of veterans reporting mental health problems, only 14% of women (in comparison with 53% of men) used VHA outpatient services (Hoff & Rosenheck, 1998). This is particularly striking because female veterans report poorer emotional health than do male veterans (Skinner et al., 1999). It has been hypothesized that the particularly personal, sensitive nature of mental health issues combined with women's extreme minority status among VHA patients may cause some women to feel uncomfortable seeking mental health care through VHA (Hoff & Rosenheck, 1998). This may be particularly true for women seeking trauma-related services after sexual assault, who find themselves in a VHA waiting room or on a ward full of male patients.

A survey of families revealed that, in comparison with spouses who were receiving medical care outside of VHA, veterans were more satisfied with their current care and were receiving more preventive services. Asked whether they would use VHA medical services if allowed to do so, 83% of spouses reported affirmatively (Jain, Avins, & Mendelson, 1998). Under certain conditions, family members are already eligible to receive health care from VHA. The most common scenarios involve families or survivors of veterans who are rated as having a "permanent and total disability," who died from their service-connected disabilities, or who were totally disabled at the time of death (DVA, 2000d). Rural families might particularly appreciate the option to consolidate their family health care within a single system. The provision of care to spouses would also serve to increase the female-to-male VHA patient ratio, thus circumventing some of the barriers hypothesized to discourage female veterans from seeking mental health care at VHA facilities, noted previously.

REORGANIZATION OF THE VETERANS HEALTH ADMINISTRATION. Historically, access to VHA outpatient care was limited to veterans with service-connected disabilities or extremely low income. Inpatient care was available to most veterans. Many were eligible for outpatient care only if it was in follow-up to hospitalization. Predictably, this resulted in high utilization of expensive inpatient VHA care. From 1980 to 1990, a 7% increase in VHA hospital admissions was recorded, despite a 6% decrease in the number of veterans (Ashton et al., 1994). This increase was associated with the aging of young veterans and increased barriers to other health care.

In 1995, the then-incumbent VA Undersecretary for Health, Kenneth Kizer, outlined a plan to transform VHA to increase access, increase the ability to adjust to the evolving health care market, and contain costs. As a result, VHA's emphasis shifted from inpatient to outpatient care, and eligibility laws were changed (West, 1999).

The Veterans Health Care Eligibility Reform Act of 1996, Public Law 104-262, made virtually all veterans (wartime and peacetime) eligible for VHA care. A complex array of variables (including service-connected disability status, ex-prisoner-of-war status, type of military discharge, income level, and war-zone exposure to toxins) is used to define priority of access and to determine whether a copayment is charged and whether third-party billing will occur. Care continues to be free for service-connected disabilities. As is typical of many health plans, enrolled patients are eligible for a standard benefits package. Selected services such as dental care, glasses and hearing aids, reconstructive surgery, and infertility services carry additional eligibility requirements (DVA, 1998; see DVA, 2000d, or contact the Health Benefits Service Center at 1-877-222-8387 or www.va.gov).

For military retirees, the picture is more complicated. Military retirees (i.e., those who completed a full career in the military) were eligible for VHA care under the preceding terms. In addition, both they and their families were eligible for care at military bases, separate from VHA. Retirees are welcome to receive VHA care; however, if they do not have service-connected disabilities, their retirement pay places them in an income bracket in which they incur considerable copayments. Because of this, many retirees deliberately settled near a military base for access to free health care at base hospitals. Many of those bases have downsized or closed since the mid-1990s. A combination of insurance programs was initiated but has not proved fully satisfactory. In Congress, legislation to enhance insurance options for retirees and their families has been considered, and this effort remains in progress (Congressman R. Shows [D-Mississippi], personal communication, January 30, 2002).

To What Extent Is Travel Distance a Significant Barrier to Care? For the many years that inpatient care was the most accessible of VHA services (on the basis of eligibility restrictions), veterans from rural and frontier areas often sought multiple, concentrated services during an admission rather than commuting for outpatient care. With more restrictive admission criteria and considerable reductions in length of stay, the importance of "carrying health care to where veterans are located" (West, 1999, p. 3) is receiving increased attention.

Many veterans travel more than 100 miles each way for VHA care, farther than the distance to the most commonly used non-VHA health care facilities (Durance, Gibson, Davis-Sacks, & Homan, 1992; Mooney et al., 2000). Many of the longest commutes occur in rural areas; however, many densely populated areas are also hundreds of miles from the nearest VHA facility (Mooney et al., 2000). Deciding whether to initiate VHA care appears to be influenced by proximity; frequency of visits appears less affected by distance (Burgess & De Fiore, 1994).

Age-related data are somewhat unclear. In studies of *outpatient* utilization, researchers have found older veterans to be most deterred by distance (Burgess & De Fiore, 1994; Fortney, Booth, Blow, & Bunn, 1995). However, after other variables that covary with age were controlled, use of VHA *inpatient* medical surgical care was found to be least influenced by distance for older veterans (Mooney et al., 2000).

In comparison with the variance explained by other demographic variables, travel distance is generally found to be a minor factor in predicting VHA utilization (Mooney et al., 2000; Rosenheck & Stolar, 1998). Particularly noteworthy in light of VHA efforts to contain inpatient days of care, however, is the finding (after clinical and demographic case mix were controlled) that veterans living more than 60 miles from an outpatient clinic are 4.8 times more likely to be hospitalized for their acute psychiatric needs (Fortney, Owen, & Clothier, 1999). Similarly, distance increases the likelihood of premature (within 30 days) readmission, although nature of the illness is the most powerful predictor (Holloway, Medendorp, & Bromberg, 1990; this study was not specific for psychiatric admissions).

Why do some veterans choose VHA, even if it means traveling farther? Fontana et al. (1999) cited a national survey of veterans in which 19.4% of VA system users reported low cost as the main reason for choosing VHA. However, Mooney et al. (2000) questioned the degree to which the decision to travel long distances for treatment at a VHA facility is motivated by financial needs. They pointed to their finding that veterans older than 65 (who could receive Medicare-funded services closer to home) were least deterred by distance when seeking hospitalization.

The second most popular reason (18.4%) for choosing VHA on the survey was that VHA "provided services not found elsewhere." Additional research is needed to determine the extent to which access to various specialized services accounts for willingness to travel extreme distances. The question remains a point of Congressional interest, and updated studies of the relationship between distance and outpatient utilization have been initiated (Feussner, 1999). The findings may aid VHA's focus on bringing services closer to distant veterans.

CARRYING HEALTH CARE TO WHERE VETERANS ARE LOCATED. Various ways to bring health care closer to the veterans have been examined. Use of mobile clinics improved access but markedly increased costs (Wray et al., 1999). Other initiatives, facilitated by technological advances, have been more successful. Most pharmacy orders are now processed by mail (Brown, 1999). Transition from a paper chart to computerized medical records streamlined communication among VHA sites, community-based clinics (Roswell, 1999), and contract providers in non-VHA facilities (Brown, 1999). Teleconferencing has allowed the development of numerous satellite clinics, staffed by nurse practitioners, in which education, management, and specialty consultation are conducted electronically (Roswell, 1999; Russo, 1999). Videoconferencing is being used to gain access to interpreters, including sign language interpreters (Russo, 1999). Some sites are providing computers and telecommunication equipment to veterans' homes and evaluating whether these machines facilitate communication with clinicians (Roswell, 1999; Russo, 1999).

Kizer (1999) reported that, as a function of the restructuring of VHA, cost savings were accomplished from 1994 to 1998 by shifting of workloads from inpatient to outpatient care and reduction of staff by nearly 20%. These savings, plus revenues generated by leasing vacant ward space to other entities (Roswell, 1999), were applied to opening new community-based primary care clinics, of which there are more than 400 (Miller, 2001). These changes proved effective in increasing access, yielding a greater than 20% increase in the number of patients served (Kizer, 1999).

Only about half of community-based clinics have an on-site mental health provider, but plans are in place to increase mental health's presence through increased staffing and telehealth consultations (Kizer, 1999). VHA staff based in Salem, Virginia, reported success with a traveling team composed of a psychiatrist, a licensed practical nurse, and two mental health technicians (Workman, Short, Turner, & Douglas, 1997). They operate eight satellite clinics located 55 to 105 miles from the medical center in American Legion or Veterans of Foreign Wars halls, churches, and so forth.

Veterans Health Administration Specialized Care for Posttraumatic Stress Disorder

When Vietnam War veterans began returning from combat, there was no such thing as *posttraumatic stress disorder* in the diagnostic nomenclature. Based in large part on the volume of trauma reactions seen in the returning veteran population, however, PTSD was soon included in the *Diagnostic and Statistical Manual of Mental Disorders,* third edition (*DSM–III;* American Psychiatric Association, 1980), and subsequent revisions. Much of the pioneering work on the assessment and treatment of PTSD was conducted by VHA, and VHA continues to provide leadership in this area. VHA's National Center for PTSD coordinates major educational, clinical, and research programs. Staff members consult on many international projects, and the Published International Literature On Traumatic Stress (PILOTS) bibliographical database is integral to the work of PTSD specialists worldwide (see http://www.ncptsd.org).

Years ago, it was argued that veterans —especially in rural areas—did not have access to specialized PTSD treatment without traveling long distances (Sandrick, 1990). Although distance remains a barrier in many locales, access is much greater today than in 1990. By 1998, the VHA operated 141 inpatient, residential, and outpatient specialized PTSD programs nationwide, including some specifically for female veterans (Fontana et al., 1999). In addition, the VHA network of Vet Centers (i.e., outpatient counseling centers for sexually assaulted and wartime veterans) increased to 205 sites (DVA, 2000a). Originally organized as peer-counseling centers, Vet Centers today are almost entirely staffed by licensed counselors. Also, in areas distant from VHA facilities, veterans may receive a limited number of free sessions from private-sector providers who are on contract with the VHA (DVA, 2000c).

The VHA utilization patterns for veterans with PTSD are unique. Since the development of specialized PTSD programs, Vietnam War veterans (who had historically underutilized VA services partly because of perceptions of disenfranchisement from "the system"; McFall, Fontana, & Rosenheck, 1999) are now *more* likely to seek PTSD care through VHA than through non-VA mental health services (Rosenheck & Fontana, 1995). Data from Fontana et al. (1999) indicated that 62% of veterans who had service-connected PTSD used VHA mental health care in 1998. Predictably, most patients enrolled in VHA PTSD clinics are seeking care for combat trauma. However, 7% are seeking help for sexual trauma and 9% for other types of trauma.

An outreach intervention designed to engage the 38% who are rated disabled by PTSD but had not been using VHA services was evaluated in Seattle (McFall, Malte, Fontana, & Rosenheck, 2000). Through a letter and phone call, outreach personnel engaged 23% of contacted veterans for an initial visit and 19% of contacted veterans for repeat visits. All those in the sample lived within a 50-mile radius of the medical center. The impact of such interventions in rural and frontier areas remains to be tested.

POSTTRAUMATIC STRESS DISORDER AND PRIMARY CARE. It is well documented that PTSD is associated with increased medical concerns (Schnurr, 1996; Wagner, Wolfe, Rotnitsky, Proctor, & Erickson, 2000). However, a diagnosis of PTSD (or schizophrenia or substance abuse) has been found to be predictive of *lower* rather than higher utilization of VHA medical services (Druss & Rosenheck, 1997). Screening for serious mental illness in primary care clinics is an excellent way to identify undiagnosed cases. Paper-and-pencil screenings identified 24% of VHA medical patients as likely to have PTSD; fewer than one third of identified patients had sought psychiatric care (Blake et al., 1990).

To address these issues, a national planning summit convened in September 1999 (DVA, 2000e). The summit report suggested that 20% of patients with PTSD could be treated in a primary care setting, particularly with increased integration of mental health and primary care personnel through either membership in the primary care team or increased consultation. The advantages for veterans living in remote areas were emphasized, because increased integration of medical and psychiatric care could reduce or consolidate appointments, thus decreasing travel time for the patient and reimbursement costs for the system.

REACHING OUT TO MEMBERS OF FAMILIES OF VETERANS WITH POSTTRAUMATIC STRESS DISORDER. As in other health care organizations, VHA clinicians routinely strive to include family members in the treatment plan. Although this is true across disorders, some particular considerations apply in the case of PTSD. PTSD has been found to have a significant negative impact on families; the emotional numbing symptom component presents the greatest challenge to interpersonal relationships (Glynn et al., 1999; Riggs, Byrne, Weathers, & Litz, 1998). Families report a high degree of emotional burden (Beckham, Lytle, & Feldman, 1996; Glynn et al., 1999). Conversely, domestic conflict was found to be the most frequent cause of veterans' crisis phone calls to counselors in an Australian sample (Bryant, 1998)—a finding consistent with my clinical observations at VA facilities in the southern and northeastern United States. In addition, a British study has shown that criticism and hostility from family members are predictive of poorer PTSD treatment outcome for the patient (Tarrier, Sommerfield, & Pilgrim, 1999). In spite of the distress suffered by both patients and their families, however, efforts to engage families in treatment are not always successful. Glynn et al. (1999) found that, even when the PTSD patient was already engaged in the treatment program, 32%–35% of families declined adjunctive behavioral family therapy. Higher levels of PTSD-related avoidance behavior and emotional numbing on the part of the veteran were statistically associated with family refusal of therapy. However, family members cited work schedules and transportation as the primary reasons for not participating.

A particularly creative series of family service projects, many accomplished through public–private partnerships, was funded by an out-of-court settlement between manufacturers of herbicides (such as Agent Orange) and

Vietnam War veterans who claimed that the herbicides caused physical injuries to themselves and, as a result of genetic damage, their children. Projects spanned all 50 states and the District of Columbia. These projects are described in a superb text edited by Rhoades, Leaveck, and Hudson (1995). Sensitivity to the distinct needs of families coping with PTSD was highlighted, and customization of services for each local culture was seen to be crucial. Rhoades et al. observed that family members often made the initial contact on behalf of the veteran and were frequently responsible for helping the veteran overcome barriers to care by exploring care options, providing transportation, and so forth. The importance of increasing family-centered service was emphasized repeatedly across projects.

Currently, the VHA South Central Medical Illness Research, Education and Clinical Center (MIRECC) is developing several multisite projects to examine family members' understanding of PTSD and their perceptions of treatment needs. The goals are to examine barriers to and catalysts for family involvement in veterans' care across the predominantly rural mid-South region and to customize interventions accordingly. Patient feedback has already indicated that travel distance and scheduling options are major factors influencing the decision of families to engage in educational or therapy sessions, or both, offered by VHA (Lyons & Root, 2001). Thus, a cognitive and emotional coping-skills group for families is being converted to home study workbooks, supplemented by clinical telephone contacts. A randomized telephone survey of veterans' families is underway to identify additional barriers and solicit family input regarding treatment needs and interests.

Conclusions and Recommendations

VHA has undergone a major overhaul to increase access and control costs. New initiatives continue. An independent study was conducted by members of the American Legion (2000) through veteran town hall meetings and focus groups, review of VHA data, and consultation with other organizations. Results show that many of the VHA reform goals have been successful. Quality of care was rated "excellent" and was reported as the main reason for maintaining VHA as a separate health care organization. Efficiency and patient satisfaction were rated "good," with satisfaction steadily improving. What is better for most veterans, however, may be worse for some. What improves one problem sometimes inadvertently creates another. Concerns that have specific implications for rural veterans include continuity of care, geographical access, and sensitivity to travel burdens.

Protect Continuity of Care

VHA is trying to bring each treatment component closer to veterans' homes. This increases the risk for fragmentation of care, inasmuch as some services are provided centrally and others at community or satellite sites. Continuity of therapists, made possible by low staff turnover, is cited as a valued strength of community-based care in some rural areas (Husted & Jorgens, 2000). VHA has implemented case manager and primary provider models to increase continuity within the VHA. However, the sweeping changes have resulted in many staff reassignments and departures. If staff turnover and frequent reassignments persist, continuity of care will be compromised. According to the American Legion (2000) study, VA organizational stability is rated as "fair." Maintaining its experienced workforce in the presence of increasing workload and shrinking resources was identified as a major challenge facing VA.

Continue Efforts to Reduce Geographical Access Disparities

Reductions in inpatient services have freed monies to expand outpatient services both at VHA medical centers and at community-based clinics. However, closer services increase access only if they are *close enough* to make the commute feasible. Otherwise, the former option of receiving multiple services during periodic hospitalizations is sacrificed without any corresponding gain for distant patients. In the American Legion (2000) study, a rating of "poor" was conferred with regard to access to services. The researchers in the study noted that geographical disparity continues, particularly with regard to long-term psychiatric care, specialty residential care for substance abuse and PTSD, and the extent to which new community-based clinics include mental health services. The wait for an appointment in many specialty clinics was also found to exceed the VHA 30-day standard, which contributed to the poor access rating. Thus, efforts to increase access must remain a priority.

Increase Protocol Flexibility to Reduce Travel Burden

Standardized treatment protocols and national VHA performance monitors are designed to promote excellence. However, some protocols have had unintended negative consequences for the veterans living farthest from their VHA medical center. For example, one monitor requires that a VHA follow-up visit occur within 30 days of each discharge. Another monitor requires that an updated global assessment of functioning be logged by VHA staff for each mental health patient every 3 months. Such monitors are clinically relevant for patients who receive their care primarily at the VHA medical center. In the case of distant veterans, however, the follow-up plans are often designed to capitalize on coordination with providers in the patient's community. Thus, compliance with the mandatory monitors creates the burden of clinically unnecessary trips to the VHA medical center, which was clearly not the original intent (Rosse & Deutsch, 2000). VHA leaders are therefore exploring the possibility of crediting telephone contacts or waiving these VHA performance standards when non-VHA or external VHA-contract providers (rather than programs within VHA medical centers) are the primary follow-up sources.

In summary, continuing efforts to maximize quality and efficiency place high demands on the VHA. However, a moment's reflection on the working conditions that combat veterans endured for the benefit of their country helps place the challenge in perspective. As a nation, we clinicians (and all Americans) need to honor the promise made to veterans by ensuring the best possible access to high-quality care.

References

American Legion. (2000). *The American Legion monitors VA healthcare value for veterans.* Retrieved June 19, 2000, from http://www.legion.org/valuereport.htm

American Psychiatric Association. (1980). *Diagnostic and statistical manual for mental disorders* (3rd ed.). Washington, DC: Author.

Ashton, C. M., Petersen, N. J., Wray, N. P., & Yu, H. J. (1998). The Veterans Affairs medical care system: Hospital and clinic utilization statistics for 1994. *Medical Care, 36,* 793–803.

Ashton, C. M., Weiss, T. W., Petersen, N. J., Wray, N. P., Menke, T. J., & Sickles, R. C. (1994). Changes in VA hospital use 1980–1990. *Medical Care, 32,* 447–458.

Beckham, J. C., Lytle, B. L., & Feldman, M. E. (1996). Caregiver burden in partners of Vietnam War veterans with posttraumatic stress. *Journal of Consulting and Clinical Psychology, 64,* 1068–1072.

Blake, D. D., Keane, T. M., Wine, P. R., Mora, C., Taylor, K. L., & Lyons, J. A. (1990). Prevalence of PTSD symptoms in combat veterans seeking medical treatment. *Journal of Traumatic Stress, 3,* 15–27.

Brown, J. (1999). VA health care and the marketplace. In *Proceedings of veterans' health care: Building for tomorrow.* First annual conference of the Foundation for Veteran's Health Care. Washington, DC: U.S.MEDICINE. Retrieved June 1, 2000, from http://www.federalmedicine.com /tscript.html

Bryant, R. A. (1998). An analysis of calls to a Vietnam veterans' telephone counseling service. *Journal of Traumatic Stress, 11,* 589–596.

Burgess, J. F., Jr., & De Fiore, D. A. (1994). The effect of distance to VA facilities on the choice and level of utilization of VA outpatient services. *Social Science & Medicine, 39,* 95–104.

Department of Veterans Affairs. (DVA; 1998). *Eligibility reform—The right care, the right time, the right place, right now: Employee handbook.* Jackson, MS: Author.

Department of Veterans Affairs. (DVA; 2000a). Gateway to VA healthcare. Retrieved June 1, 2000, from http://www.va.gov/About_VA/Orgs/VHA/index.htm

Department of Veterans Affairs, Assistant Secretary for Planning and Analysis, Office of the DAS for Program and Data Analyses. (DVA; 2000b, March). *The changing veteran population, 1990–2020.* Washington, DC: Author.

Department of Veterans Affairs, Health Services Research & Development Service. (DVA; 2000c, January). Rural health—Improving access to improve outcomes. *HSR&D Management Brief, 13,* 1–3.

Department of Veterans Affairs, Office of Public Affairs (DVA; 2000d). *Federal benefits for veterans and dependents* (Department of Veterans Affairs Publication No. S/N 051-000-00220-2). Washington, DC: U.S. Government Printing Office.

Department of Veterans Affairs, PTSD/Primary Care Executive Working Group (DVA; 2000e). *VA PTSD/primary care summit meeting report: Integrating PTSD services into primary care settings. Results of the first VA PTSD/primary care summit meeting, San Francisco* (Unpublished report). (Available from Dr. Gregory Leskin, VA Palo Alto Health Care System, 795 Willow Road, Menlo Park, CA 94025.)

Druss, B. G., & Rosenheck, R. A. (1997). Use of medical services by veterans with mental disorders. *Psychosomatics, 38,* 452–458.

Durance, P. W., Gibson, T. B., Davis-Sacks, M. L., & Homan, R. K. (1992). Multifacility utilization by the chronically mentally ill in the Department of Veterans Affairs. *Journal of Mental Health Administration, 19,* 178–194.

Feussner, J. R. (1999, December 22). Department of Veterans Affairs memorandum from chief research and development officer acting under secretary for health. Washington, DC: Department of Veterans Affairs.

Fontana, A., Rosenheck, R., Spencer, H., Gray, S., & DiLella, D. (1999). *The long journey home VII: Treatment of posttraumatic stress disorder in the Department of Veterans Affairs: Fiscal year 1998 service delivery and performance.* West Haven, CT: U.S. Department of Veterans Affairs Northeast Program Evaluation Center.

Fortney, J. C., Booth, B. M., Blow, F. C., & Bunn, J. Y. (1995). The effects of travel barriers and age on the utilization of alcohol treatment aftercare. *American Journal of Drug and Alcohol Abuse, 21,* 391–406.

Fortney, J. C., Owen, R., & Clothier, J. (1999). Impact of travel distance on the disposition of patients presenting for emergency psychiatric care. *Journal of Behavioral Health Services Research, 26,* 104–108.

Glynn, S. M., Eth, S., Randolph, E., Foy, D. W., Urbaitis, M., Boxer, L., et al. (1999). A test of behavioral family therapy to augment exposure for combat-related posttraumatic stress disorder. *Journal of Consulting and Clinical Psychology, 67,* 243–251.

Hoff, R. A., & Rosenheck, R. A. (1997). Utilization of mental health services by women in a male-dominated environment: The VA experience. *Psychiatric Services, 48,* 1408–1414.

Hoff, R. A., & Rosenheck, R. A. (1998). Female veterans' use of Department of Veterans Affairs health care services. *Medical Care, 36,* 1114–1119.

Holloway, J. J., Medendorp, S. V., & Bromberg, J. (1990). Risk factors for early readmission among veterans. *Health Services Research, 25,* 213–237.

Husted, J., & Jorgens, A. (2000). Population density as a factor in the rehospitalization of persons with serious and persistent mental illness. *Psychiatric Services, 51,* 603–605.

Iglehart, J. K. (1996). Reform of the Veterans Affairs health care system. *New England Journal of Medicine, 335,* 1407–1411.

Jain, S., Avins, A. L., & Mendelson, T. (1998). Preventive health services and access to care for male veterans compared with their spouses. *Western Journal of Medicine, 168,* 499–503.

Kazis, L. E., Miller, D. R., Clark, J., Skinner, K., Lee, A., Rogers, W., et al. (1998). Health-related quality of life in patients served by the Department of Veterans Affairs: Results from the Veterans Health Study. *Archives of Internal Medicine, 158,* 626–632.

Kazis, L. E., Ren, X. S., Lee, A., Skinner, K., Rogers, W., Clark, J., et al. (1999). Health status in VA patients: Results from the Veterans Health Study. *American Journal of Medical Quality, 14,* 28–38.

Kizer, K. W. (1995). *Vision for change: A plan to restructure the Veterans Health Administration.* Washington, DC: U.S. Department of Veterans Affairs. Retrieved June 1, 2000, from http://www.va.gov/About_VA/Orgs/VHA/index.htm

Kizer, K. W. (1999). Remarks. In Hon. G. V. Montgomery (Moderator), Session Four: From budgets to crutches, Capitol Hill always has a say. In *Proceedings of veterans' health care: Building for tomorrow* (pp. 69–75). First annual conference of the Foundation for Veteran's Health Care. Washington, DC: U.S. MEDICINE. Retrieved June 1, 2000, from http://www.federalmedicine.com/tscript.html

Lyons, J. A., & Root, L. P. (2001). Family members of the PTSD veteran: Treatment needs and barriers. *National Center for Posttraumatic Stress Disorder Clinical Quarterly, 10*(3), 48–52.

McFall, M., Fontana, A., & Rosenheck, R. (1999). Current admission and exclusion criteria used by specialized intensive PTSD programs. In A. Fontana, R. Rosenheck, H. Spencer, S. Gray, & D. DiLella (Eds.), *The long journey home VII: Treatment of posttraumatic stress disorder in the Department of Veterans Affairs: Fiscal year 1998 service delivery and performance* (pp. 167–188). West Haven, CT: U.S. Department of Veterans Affairs Northeast Program Evaluation Center.

McFall, M., Malte, C., Fontana, A., & Rosenheck, R. A. (2000). Effects of an outreach intervention on use of mental health services by veterans with posttraumatic stress disorder. *Psychiatric Services, 51,* 369–374.

Miller, L. J. (2001, June). Improving access to care in the VA health system: A progress report. *VA Health Services Research and Development Forum,* pp. 1–2.

Mooney, C., Zwangziger, J., Phibbs, C. S., & Schmitt, S. (2000). Is travel distance a barrier to veterans' use of VA hospitals for medical surgical care? *Social Science & Medicine, 50,* 1743–1755.

Rhoades, D. K., Leaveck, M. R., & Hudson J. C. (1995). *The legacy of Vietnam veterans and their families—Survivors of war: Catalysts for change* (Agent Orange Class Assistance Program, Publication No. SN 028-004-00090-7). Washington, DC: U.S. Government Printing Office.

Riggs, D. S., Byrne, C. A., Weathers, F. W., & Litz, B. T. (1998). The quality of the intimate relationships of male Vietnam veterans: Problems associated with posttraumatic stress disorder. *Journal of Traumatic Stress, 11,* 87–101.

Rosenheck, R., & Fontana, A. (1995). Do Vietnam era veterans who suffer from posttraumatic stress disorder avoid VA mental health services? *Military Medicine, 160,* 136–142.

Rosenheck, R., & Massari, L. (1993). Wartime military service and utilization of VA health care services. *Military Medicine, 158,* 223–228.

Rosenheck, R., & Stolar, M. (1998). Access to public mental health services: Determinants of population coverage. *Medical Care, 36,* 503–512.

Rosse, R. B., & Deutsch, S. I. (2000). Use of the Global Assessment of Functioning (GAF) scale in the VHA: Moving toward improved precision. *Veterans Health System Journal, 5*(4), 50–58.

Roswell, R. H. (1999). Address. In J. Brown (Moderator), Session One: VA health care and the marketplace. In *Proceedings of veterans' health care: Building for tomorrow* (pp. 11–16, 19, 21–25). First annual conference of the Foundation for Veteran's Health Care. Washington, DC: U.S. MEDICINE. Retrieved March 17, 2001, from http://www.federalmedicine.com /tscript.html

Russo, H. (1999). Address. In A. H. Wilson (Moderator), Session Three: Decentralization of health care and the role of information technology. In *Proceedings of veterans' health care: Building for tomorrow* (pp. 41–47). First annual conference of the Foundation for Veteran's Health Care. Washington, DC: U.S. MEDICINE. Retrieved March 17, 2001, from http://www.federalmedicine.com/tscript.html

Sandrick, K. (1990). Expanded delivery system needed for post-traumatic stress. *Hospitals, 64*(11), 44–45.

Schnurr, P. P. (1996). Trauma, PTSD, and physical health. *PTSD Research Quarterly, 7*(3), 1–6.

Shows, R. (2000). *Summary of H. R. 2966, The Keep Our Promise to America's Military Retirees Act: A bill to restore earned health care coverage to retired members of the uniformed services.* Retrieved June 1, 2000, from http://www.house.gov/shows/HR2966-Summary.htm

Skinner, K., Sullivan, L. M., Tripp, T. J., Kressin, N. R., Miller, D. R., Kazins, L., et al. (1999). Comparing the health status of male and female veterans who use VA health care: Results from the VA Women's Health Project [Electronic version]. *Women & Health, 29*(4), 17–33. Abstract retrieved March 17, 2001, from http://www.ncbi.nlm.nih.gov/pubmed

Stearns, C. (1999). Address. In Hon. G. V. Montgomery (Moderator), Session Four: From budgets to crutches, Capitol Hill always has a say. In *Proceedings of veterans' health care: Building for tomorrow* (pp. 57–64). First annual conference of the Foundation for Veteran's Health Care. Washington, DC: U.S. MEDICINE. Retrieved March 17, 2001, from http://www.federalmedicine.com/tscript.html.

Strauss, G. D., Sack, D. A., & Lesser, I. (1985). Which veterans go to VA psychiatric hospitals for care: A pilot study. *Hospital and Community Psychiatry, 36,* 962–965.

Sunshine, J. H., Witkin, M. J., Atay, J. E., & Manderscheid, R. W. (1991, June). Mental health services of the Veterans Administration, United States, 1986 [Abstract]. *Mental Health Statistical Note, 197,* 1–17. Retrieved June 1, 2000, from http://www.ncbi.nlm.nih.gov/pubmed

Tarrier, N., Sommerfield, C., & Pilgrim, H. (1999). Relatives' expressed emotion (EE) and PTSD treatment outcome. *Psychological Medicine, 29,* 801–811.

Virgo, K. S., Price, R. K., Spitsnagel, E. L., & Ji, T. H. (1999). Substance abuse as a predictor of VA medical care utilization among Vietnam veterans [Abstract]. *Journal of Behavioral Health Services Research, 26,* 126–139. Retrieved June 1, 2000, from http://www.ncbi.nlm.nih.gov /pubmed

Wagner, A. W., Wolfe, J., Rotnitsky, A., Proctor, S. P., & Erickson, D. J. (2000). An investigation of the impact of posttraumatic stress disorder on physical health. *Journal of Traumatic Stress, 13,* 41–55.

Weiss, T. W., & Ashton, C. M. (1994). Access of women veterans to Veterans Affairs hospitals [Abstract]. *Women & Health, 21*(2–3), 23–38. Retrieved June 2, 2000, from http://www.ncbi.nlm.nih.gov/pubmed

West, T. G., Jr. (1999). Keynote address. In *Proceedings of veterans' health care: Building for tomorrow* (pp. 1–7). First annual conference of the Foundation for Veteran's Health Care. Washington, DC: U.S. MEDICINE. Retrieved June 1, 2000, from http://www.federalmedicine.com /tscript.html

Workman, E. A., Short, D., Turner, R., & Douglas, W. (1997). A 30-year progress report on a VA satellite clinic program. *Psychiatric Services, 48,* 1582–1583.

Wray, N. P., Weiss, T. W., Menke, T. J., Gregor, P. J., Ashton, C. M., Christian, C. E., et al. (1999). Evaluation of the VA mobile clinics demonstration project. *Journal of Healthcare Management, 44,* 133–147.

18

Ethnicity and Rural Status in Behavioral Health Care

Carol A. Markstrom, B. Hudnall Stamm,
Henry E. Stamm IV, S. Megan Berthold, and
Paulette Running Wolf

Rural areas tend to be less culturally diverse than urban areas (Williams & Ruesink, 1998). However, there is a varied composition of peoples and increasing ethnic diversity. Some rural communities consist of almost a single ethnic group; others are predominantly EuroAmerican. Some rural ethnic groups live in enclaves dominated by cultural traditions of one group; some reflect greater diversity. In others, the cultural heritage is obscured but drives the values and activities of the community.

In many ethnic communities, the interaction with EuroAmerican culture has resulted in a reduction in resources and the imposition of cultural scars. There are growing numbers of refugee communities in rural areas, some European and others from a variety of racial and ethnic backgrounds. Most fleeing refugees have experienced extreme stressors such as exposure to warfare, fear for their lives, starvation, sleep deprivation, the deaths of those around them, and sexual and physical assault. Upon arrival in their host countries, they face lingual, racial, and cultural barriers and, in general, initial lower economic status. Recognition of the scars of fleeing from their homelands may come slowly, if at all (Marsella, Bornemann, Ekblad, & Orley, 1994).

In the first section of this chapter, we address general factors that aggravate and serve as barriers to adequate behavioral health care for minorities. In the next section, we acquaint the reader with salient cultural characteristics of four ethnic groups in the United States: African Americans, Latinos and Latinas, American Indians and Alaska Natives, and Asians. We also provide information on working with refugees, because many ethnic groups are part of the greater refugee community. In the final section, we provide specific suggestions for working with ethnic groups in rural areas.

Dr. Markstrom can be reached at College of Agriculture, Forestry and Consumer Science, Family and Consumer Science, Allen Hall 704 G, P.O. Box 6124, Morgantown, WV 26506. E-mail: mark@wvnvm.wvnet.edu

Ethnic Communities in the United States

It is not possible to adequately address all ethnic and racial groups in a short chapter such as this. Our purpose in this chapter is to highlight some of the possible issues. True cultural competency arises from scholarly effort, genuine caring, openness to change, and experience.

Factors Aggravating Effective Behavioral Health Care for Ethnic Groups

POVERTY AND ETHNICITY. Poverty interacts with rural status and affects health outcomes for ethnic minorities. Racial and ethnic disparities in socio-economic status (SES) may lead to unequal representation of some groups in with lower SES (McLoyd, 1998; Taylor, 1997). Duncan (1991) observed that racial and ethnic minorities are especially susceptible to lasting poverty. According to a 3-year average calculated by the Bureau of the Census (from 1997 to 1999), the poverty rate among American Indians and Alaska Natives was 25.9%; poverty rates among African Americans and Hispanics were 25.4% and 25.1%, respectively; and poverty rates among Asians and Pacific Islanders (as a group) and non-Hispanic White persons were 12.4% and 8.2%, respectively. The study also revealed findings for annual income (1997–1999): Asians and Pacific Islanders had the highest median household income ($48,614), and non-Hispanic White persons had the second highest ($43,278). For other groups, the median incomes of American Indians and Alaska Natives, Hispanics, and African Americans were $30,874, $29,110, and $26,608, respectively (U.S. Bureau of the Census, 2000c). Unequal or restricted access to resources compounds the stress of coping with lower SES. According to Clark, Anderson, Clark, and Williams (1999), who argued from a biopsychosocial model, psychological and physiological reactions to racism might lead to adverse health outcomes, such as depression and susceptibility to physical illness. In short, racism, poverty, and rural residence affect behavioral health.

BARRIERS TO BEHAVIORAL HEALTH CARE FOR RURAL MINORITIES. Members of ethnic groups use health care services at a lower level than do White persons (Giachello & Arrom, 1997). For members of most rural ethnic groups, there are few culturally based clinics and services and even fewer culturally competent providers. In contrast, ethnic groups in urban areas are more likely to have access to culturally based services. Furthermore, some disorders are more prevalent among certain ethnic groups, and professionals who are not culturally sensitive may not know this. In short, in rural areas, health care systems are less likely to be flexible in meeting the needs of people with different cultural practices and languages (Giachello & Arrom, 1997).

Lack of privacy in small towns and strong extended family ties of some ethnic groups may lead to fears of being stigmatized and a reluctance of individuals to seek appropriate services. Some minority groups have a culture of modesty that for them is more salient than the general White culture, which makes it more difficult for them to overcome privacy barriers. Health education may be directed toward the wrong member of the family and may thus be ineffective. These barriers affect ethnic groups in varying degrees. In the following section, we summarize some cultural characteristics of ethnic groups.

Ethnic Groups

Belief, tradition, experience, and knowledge influence health-seeking behavior. What constitutes health risks, or even the definition of illness, varies according to culture. Culture, therefore, *must* be understood (Nader, Dubrow, & Stamm, 1999; Toumishey, 1993). However, it should be noted that there is within-group diversity and not all characteristics fit every member of a group.

AFRICAN AMERICANS. There are 33.9 million African Americans in the United States, constituting 12.8% of the population (U.S. Bureau of the Census, 1998). Most African Americans reside in the southern United States, and many of those live in rural areas (Wilkinson, 1999). African Americans have a rural legacy that is attached historically to slavery, farming, and the land (DeGenova, 1997). However, with changes in the economic structure in the South after the Civil War, many African Americans, particularly men, migrated to northern cities. These shifts in living patterns changed the family structure (Tully, 1999).

Strong kinship bonds. The extended family is a major source of social support, with characteristics of frequent contact, geographical proximity, and a strong kinship bonds (e.g., Gibbs, 1998; Hatchett & Jackson, 1999; Munsch & Wampler, 1993; Taylor, 1996; Tully, 1999). The slave experience forced Black people to turn to a wider network for support and reinforced the importance of family. The African American family persisted because of its strong kinship and multigenerational kinship networks. African American woman-headed households, which have been common since before the Civil War, have been noted in the literature as a legitimate family form (Sudarkasa, 1999). The extended family is a coping system (Harrison, Wilson, Pine, Chan, & Buriel, 1994). Taylor and Roberts (1995) found that familial social support of African American parents had indirect positive effects on parenting. However, the expectation of strong social support from families can lead to psychological distress when that support is not forthcoming (Taylor, 1996). Friends, neighbors, church members, and coworkers are highly valued and increase the social capital of a family (Taylor, Hardison, & Chatters, 1996). Neighborhood social capital is associated with less depression among African American adolescents (Stevenson, 1998).

Distinctions in men's and women's roles. As noted, African American families frequently are woman-headed households. The absence of men from these families, both historically and currently, can be linked to various factors. The slavery system probably had the most disastrous effects on the family because marriage was restricted and families were separated. Men lost their status in the household; slave-owners controlled the destiny of their lives and families (Hines & Boyd-Franklin, 1996; Tully, 1999). As a result, Black men were powerless to support and protect their families for more than 250 years.

After slavery ended, Black men in search of work migrated from rural southern farm communities to urban areas. Thus, for many African American households, both rural and urban, women have assumed the breadwinning and caretaking roles, with minimal assistance from husbands or elder men in the family (Tully, 1999).

Strong religious orientation. Religion has been the major formal institution in African American society and is both a social and personal resource (Ellison, 1993; Gibbs, 1998; Hines & Boyd-Franklin, 1996; McDavis, Parker, & Parker, 1995). The church or other religious institution offers guidance or assistance in negotiating many difficulties that arise over the course of a life span and in relation to experiences of being a racial minority (e.g., prejudice and discrimination). Religion and religious institutions serve as major sources of support during times of crises for African Americans (Wyche & Rotheram-Borus, 1990). Associated positive health outcomes emerge, as shown by Moore and Glei (1995), who found that Black participants scored higher than White participants on the Positive Well-Being Index; the higher scores were specifically attributed to greater religiosity and concern for correcting social inequalities. Health promotion programs commonly occur within black churchs and religious organizations. These programs present information on medical care access, reimbursement, and disease prevention (Sutherland, Barber, Harris, & Cowart, 1992).

LATINOS AND LATINAS. The 28.4 million Hispanics or Latinos and Latinas in the United States account for 10.8% of the population (U.S. Bureau of the Census, 1998b). There are regional differences in living patterns among the various Latino and Latina groups: They represent great diversity in national and ethnic origins, social class, language and dialect, history, immigration and citizenship status, degree of acculturation, and location in the United States. For instance, most Mexican Americans live in the southwestern United States; 40% live in small urban and rural communities (Ramirez, 1998). In contrast, Puerto Ricans tend to live in eastern urban areas (Wilkinson, 1999). The comments in this chapter apply specifically to Mexican Americans, but they share some features with other Latino and Latina groups, such as Puerto Ricans, Cubans, Salvadorans, and people of Central or South American origin (Valdez, Giachello, Rodriguez-Trias, Gomez, & de la Rocha, 1993). A fuller assessment of the health care needs, especially with regard to trauma, is found in Vélez-Ibáñez and Parra (1999).

Strong kinship bonds. Latinos and Latinas also have a lengthy history of multigenerational kinship bonds. "Familialism" represents the strong identification with and loyalty and attachment to family (DeGenova, 1997; Pinzon & Perez, 1997; Vélez-Ibáñez & Parra, 1999). Because practitioners are more inclined to treat individuals than extended families, the family may play a role in service planning. Interventions must account for all family members, including children. Parents tend to be warm and nurturing with their children and are highly protective. Parenting may be more relaxed with younger children, but adolescents are expected to take on significant household responsibilities (Ramirez, 1998).

Distinctions in men's and women's roles. Latino and Latina culture is characterized by sex-typed masculine and feminine characteristics, termed *machismo* and *marianismo* (Pinzon & Perez, 1997). Boys and girls are socialized into their appropriate roles at young ages (Ramirez, 1998), but the differentiation becomes more pronounced in adolescence (DeGenova, 1997). Machismo, the "essence or soul of masculinity" (Mosher & Tomkins, 1987, p. 65), traditionally elevates men as heads of the family structure. Boys are given more liberties, with tolerance for loud and aggressive behavior. Conversely, *marianismo* promotes chastity and family-oriented behavior among women. Girls are taught to be feminine and demure and to stay close to home. In view of the greater freedoms of women in contemporary American culture, conflict with marianismo may emerge. Machismo has both positive and negative aspects. DeGenova (1997) noted that some of the positive aspects include bravery, courage, self-defense, respect, and pride. Less desirable attributes include suppression of emotions, cognitions, and behaviors that are more "feminine." This behavior may result in social, mental, and physical health problems. The degree of machismo is lessening, however, as women gain status through employment outside of the home (Ramirez, 1998).

Strong religious orientation. Latino and Latina culture also includes a religious component that is similar to African American religious life. Typically, rather than investment in faith and social life into, for example, an indigenous Protestant Black church, religion is linked to the Roman Catholic faith (Pinzon & Perez, 1997), often in combination with peasant or folk beliefs (DeGenova, 1997). This blending of Catholicism and peasant or folk religion may make it necessary for health care providers to include religious conceptions and perhaps religious folk healers when planning medical, psychosocial, or community interventions for members of this ethnic group (Vélez-Ibáñez & Parra, 1999).

Migrant workers. Migrant and seasonal farmworkers form a special subgroup of rural Latinos and Latinas. To illustrate the extent of potential problems, Kupersmidt and Martin (1997) reported that 66% of the children of these families had one or more psychiatric diagnoses. Illnesses, lack of immunization, and poor nutritional patterns aggravate these conditions. Labor laws for agricultural work allow many of these children to work in the fields. Factors that may place this group at special risk include the migratory living and work pattern, chronic poverty and chronic homelessness, unhealthy living conditions, unsafe and unsanitary working conditions in the field, and temporary housing that violates housing codes (Kupersmidt & Martin, 1997). Farm workers rarely have health care coverage or even access to care. Even if there are clinics offering free care, some Latinos and Latinas may be afraid to seek care for fear of being reported to immigration authorities. The migratory living pattern precludes stability in schools, connections to community organizations, having one family physician who knows the family well, and so forth.

INDIGENOUS PEOPLES OF NORTH AMERICA. Native North America encompasses a tremendous diversity of peoples and cultures, with over 550 federally recognized tribes and 2 million people. What follows is a brief introduction (see

Stamm & Stamm, 1999, for a broader analysis). In 1990, of Alaska Natives, American Indians, and Native Hawaiians, nearly half lived in the western part of the United States, 29% in the South, 17% in the Midwest, and 6% in the Northeast. About 43% of the American Indian and Alaska Native populations live on reservation or trust lands (Paisano, 1999). Between 1990 and 2000, the American Indian and Alaska Native resident population grew by 17.9%, exceeding the national growth rate of 10.7% (U.S. Bureau of the Census, 2000b). By 2050, the Native American and Alaska Native population is expected to grow faster than the White or African American population and more slowly than the Hispanic or Asian and Pacific Islander population (U.S. Bureau of the Census, 2000a).

The Indian Health Service (IHS), a federal agency within the U.S. Department of Health and Human Services, is the principal provider of health care for American Indians and Alaska Natives and currently provides services to approximately 1.5 million of the 2 million persons living mostly on reservations (IHS, 2000; U.S. Department of the Interior, 1994). Health services are administered though IHS facilities and, as a result of Public Law 93-638, through block grants to tribally operated facilities. IHS is the only health care for many American Indian and Alaska Native people and is the primary mental health provider in many communities. Despite treaty obligations for the government to provide acceptable health care to American Indians and Alaska Natives, a lack of adequate federal funding is a major barrier.

Strong kinship bonds. As is true of the other groups, American Indians have a very integral family life (LaFromboise & Low, 1998; Stamm & Stamm, 1999). Loyalty to family is of utmost importance. The extended family takes an active role in parenting; aunts and uncles serve as secondary parents, and grandparents share tasks, too. Children are highly valued and respected. Creativity is encouraged (DeGenova, 1997), and at young ages, children are integrated into adult social activities, such as powwows and other ceremonial activities. A major concern for many American Indian and Alaska Native parents is that their cultural heritage will be lost as their offspring leave the reservations or native villages (see DeGenova, 1997).

Distinctions in men's and women's roles. Both men's and women's roles are accepted and respected in American Indian culture. There has been greater continuity, however, in women's roles. American Indian women traditionally served as caretakers of children and households (including elders). Women still have primary responsibility for childcare and the household. In contrast, the traditional roles for Native men—that of warrior and hunter— have been disrupted. For many, the role of warrior has been translated into public or military service. Thus, great respect is shown to men who serve their community and country, from tribal leaders to veterans from World War II to veterans from Desert Storm (DeGenova, 1997).

Men also had traditional roles, depending on the tribe, of hunting, fishing, or building. Today, these positions have translated into working in professions such as logging and ranching. Taking care of livestock and participating in rodeos are common activities of many American Indians in the western United

States. In addition, jobs in helping professions, such as teaching, health care, and alcohol and drug treatment, are consistent with traditional roles of medicine men. Storytelling, too, is a traditional skill that has translated to the contemporary role of educator.

Strong religious orientation. Spirituality pervades all aspects of existence for American Indians and is not compartmentalized from other domains of life. There is a high degree of respect for nature and natural things that is reflected in their spiritual beliefs. However, variability exists in how religion is practiced. Some American Indians may practice traditional tribal spirituality, some Christianity, and others a combination of the two (DeGenova, 1997; Stamm & Stamm, 1999). Regardless of the nature of the American Indians' and Alaska Natives' belief systems, notions of mental health are not separated from physical health or spiritual health. Some IHS facilities accommodate traditional forms of healing. Health care workers need to recognize this affinity between spirituality and healing in order to be effective in most American Indian and Alaska Native communities (Stamm & Stamm, 1999).

ASIAN AMERICANS AND PACIFIC ISLANDERS. There are 9.7 million Asian Americans and other Pacific Islanders living across the United States who account for 3.7% of the population (U.S. Bureau of the Census, 1998), concentrated mostly in California (Wilkinson, 1999). Many of the Asian Americans today are third- and fourth-generation Americans who have Japanese or Chinese ancestry. Since the end of the Vietnam War, increasing numbers have been refugees or immigrants from Cambodia, Laos, and Vietnam. As refugees or recent immigrants, persons from Southeast Asia in the United States have different life experiences than those with longer histories in the United States. For detailed examination of Asian Americans from Southeast Asia, see Gerber, Nguyen, and Bounkeua (1999). What follows is a portrayal of the recent immigrants from Southeast Asia.

Strong kinship bonds. In Asian countries, elderly persons were treated with respect and obeyed by younger persons. Farming communities often included members of extended family networks. Often, however, elderly persons were illiterate in their written language of origin, especially those from rural regions. This has had direct bearing on the nature of kinship and familial relationships. Because children attend American schools, they find themselves exposed to the more individualistic American culture and often gain power as they serve as translators for their parents (Smith-Hefner, 1999). According to Gerber et al. (1999), these changes have created true "generation gaps" between the older, more traditional parent generation (the immigrants) and their Americanized children.

Distinctions between men's and women's roles. American life causes adjustment difficulties. Men and women find themselves in nontraditional roles. Traditionally, Southeast Asian men were the primary breadwinners for their families, and for farmers, land ownership was a mark of status. In the United States, many Southeast Asian women work outside the home, finding employment more quickly than their husbands, which thereby disrupts the family role relationships. This power shift, coupled with illiteracy and a new language, is particularly devastating in men's lives. The feeling of debasement affects even those from middle- or upper-class backgrounds, because they rarely find similar opportunities in the United States. As a result, many refugee and immigrant families from Southeast Asia have suffered pervasive life disruptions, the development of adversarial relations between husbands and wives, and loss of the social support that normally would have come from their extended family communities (Gerber et al., 1999).

Strong religious orientation. Persons from Southeast Asia hold a variety of religious beliefs, including Buddhism, Hinduism, animism, Confucianism, and Taoism. As with the other ethnic groups, these beliefs have profoundly affected understandings of modes of living, causes of illness, and treatment (see Kitigawa, 1989; Overmeyer, 1986; Reat, 1994). According to many people from Southeast Asia, illness is brought on by a god or spirit as an indication of the person's past misdeeds or perhaps an offense against a malicious spirit. In such a case, the person would seek out a monk, priest, or spiritual traditional healer, not a Western health care worker, to alleviate the illness, or the person might pray at an ancestral altar for intervention by ancestral spirits. Western practitioners need to recognize that such clients may be seeking additional sources of healing (Gerber et al., 1999). Alternatively, the client or patient may seek intervention from a Western practitioner when other avenues of healing fail.

REFUGEE GROUPS. Refugees have been forced to flee their countries to escape persecution based on race, religion, nationality, membership in a particular social group, or political opinion (Marsella et al., 1994; United Nations Conference of Plenipotentiaries on the Status of Refugees and Stateless Persons, 1951). Between 5% and 35% of refugees and asylum seekers arriving in the United States are survivors of torture (Elsass, 1997; Office of Refugee Resettlement, 1997). The United States has the highest number of resettled refugees in the world (1,146,400), including half of all those resettled by the United Nations High Commissioner for Refugees (1998). Many refugees go to urban areas, often where there are well-developed ethnic enclaves and support networks, but the number of refugees in rural areas in the United States has increased since 1990.

The refugee experience is traumatizing, with multiple events leading to flight (Marsella et al 1994; van der Veer, 1998). Loved ones who were sources of social support are left behind. Many refugees have experienced traumas such as attacks, robberies, beatings, and rapes during their escape. Some have endured violence in refugee camps (Berthold, 1998, 2000; Mollica et al., 1991).

Upon relocation in the United States, many refugees live in poor inner-city neighborhoods, often with high levels of community violence and racial tension (Berthold, 1998). They may experience periods of homelessness or move frequently. It is not uncommon for refugees to move from cities to rural areas in the hope of finding increased safety and peace or expanded job opportunities. Because of a host of cultural factors and the nature of their experiences, refugees often are reluctant to discuss their trauma with others unless they have established a relationship of trust (van der Veer, 1998). If health professionals fail to establish a trusting relationship and inquire about the trauma history, they are likely to overlook or even misdiagnose physical and psychological problems resulting from exposure to trauma. In working with refugee clients, it is important to be familiar with approaches to healing in *their* cultures and to assess the extent to which clients believe in these approaches. Sue and Zane (1995) stressed that to be credible in the eyes of the client, (a) the therapist's conceptualization must be congruent with the belief system of the client, (b) problem resolution must be culturally compatible and acceptable, and (c) the goals of treatment must be shared.

Many rural communities lack adequate resources as well as legal and community support to provide needed services to refugees. Furthermore, refugees may not have English proficiency and knowledge of resources to navigate the institutional systems that are available. It may be particularly distressing for some in remote areas who have difficulties obtaining ethnic foods and in locating places to worship and who are isolated from others who share their language, culture, and experiences. Creative and collaborative interagency and community-based strategies are essential for addressing these challenges. It is important to note that in order to survive multiple traumatic experiences, refugees tend to have positive attributes and psychological strengths, to be incredibly resourceful, and to be resilient. Service providers should acknowledge and draw upon these qualities when empowering and serving these people.

Conclusions and Recommendations

Apply a Model of Social Capital Resources to Rural Behavioral Health Care for Ethnic Groups

J. S. Coleman (1988; J. Coleman, 1990) proposed a model of social capital in which resources needed for optimal development are designated. Social capital encompasses physical, human, and social components. Castle (1998) reconceptualized Coleman's notions of social capital to apply to rural places and people and defined social capital as group connections that enhance individual production and efforts. The ability to give and receive social support is a form of social capital, and social support is related to more optimal psychosocial and health outcomes (Flach, 1988; Garmezy, 1983; Seiffge-Krenke, 1995; Werner & Smith, 1982). Social capital is a resource; those who accumulate it may be more deeply involved in their networks and communities (Furstenberg & Hughes, 1995). It is conceived as a force that builds cooperation, trust, understanding, and empathy (Newton, 1997), moving people from self-centeredness to orientations toward others, community, and the common good.

Utilize the Resources in the Therapeutic Process, Particularly Among Ethnic Groups

It is recommended, therefore, that behavioral health care practitioners working with ethnic groups in rural communities use social capital in the therapeutic process. For instance, McAuley (1998) noted the value of neighborliness in

rural African American communities. Neighborliness is an indigenous phenomenon in many rural communities that can be capitalized on. Parallel
services—that is, services that draw on community resources (social capital)—
may be adaptive substitutes or sited in conjunction with more formal mental
health agencies (see also Stamm & Friedman, 2000).

Although too much social involvement and dependence can be labeled
enmeshment, it is necessary to recognize that the stronger social ties of some
ethnic groups can be adaptive and normative to the culture. Hence, mental
health care providers must carefully determine what is culturally appropriate
in terms of closeness, family influence, and family obligation versus what may
be used as an excuse to control and abuse others.

Develop Adequate Data to Understand Health Disparities Across Ethnicity

In order to reduce the health disparities of ethnicity, there must be adequate
data available on health status, patterns of use, health care financing, and
outcomes. It is essential to gain community involvement in data collection on
health issues and the proper interpretation and application of data. Health
policy and practices should recognize the need to develop policies to provide
comprehensive health services, the need for universal health care to serve the
high number of underinsured people in rural and minority populations, and
the use of prevention efforts for all patients. Some considerations in the area
of health delivery systems include the need for linguistically and culturally
appropriate services that include the needs and input of the community and
that are accessible to rural minorities.

Incorporate Unique Cultural Norms Into Specific Ethnic Groups' Health Care Culture

Culturally competent care includes developing methods for incorporating into
health care programs the unique characteristics of a given ethnic group and,
furthermore, a format for disseminating those cultural norms to new practitioners within the system. Workshops and programs that inform practitioners
about cultural differences and how to involve or integrate themselves into a
specific culture would be very helpful. To provide effective behavioral health
care to ethnic groups in rural areas, it is necessary to understand the special
issues related to rural and minority status. Practitioners must examine how
societal factors of racism have affected the ethnic group. Practitioners should
also make a conscientious effort to learn the values, beliefs, practices,
language, and verbal and nonverbal communication patterns of the ethnic
groups they serve. It helps practitioners to have awareness and appreciation
of their own ethnic backgrounds in order to gain an appreciation of others' differences. Because of the variation within the United States, this can be a difficult task. As part of a quest for self-awareness, practitioners should examine
their own prejudices and stereotypes about other groups. They should
remember that within-group diversity is sometimes greater than between-
group diversity.

References

Berthold, S. M. (1998). *The effects of exposure to violence and social support on psychological and behavioral outcomes among Khmer refugee adolescents.* Unpublished doctoral dissertation, University of California, Los Angeles.

Berthold, S. M. (2000). War traumas and community violence: Psychological, behavioral, and academic outcomes among Khmer refugee adolescents. *Journal of Multicultural Social Work, 8*(1/2), 15–46.

Castle, E. M. (1998). A conceptual framework for the study of rural places. *American Journal of Agricultural Economics, 80,* 621–631.

Clark, R., Anderson, N. B., Clark, V. R., & Williams, D. R. (1999). Racism as a stressor for African Americans: A biopsychosocial model. *American Psychologist, 54,* 805–816.

Coleman, J. (1990). *Foundations of social theory.* Cambridge, MA: Belknap.

Coleman, J. S. (1988). Social capital in the creation of human capital. *American Journal of Sociology, 94*(Suppl. 95), S95–S120.

DeGenova, M. K. (1997). *Families in cultural context: Strengths and challenges in diversity.* London: Mayfield.

Duncan, G. (1991). The economic environment of childhood. In A. C. Huston (Ed.), *Children in poverty* (pp. 23–50). New York: Cambridge University Press.

Ellison, C. G. (1993). Religious involvement and self-perception among Black Americans. *Social Forces, 71,* 1027–1055.

Elsass, P. (1997). *Treating victims of torture and violence: Theoretical, cross-cultural, and clinical implications.* New York: New York University Press.

Flach, F. (1988). *Resilience: Discovering a new strength at times of stress.* New York: Fawcett Columbine.

Furstenberg, F. F., & Hughes, M. E. (1995). Social capital and successful development among at-risk youth. *Journal of Marriage and the Family, 57,* 580–592.

Garmezy, N. (1983). Stressors of childhood. In N. Garmezy & M. Rutter (Eds.), *Stress, coping, and development in children* (pp. 43–84). New York: McGraw-Hill.

Gerber, L., Nguyen, O., & Bounkeua, P. K. (1999). Working with Southeast Asian people who have migrated to the United States. In K. Nader, N. Dubrow, & B. H. Stamm (Eds.), *Honoring differences: Cultural issues in the treatment of trauma and loss.* Philadelphia: Taylor & Francis.

Giachello, A. L., & Arrom, J. O. (1997). Health service access and utilization among adolescent minorities. In D. K. Wilson, J. R. Rodrigue, & W. C. Taylor (Eds.), *Health-promoting and health-compromising behaviors among minority adolescents* (pp. 303–320). Washington, DC: American Psychological Association.

Gibbs, J. T. (1998). African American adolescents. In J. T. Gibbs, L. N. Huang, & Associates (Eds.), *Children of color: Psychological interventions with culturally diverse youth* (pp. 171–214). San Francisco: Jossey-Bass.

Harrison, A. O., Wilson, M. N., Pine, C. J., Chan, S. Q., & Buriel, R. (1994). Family ecologies of ethnic minority children. In G. Handel & G. G. Whitchurch (Eds.), *The psychosocial interior of the family* (pp. 187–209). New York: Walter de Gruyter.

Hatchett, S. J., & Jackson, J. S. (1999). African American extended kin system. In H. P. McAdoo (Ed.), *Family ethnicity: Strength in diversity* (2nd ed., pp. 171–190). Thousand Oaks, CA: Sage.

Hines, P. M., & Boyd-Franklin, N. (1996). African American families. In M. McGoldrick, J. Giordano, & J. K. Pearce (Eds.), *Ethnicity and family therapy* (2nd ed., pp. 66–84). New York: Guilford.

Indian Health Service. (2000). *Fact sheet.* Retrieved March 19, 2001, from http://www.ihs.gov

Kitigawa, J., & Cummings, M. (1989). *Buddhism and Asian history.* New York: Macmillan.

Kupersmidt, J. B., & Martin, S. L. (1997). Mental health problems of children of migrant and seasonal farm workers: A pilot study. *Journal of the American Academy of Child and Adolescent Psychiatry, 36,* 224–232.

LaFromboise, T. D., & Low, K. G. (1998). American Indian children and adolescents. In J. T. Gibbs, L. N. Huang, & Associates (Eds.), *Children of color: Psychological interventions with culturally diverse youth* (pp. 112–142). San Francisco: Jossey-Bass.

Marsella, A. J., Bornemann, T., Ekblad, S., & Orley, J. (Eds.). (1994). *Amidst peril and pain: The mental health and well-being of the world's refugees.* Washington, DC: American Psychological Association.

McAuley, W. J. (1998). Historical and contextual correlates of parallel services for elders in African American communities. *The Gerontologist, 38,* 445–455.

McDavis, R. J., Parker, W. M., & Parker, W. J. (1995). Counseling African Americans. In N. Vacc, S. DeVaney, & J. Wittmer (Eds.), *Experiencing and counseling multicultural and diverse populations* (3rd ed., pp. 217–250). Bristol, PA: Accelerated Development.

McLoyd, V. C. (1998). Socioeconomic disadvantage and child development. *American Psychologist, 52,* 185–204.

Mollica, R. F., Poole, C., & Tor, S. (1998). Symptoms, functioning, and health problems in a massively traumatized population: The legacy of the Cambodian tragedy. In B. P. Dohrenwend (Ed.), *Adversity, stress and psychopathology,* (p. 34–51). London: Oxford University Press.

Moore, K. A., & Glei, D. (1995). Taking the plunge: An examination of positive youth development. *Journal of Adolescent Research, 10,* 15–40.

Mosher, D. L., & Tomkins, S. S. (1987). Scripting the macho man: Hypermasculine socialization and enculturation. *Journal of Sex Roles, 26,* 60–84.

Munsch, J., & Wampler, R. S. (1993). Ethnic differences in early adolescents' coping with school stress. *American Journal of Orthopsychiatry, 63,* 633–646.

Nader, K., Dubrow, N., & Stamm, B. H. (Eds.). (1999). *Honoring differences: Cultural issues in the treatment of trauma and loss.* Philadelphia: Taylor & Francis.

Newton, K. (1997). Social capital and democracy. *American Behavioral Scientist, 40,* 575–586.

Office of Refugee Resettlement. (1997). *Making a difference. FY 1997 annual report to Congress.* Washington, DC: Author.

Overmeyer, D. (1986). *Religions of China.* San Francisco: Harper & Row.

Paisano, E. L. (1999). *The American Indian, Eskimo, and Aleut population.* Washington, DC: U.S. Bureau of the Census. Retrieved March 4, 2001 from http://www.census.gov/population /www/pop-profile/amerind.html

Pinzon, H. L., & Perez, M. A. (1997). Multicultural issues in health education programs for Hispanic-Latino populations in the United States. *Journal of Health Education, 28,* 314–316.

Ramirez, O. (1998). Mexican American children and adolescents. In J. T. Gibbs, L. N. Huang, & Associates (Eds.), *Children of color: Psychological interventions with culturally diverse youth* (pp. 215–239). San Francisco: Jossey-Bass.

Reat, N. (1994). *Buddhism: A history.* Berkeley, CA: Asian Humanities Press.

Seiffge-Krenke, I. (1995). *Stress, coping, and relationships in adolescence.* Mahwah, NJ: Erlbaum.

Smith-Hefner, N. J. (1999). *Khmer American: Identity and moral education in a diasporic community.* Berkeley, CA: University of California Press.

Stamm, B. H., & Friedman, M. J. (2000). Cultural diversity in the appraisal and expression of traumatic exposure. In A. Shalev, R. Yehuda, & A. McFarlane, *International handbook of human response to trauma* (pp. 69–85). New York: Plenum Press.

Stamm, B. H., & Stamm, H. E., (1999). Ethnocultural aspects of trauma and loss in Native North America. In K. Nader, N. Dubrow, & B. H. Stamm (Eds.), *Honoring differences: Cultural issues in the treatment of trauma and loss* (pp. 50–69). New York: Brunner-Rutledge.

Stevenson, H. C. (1998). Raising safe villages: Cultural-ecological factors that influence the emotional adjustment of adolescents. *Journal of Black Psychology, 24,* 44–59.

Sudarkasa, N. (1999). African American females as primary parents. In H. P. McAdoo (Ed.), *Family ethnicity: Strength in diversity* (2nd ed., pp. 191–200). Thousand Oaks, CA: Sage.

Sue, S., & Zane, N. (1995). The role of cultural techniques in psychotherapy: A critique and reformulation. In N. R. Goldberger & J. B. Veroff (Eds.), *The culture and psychology reader* (pp. 767–788). New York: New York University Press.

Sutherland, M., Barber, M., Harris, G., & Cowart, M. (1992). Health promotion in southern rural black churches: A program model. *Journal of Health Education, 23,* 109–111.

Taylor, R. D. (1996). Adolescents' perceptions of kinship support and family management practices: Association with adolescent adjustment in African American families. *Departmental Psychology, 32,* 687–694.

Taylor, R. D. (1997). The effect of economic and social stressors on parenting and adolescent adjustment in African-American families. In R. W. Taylor & M. C. Wang (Eds.), *Social and emotional adjustment and family relations in ethnic minority families* (pp. 35–52). Mahwah, NJ: Erlbaum.

Taylor, R. D., & Roberts, D. (1995). Kinship support and maternal and adolescent well-being in economically disadvantaged African-American families. *Child Development, 66,* 1585–1597.

Taylor, R. J., Hardison, C. B., & Chatters, L. M. (1996). Kin and nonkin as sources of informal assistance. In H. W. Neighbors & J. S. Jackson (Eds.), *Mental health in Black America* (pp. 130–145). Thousand Oaks, CA: Sage.

Toumishey, H. (1993). Multicultural healthcare: An introductory course. In R. Masi, L. Mensah, & K. McLeod (Eds.), *Health and cultures: Exploring the relationships* (pp. 113–138). Oakville, Ontario, Canada: Mosaic Press .

Tully, M. A. (1999). Lifting our voices: African American cultural responses to trauma and loss. In K. Nader, N. Dubrow, & B. H. Stamm, (Eds.), *Honoring differences: Cultural issues in the treatment of trauma and loss* (pp. 23–47). Philadelphia: Taylor & Francis.

United Nations Conference of Plenipotentiaries on the Status of Refugees and Stateless Persons. (1951). Convention relating to the Status of Refugees Adopted on 28 July 1951 by the United Nations Conference of Plenipotentiaries on the Status of Refugees and Stateless Persons convened under General Assembly resolution 429 (V) of 14 December 1950 entry into force 22 April 1954, in accordance with article 43. Retrieved March 25, 2001, from http://www.unhchr.ch /html/menu3/b/o_c_ref.htm

United Nations High Commissioner on Refugees. (1998). *Report and fact sheet.* Retrieved March 4, 2001, from http://www.unhcr.ch/world/amer/usa.htm

U.S. Bureau of the Census. (1998). *Current population reports, series P23-194, population profile on the United States: 1997.* Washington, DC: U.S. Government Printing Office.

U.S. Bureau of the Census. (2000a). *Census Bureau projects doubling of nation's population by 2100.* Retrieved March 25, 2001, from http://www.census.gov/Press-Release/www/2000/cb00-05.html

U.S. Bureau of the Census. (2000b). *Resident population estimates of the United States by sex, race, and Hispanic origin.* Retrieved March 25, 2001, from http://www.census.gov/population /estimates/nation/intfile3-1.txt

U.S. Bureau of the Census. (2000c). *Poverty rate lowest in 20 years, household income at record high, Census Bureau reports.* Retrieved March 25, 2001, from http://www.census.gov/Press-Release/www/2000/cb00-158.html

U.S. Department of the Interior, Bureau of Reclamation. (1994). *Indian Self-Determination and Education Assistance Act of 1975* (P.L. 93-638; 88 Stat. 2203; 42 USC 450-458). Retrieved March 19, 2001, from http://www.usbr.gov/laws/isdeea.html

Valdez, R. B., Giachello, A., Rodriguez-Trias, H., Gomez, P., & de la Rocha, C. (1993). Improving access to healthcare in Latino communities. *Public Health Reports, 108,* 534–539.

van der Veer, G. (1998). *Counseling and therapy with refugees and victims of trauma: Psychological problems of victims of war, torture and repression* (2nd ed.). New York: John Wiley.

Vélez-Ibáñez, C. G., & Parra, C. G. (1999). Trauma issues and social modalities concerning mental health concepts and practices among Mexicans of the southwest United States with reference to other Latino groups. In K. Nader, N. Dubrow, & B. H. Stamm (Eds.), *Honoring differences: Cultural issues in the treatment of trauma and loss* (pp. 76–97). Philadelphia: Taylor & Francis.

Werner, E. E., & Smith, R. S. (1982). *Vulnerable but invincible: A longitudinal study of resilient children and youth.* New York: Adams.

Wilkinson, D. (1999). Reframing family ethnicity in America. In H. P. McAdoo (Ed.), *Family ethnicity: Strength in diversity* (2nd ed., pp. 15–60). Thousand Oaks, CA: Sage.

Williams, R., & Ruesink, D. C. (1998). The changing rural family and community: Implications for congregational ministry. *Journal of Family Ministry, 12,* 6–21.

Wychc, K. F., & Rothcram-Borus, M. J. (1990). Suicidal behavior among minority youth in the United States. In A. R. Stiffman & L. E. Davis (Eds.), *Ethnic issues in adolescent mental health* (pp. 323–338). Thousand Oaks, CA: Sage.

Index

About the Editor

B. Hudnall Stamm, educated in psychology and statistics at Appalachian State University (BS, MA) and the University of Wyoming (PhD), is a research professor as well as the director of telehealth and the deputy director of the Idaho State University Institute of Rural Health. Previous appointments include positions with the VA National Center for Posttraumatic Stress Disorder, Dartmouth Medical School, and the University of Alaska, Anchorage. Working primarily with rural underserved peoples, Stamm focuses on health policy, cultural trauma, and work-related traumatic stress. Stamm is the author of numerous professional documents and books, including *Measurement of Stress, Trauma and Adaptation* (1995), *Cultural Issues and the Treatment of Trauma and Loss* (with Nader and Dubrow, 1999), and *Secondary Traumatic Stress* (1995/1999). Stamm's work is used in over 30 countries and many diverse fields, including health care, disaster response, news media, and the military. See www.isu.edu/~bhstamm and www.isu.edu/irh for more information.

DATE DUE

7/30/05		